Therapeutic Communication for Health Professionals

Third Edition

Cynthia Herbert Adams, Ph.D.
Licensed Psychologist and Professor Emeritus

Peter D. Jones, M.D., MBA
Internal Medicine

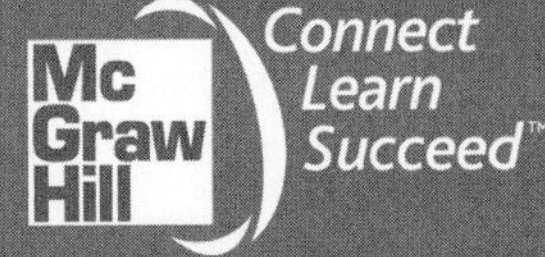

The McGraw·Hill Companies

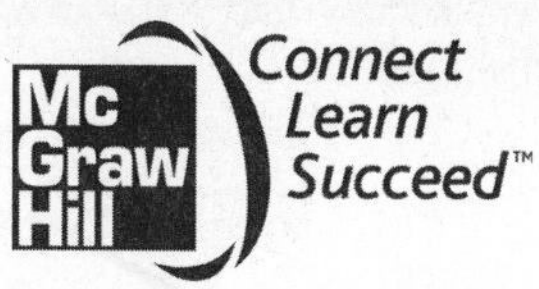

THERAPEUTIC COMMUNICATION FOR HEALTH PROFESSIONALS

Published by McGraw-Hill, a business unit of The McGraw-Hill Companies, Inc., 1221 Avenue of the Americas, New York, NY, 10020.

Some ancillaries, including electronic and print components, may not be available to customers outside the United States.

This book is printed on acid-free paper.

2 3 4 5 6 7 8 9 0 QDB/QDB 1 0 9 8 7 6 5 4 3 2 1 0

ISBN 978-0-07-340208-6
MHID 0-07-340208-7

Vice president/Editor in chief: *Elizabeth Haefele*
Vice president/Director of marketing: *John E. Biernat*
Publisher: *Kenneth S. Kasee Jr.*
Senior sponsoring editor: *Debbie Fitzgerald*
Developmental editor: *Bonnie Hemrick*
Freelance developmental editor: *Andrea Edwards*
Editorial coordinator: *Parissa DJangi*
Marketing manager: *Mary B. Haran*
Lead digital product manager: *Damian Moshak*
Media development editor: *Marc Mattson*
Director, Editing/Design/Production: *Jess Ann Kosic*
Project manager: *Kathryn W. Mikulic*
Senior production supervisor: *Janean A. Utley*
Senior designer: *Anna Kinigakis*
Senior photo research coordinator: *John C. Leland*
Media project manager: *Cathy L. Tepper*
Cover design: *Anna Kinigakis*
Interior design: *Kay Lieberherr*
Typeface: *10.5/13 New Aster*
Compositor: *Aptara, Inc.*
Printer: *Quad/Graphics*
Cover credit: © *Stockbyte/Getty Images*
Credits: The credits section for this book begins on page 336 and is considered an extension of the copyright page.

Library of Congress Cataloging-in-Publication Data

Adams, Cynthia H., 1948-
Therapeutic communication for health professionals / Cynthia Herbert Adams, Peter D. Jones.—3rd ed.
p. ; cm.
Rev. ed. of: Interpersonal communication skills for health professionals / Cynthia H. Adams, Peter D. Jones. ©2000.
Includes bibliographical references and index.
ISBN-13: 978-0-07-340208-6 (alk. paper)
ISBN-10: 0-07-340208-7 (alk. paper)
1. Medical personnel and patient. 2. Communication in medicine. 3. Health counseling.
I. Jones, Peter D., M.D. II. Adams, Cynthia H., 1948- Interpersonal communication skills for health professionals. III. Title.
[DNLM: 1. Communication. 2. Professional-Patient Relations. 3. Counseling—methods.
4. Interprofessional Relations. W 21.5 A211t 2011]

R727.3.A33 2011
610.69'6—dc22

2009047856

www.mhhe.com

Brief Contents

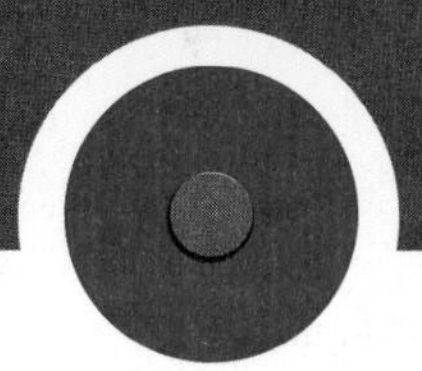

Contents

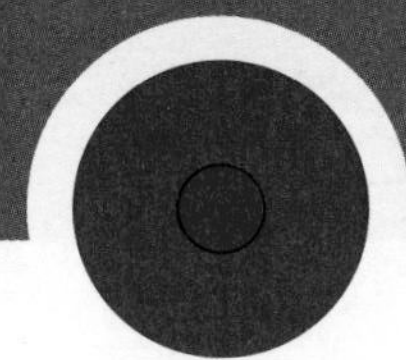

Dedication

Dedicated to the memory of Chuck Baldwin, DVM, a dedicated healer and a lover of all creatures, and to RuthAnn Lobo, whose personal courage and uplifting spirit are always an inspiration.

About the Authors

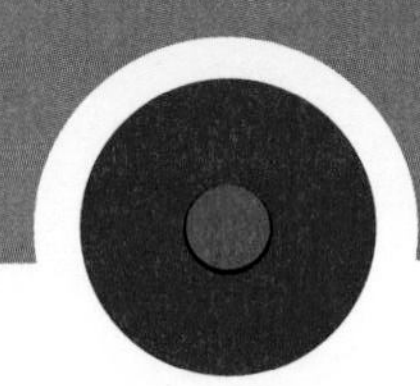

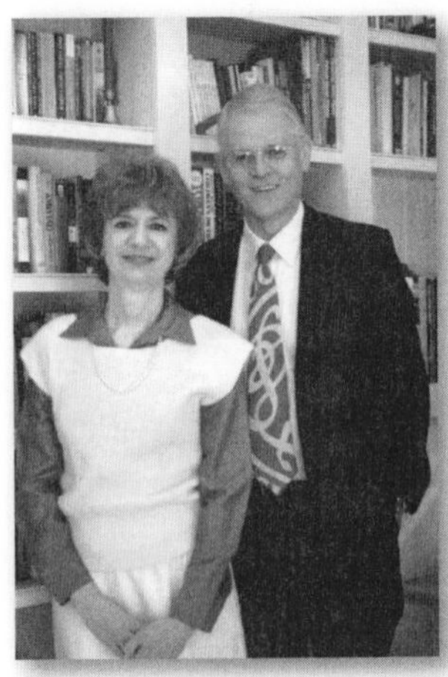

CYNTHIA ADAMS, PH.D

Cynthia Adams, a licensed psychologist, is a professor and associate vice-provost emeritus of the University of Connecticut; she taught in the former School of Allied Health. Her primary research area was eating disorders and interdisciplinary health care. She has numerous publications in this area. Following her retirement from the university, she has become certified in treating co-occurring mental health and substance abuse issues. Currently she maintains a private practice and works part-time for Natchaug Hospital in Mansfield Center, CT. Her B.S. is from the University of New Hampshire, and she earned her master's and doctorate degrees from the University of Connecticut. The idea for this textbook was based upon her lecture notes for an interdisciplinary health course in which Peter Jones, M.D. was a frequent guest lecturer. She may be reached through www.psychologicaltreatment.net.

PETER JONES, M.D.

Peter Jones graduated as a scholar in pathology from St. John's College, Cambridge, UK. He went on to medical school at Oxford University, UK, subsequently doing a dual residency in internal medicine and family practice. In 1977 he immigrated with his American wife, Ann, and three daughters to rural Connecticut, where he has practiced internal medicine for over 30 years. He became a Fellow of the American College of Physicians. His avocations include classical piano playing, flamenco and classical guitar playing, American history, numismatics, and magic. He is also a University of Connecticut MBA graduate, Phi Beta Kappa.

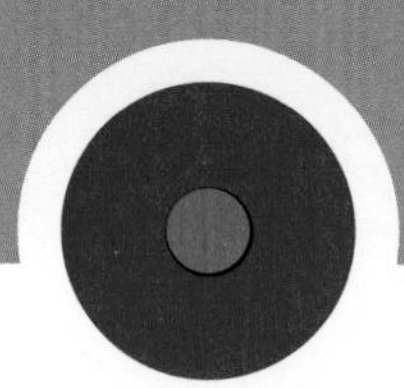

Foreword

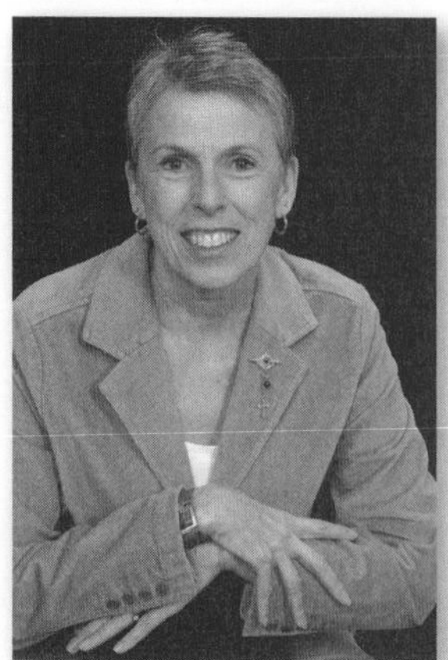

RuthAnn Lobo gives her perspective both as a patient and as the mother of a famous athlete.

Most of us have been escorted by a health care professional to a tiny cubicle where each of our defense mechanisms seems to diminish with each layer of clothing that is shed. I am grateful when radiographers, technologists, or nurses whisk me quickly from those pod-like holding areas where outdated magazines have been stripped of tantalizing recipes and a patient's thoughts are left to wander in dark and secret places.

I have personally experienced anxiety when surrounded by the space age technology of modern medicine, the threat of the gleaming stainless steel and ceramic behemoths that loom in wait and hold me hostage as they sweep closely over my body, making me wonder if their parts are secure and their nuts and bolts tightened to perfection. Then I am comforted, not by the mechanics of the experience but by the humanity of those who stand by in pastel scrubs or flowered tops, who patiently explain each step of the process and wield the tools of their trade with a soft voice, or a kind smile, or a tender touch.

As an educator and counselor with 35 years of experience and as a breast cancer survivor, I am excited to recommend this textbook for the training of future health professionals. It encompasses not only the essentials of human developmental levels but also the human factor: the essentials of communications, laws, and ethics of health and counseling practices. Basic knowledge and skill sets to reach clients come together effectively in this text.

My husband and I have raised three student/athletes, one of whom, Rebecca, is internationally recognized and a Gold Medal Olympian. We have seen many injuries resulting in contacts with every level of sports medicine from orthopedic surgeon to rehabilitation assistant. Those who left a lasting impression tended to the body but also to the mind and spirit; they knew how to comfort, inspire, understand, and motivate.

It was in December 1993 that I was diagnosed with breast cancer while Rebecca was enjoying a promising basketball career at the University of Connecticut. Thrust into the limelight by my daughter's success and a life-threatening disease, I found myself called upon to speak out for funding to support cancer awareness, research, and related health care issues. As the recipient of modern medicine, I expect my medical team to be at the top of technology. I have come to expect, as well, professionals who are careful never to breach the fine line between professionalism and intrusion but still manage through a look or a word to impart a message that says, "We are in this together." I am indebted to those who can deliver a bone scan, a mammogram, or an x-ray without the slightest suggestion that a woman missing one breast is in any way out of the norm.

Health professionals dealing with people going through these dynamic issues must be prepared at every level: This book is invaluable for their training.

– RuthAnn Lobo

Being a health professional is a noble and important calling. Health professionals at every level are involved in significant acts of healing, research, and comforting, and the need for health professionals continues to grow as America continues to age and as technology and science demand more specialized knowledge. Yet, beyond scientific knowledge, health science students need to learn the therapeutic use of counseling and communication skills and a basic understanding of human behavior and become well-informed on professional issues, which include those raised by advancing technology. Without these skills, their knowledge cannot be applied.

Further, the demographics of this country are rapidly changing and these changes necessitate a shift in cultural paradigms, health care approaches, and models as well as the emphasis of care. Understanding human behavior is complicated by evolving social pressures and diseases; and governmental roles with health care are also redefining the application of the art. Greater patient-care oversight and advances in technology create another dimension of knowledge that the health professional must glean to survive and practice his or her craft.

What Sets This Book Apart?

Therapeutic Communication for Health Professionals fills a vital need as it introduces students to the basic skills of counseling and communication that are the foundation for all interactions. Further, students will understand basic psychologic defense mechanisms that show up throughout therapeutic interaction, they will know how to deal with patients who are facing incredible losses, they will comprehend the significance of human development throughout the lifespan, and they will recognize the need to serve special populations and to apply their skills to disease prevention. Additionally, they will work and communicate well within an interdisciplinary team, apply the highest ethical standards of their chosen professions, and have the ability to recognize and respond appropriately to all forms of abuse and discrimination and to address and prevent legal issues. All of the above are placed within a multicultural context allowing the health professional to better reach all patients.

In *Therapeutic Communication for Health Professionals,* we review skills that are needed to better develop a basic understanding of the patient and an improved ability to communicate both with patients and within the health care universe. This therapeutic counseling/communications background is then overlaid with an understanding of the human issues that face most of our patients, who must deal with loss due to illness or social condition and who are in an environment that often feels hostile and frightening. Our goal is for the readers to place themselves in the patient's place to better understand how patients think and feel across multicultural lines. Additionally, the health professional is in a dynamic environment where change is constant. Comprehension of basic interdisciplinary roles, ethical standards, and legal concerns provides a framework from which change may be assessed and absorbed into the therapeutic milieu.

Therapeutic Communication for Health Professionals is composed of three main sections. **Part 1, Foundations of Counseling and Communication,** covers two chapters that provide skills referred to throughout the remainder of the text. These chapters provide the stepping stones needed to hone the skills of therapeutic communication and to relate to patients and the interdisciplinary team. No health professional should enter a clinical setting without being exposed to the baseline information this section establishes.

In **Chapter 1, Body Language and Nonverbal Communication,** the student is introduced to the value of body language, also referred to as kinesics. It describes the component parts of this nonverbal communication, which is often more honest than is verbal communication. The reader learns how to interpret the clients' body language, to send the appropriate professional message themselves, and to set a standard for ideal communication. This chapter was revised to discuss professional boundaries and the appropriate behaviors between a professional and a client, especially when there are gender differences. This version also reviews basic differences in body language between cultural groups. It contains current references and additional case studies.

Chapter 2, Basic Skills in Verbal Communication, builds on nonverbal skills and emphasizes listening skills, synthesizing the use of nonverbal skills, paraphrasing, empathizing, and using questions appropriately while remaining client focused. Paraphrasing is used to help the health provider verify what has been heard and to build rapport. The chapter then introduces empathy and assists the reader to develop and practice this skill. The use of open-ended questions is reviewed as are possible communication hazards. This chapter is expanded from the previous edition as it distinguishes empathy from sympathy, looks more closely at the concerns of overinvolvement, cautions of the danger of judging our clients, and explores how health professionals need to avoid taking patient comments personally. Finally, it offers a number of helpful research articles dealing with verbal communication.

Part 2, Foundations for Understanding Human Behavior, provides students with a comprehensive review of the psychosocial and behavioral dilemmas most common in health care today. The seven chapters in this section examine knowledge necessary to round out a professional's ability to comprehend and treat the human condition when added to the skills gained in Part 1.

Chapter 3, Basic Psychology, reviews different psychologic theories explaining human behavior: Maslow's Hierarchy of Human Needs, Pavlov,

Freud, Adler, Jung, and Gestalt therapy. More modern approaches are also reviewed, such as transactional analysis and Carl Rogers' focus on paraphrasing, empathizing, and positive regard. Understanding Freud's defense mechanisms is an important aspect of this chapter as it applies to so much human behavior.

Chapter 4, Mental Health and Adaptive Disorders, reviews clinical syndromes and underlying personality disorders. It looks at how different people respond to their symptoms or those of a family member, called "illness behavior." Illness requires adapting to different roles for optimal recovery. Illness behavior related to work is important in terms of motivation and effect. Illness may present in many different ways depending upon the personality of the patient, his or her intellect, and how his or her illness may impose limitations. Some patients use illness as a game (Eric Berne), using appointment negotiating and manipulation. Finally, we keep in mind the patient's primary and secondary relationships.

Chapter 5, Death and Dying, examines the Kübler-Ross stages of dying: denial, anger, bargaining, depression, and acceptance. In *denial,* a patient needs a psychologic buffer between what his or her mind can accept and harsh reality. The patient experiences a devastating sense of unfairness in the loss and is *angry*. *Bargaining* follows and may have some religious overtones as the patient struggles to find a way to change the diagnosis. During *depression* the patient more fully feels the pain of all forms of loss. *Acceptance* is generally a calmer stage in which the patient is facing what must be accepted. These stages are also true for losses that alter body image. *Negative euthanasia* and p*ositive euthanasia* are also defined. Finally, this chapter describes five ways in which to help the dying: listen, focus through paraphrasing, respond from your own gut, leave hope intact, and assist the family to be with the patient. Working with families and the hospice team is important to this content.

Chapter 6, Developmental Issues: Early Childhood and Adolescence, reviews early childhood and adolescent issues. Parents often expect a perfect child and have to be helped to accept a child that does not meet their expectations. Bonding is a close mutual attachment between infant and parent. Bonding and dependency lead to appropriate body schema and the development of a separate self. The young infant going through the "terrible twos" becomes negative as an expression of the child's sense of autonomy. Here the health practitioner is encouraged to use positive reinforcement and to encourage parents to do the same. Modeling and competence are further ways that young children will develop. This section closes with a discussion of developmental milestones.

Puberty causes rapid physiologic and emotional changes. Coping with these changes involves family and social support. The more different the teenager feels, the more support is required. Differentiating from parents nearly always means a struggle. No matter how good things are at home, adolescents fight for independence by rejecting what their parents offer. The more problems a child has had in the past, the more likely is difficulty during this breakaway phase. Eating disorders and other risky behaviors are reviewed. Families survive best when providing long-term stability and offering adolescents emotional support; rewards should be on the basis of responsible behavior.

Chapter 7, Developmental issues: Senescence, details elder issues. Older people have a wealth of experience that historically has been respected. Seventy-six million baby boomers will soon retire. Although age brings increasing loss of biologic adaptability, the great majority of the elderly still cope well with life's problems, leading fulfilling lives. However, disengagement theory states the elderly sever friendships as part of a general disengagement from society. Stigma is associated with retirement, economic loss, social isolation, touching, and sex in the elderly. Illness is increasingly common among the elderly. Because dementia is the most common reason for institutionalization, it is given special attention. The elderly have to deal with loss, and as they face their own demise, they may choose to have advance directives, including a living will. End-of-life decisions are frequently disregarded by health care agents when the situation demands "comfort measures only."

Chapter 8, Addiction, discusses the problem of addiction—substance abuse, or chemical dependency, and smoking—with emphasis on alcoholism. It defines addiction, dependence, habituation, and tolerance and cites the addict's need to continue the substance abuse as stronger than the consequences of use. The causes of addiction are reviewed, including a biologic predisposition. Also reviewed are the psychologic responses common to most abusers, the response to peer pressure for substance misuse, and cultural links to abuse that may also be hereditary. The chapter also focuses on the classifications of addictive drugs and points out the current problem of extensive misuse of prescription drugs exceeding all street drug use except marijuana, as was exemplified by Michael Jackson's tragic death. This section has added a discussion on the medical use of marijuana and discusses the issues related to legalization of marijuana.

The prevention and treatment of substance abuse is described, including approaches to youth who have never tried drugs and efforts to target at-risk students to help prevent drug use. Narcotics Anonymous helps these addicts as AA assists the alcoholic. Motivational interviewing, cognitive behavioral therapy, and most of the therapies used for alcoholics will help all addicts. Methadone and Suboxone are two pharmacologic treatments which assist the opioid addict (heroin) from relapsing.

Smoking is the most common preventable cause of death in the United States today. Smokers give up on average 14 years of life for their habit, suffer many ailments, and risk the health of infants exposed to smoke. Smoking costs the American consumer $76 billion dollars a year in health costs and $92 billion in lost productivity and earnings. Clients should be encouraged to attend smoking cessation programs, perhaps hypnotherapy or acupuncture clinics, review literature, use a nicotine patch or gum to help with the addiction, or try other medications and counseling.

Chapter 9, The Role of Counseling in Prevention, begins with a definition of counseling and demonstrates the evolution of communication skills into good counseling techniques by introducing the *influencing response*. This section has also added a review of health-related occupations based on counseling skills. Both mental health and physical health are discussed in terms of risk factors that counseling may mediate, with emphasis on a preventive model. Risk factors are viewed in three major categories: genetic programming, environmental conditions, and lifestyle factors. The national epidemic of obesity and metabolic syndrome are used to synthesize the application of this preventive model. The final section of this chapter reviews motivational strategies: (1) AIM, which stands for awareness, information, and motivation, (2) the transtheoretical model of change (TTM), and (3) the application of the TTM model, which is known as motivational interviewing.

Part 3, Issues for Heath Professionals, offers five chapters that focus on the professional's knowledge base and the skills needed by a competent health practitioner to act as a professional. This covers good inter- and intradisciplinary communications and the ethical and legal savvy a practitioner must have in these times. Knowledge of technology and its responsibilities, the professionals' role in abuse and discrimination, and a compelling case for the necessity of a multicultural perspective are presented.

Chapter 10, Interdisciplinary Communication, states the role of health care providers is always evolving. Health professionals are more involved in management, communication, and computers. Communication is vital for both intra and interdisciplinary communication. Health professional roles are defined by the patient, the job description, professional specialty training, provider perception, and liability concerns. As patients see different health professionals, the terms consultant, collaborator and referral source need to be defined. The aspiring health professional needs to be skilled not only at communicating with patients but also with other health professionals, and, increasingly, in handling information technology. Important acronyms for computerized systems are defined. The American Recovery and Reinvestment Act of 2009 is influencing implementation of computerization in both health professionals' offices and in hospitals.

Chapter 11, Professional Ethics, defines ethics as a set of guidelines for professionals that are designed to ensure public rights. Consequences for a breach of ethics can be imposed by professional organizations. These consequences are different from the punishments typically handed down for legally defined misconduct. The relationship between the health professional and the patient is discussed in terms of beneficence, nonmalfeasance, autonomy, and justice. All health professional organizations charge their members with basic responsibilities to the public in 10 areas: professional responsibility, competence, moral and legal standards, public statements, confidentiality, welfare of the consumer, professional relationships, assessment techniques, use of animals, and. research with human subjects. Understanding these principles can increase the health professional's skill in making ethical judgments. Themes such as prior informed consent and the risks/benefits ratio are key concepts for future health professionals to understand. HIPAA guidelines and standards inform health professionals of how to manage information while simultaneously protecting patients' rights. A practice that is HIPAA compliant is one that practices a highly ethical standard. Many ethical dilemmas are reviewed.

Chapter 12, Abuse, Impairment, and Discrimination, presents several examples of abuse: elder, spouse, and sexual. All forms of abuse are subjects of various federal and state laws with similar content. Mental impairment may involve incompetence, lack of insight, or developmental delay. The many forms of sexual abuse are presented, including protocols for dealing with the rape victim. Abusers need professional help, as well as the abused. Most abused people are in dependent roles. When the abuse is of sufficient severity to threaten the immediate or future mental or physical health of a person, then the abused patient must be protected. Mental impairment is divided into emotional, social, and cultural issues, including the concepts of discredited and discreditable stigma. Prejudice is contrasted with discrimination. Disability involving four major areas—medical, social, educational, and vocational—is a major area for specialization of a number of allied health professionals. The provisions of the Americans with Disabilities Act are presented.

Chapter 13, Legal Concerns, states only those who have prepared by virtue of educational training, who have not committed a felony, who have good character references, and who have proper clinical training may be licensed. Certification and registration also offer access to professional status and privileges. Accreditation is a process of approving educational training programs for health professionals. The power inherent in this approval process has made accreditation a historically political tool. Legal controls like licensure work best in tandem with the ethical controls of the various health professional associations. Malpractice is defined, and the authors point out that the most common cause of suits is a lack of relationship or breakdown of the relationship between patient and health professional. Communication and documentation are the cornerstones of preventing malpractice suits.

Chapter 14, Multicultural Health Issues, is a new chapter in this textbook. It provides a brief historical perspective on ethnic, cultural, and racial issues within the United States. It defines the term culture to include beliefs, practices, religion, language, music, sports, laws, taboos, and much more beyond ethnic identity. Many relevant terms are defined within a context of inclusion. The considerations raised may be applied to gender differences and to those with disabilities. The reader will see the cultural and familial influences on health and develop an appreciation of the importance of cultural competence among providers. An overview of ethnocentricity is provided as well as an overview of popular alternative medicine practices and mental health concerns. It is believed that all of health care profits by learning from other cultures even though their practices may be non–evidence based. It is also necessary to understand the belief systems of our clients in order to reach them for appropriate treatment. This is imperative to becoming culturally competent.

This chapter synthesizes the impact of demographic trends and how current and future populations' base needs will require specific consideration for both physical and mental health issues. Most importantly this chapter assists the reader to look at his or her own ability to make a difference, individually and through institutions. The chapter borrows from social psychology to examine how individuals make generalizations through impression formation and attribution theory. Strategies are discussed for making a more meaningful impact on the health care needs of Americans irrespective of race, ethnicity, color, religion, language, gender, disability, sexual preference, or gender identity, requiring that providers become involved with the communities they wish to serve.

New to the Third Edition

- An entire chapter on multiculturalism was added to help students gain insight into cultural differences in the health care setting and how to handle them.
- References and examples are updated with current health statistics and information.
- Learning Outcomes are updated using Bloom's Taxonomy.
- Key Terms are included in each chapter opener.
- Case studies illustrate common scenarios that the student might see in health care settings, and each case study has at least one question tied to it in order to encourage the student to think critically about communication and its implications.
- The Chapter Review includes References and Additional Readings so the student can easily find a resource to expand upon a concept that might need further clarification.
- Key Points boxes define and expand upon important terms or concepts.

Supplements

McGraw-Hill Higher Education Online Learning Center

- Access the Online Learning Center at **www.mhhe.com/adamscommunication3e.**
- Quizzes for each chapter supplement the end-of-chapter reviews in the textbook.
- Flashcards containing key terms and definitions taken from each chapter enable the student to self-test throughout the course.
- A thorough PowerPoint® slide presentation for every chapter makes the teaching and learning experience exciting and is available to students for the visual learner to be able to pace him or herself through the text material.
- An Instructor's Manual contains a chapter overview, key term review, answer keys, and additional activities and class assignments for every chapter.
- McGraw-Hill's EZ-Test Test Generator is an electronic testing program that allows instructors to create tests from book-specific items. It accommodates a wide range of question types, and instructors may add their own questions. Multiple versions of the test can be created, and any test can be exported for use with course management systems such as WebCT, BlackBoard, or PageOut. EZ-Test Online is a new service and gives you an online place to easily administer the exams and quizzes you create with EZ-Test. The program is available for Windows and Macintosh environments.
- At least one video vignette accompanies each chapter to illustrate important concepts in therapeutic communication. A series of questions is presented after each vignette to reinforce the learning outcomes of the respective chapters.

Acknowledgments

Therapeutic Communication for Health Professionals must begin by thanking our editors, especially Andrea Edwards, for her superb editing, patience, and kindness while keeping us on track; Bonnie Hemrick for moving the project along; and Debbie Fitzgerald for her original faith in us and the project and for her fairness in multiple conference calls!

We are most grateful to Sally Fraley, a health professional in her own right, who stepped out of this role to provide numerable high-tech services to these low-tech authors and used her artistic flare to help select the art for this text. Her technical expertise and coverage 24/7 kept the project on target and relieved much stress. She is a good friend as well.

Pamela Roberts, Ed.D, P.T., deserves thanks as her work on developmental issues for infants and children has withstood each edition of this text. Her original work was appropriate, important, and beneficial to the education of health professionals.

RuthAnn Lobo, the dearest of friends, is a person who deals with multiple levels of health care. She believed in this book and wrote a sensitive and compassionate foreword that introduces the reader to the importance of the human side of illness and disease. We dedicate this book to her and to all who struggle with health issues.

We also dedicate this book to our spouses, Roger Adams and Ann Jones, who have had to fare many hours without us and take on additional chores while we were rewriting this textbook. Further, this book is dedicated to Peter's children, Ashley, Rebecca, and Alexandra, and his grandson Marcos; to Andrew Adams, a writer who had faith that his mother could manage one more book and whose own work was always an inspiration; and to Alana Fritsch, with love.

Finally, this book is a tribute to the institutions where the authors have worked and so have learned about the real meaning of patient care and the value of communication: the University of Connecticut, Windham Community Memorial Hospital, Perception Programs, Inc., and Natchaug Hospital. These experiences have taught us well.

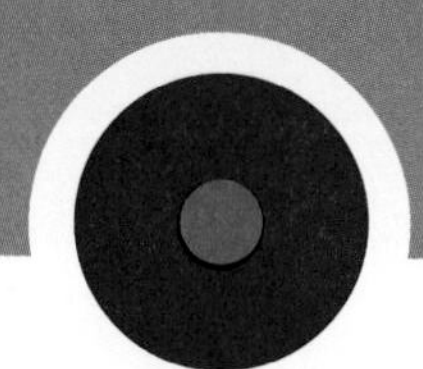

Reviewers

Sandra Affenito, PhD, RD, CDN
Department of Nutrition
Saint Joseph College
West Hartford, Connecticut

Dr. Hooshiyar Ahmadi
Medical Assisting
Remington College
Frisco, Texas

Cindi Brassington, BS, MS, CMA
Professor of Allied Health
Quinebaug Valley Community College
Danielson, Connecticut

Janet Davis, BSN, MS, MBA, PhD
School of Nursing and Health Sciences
Robert Morris College
Chicago, Illinois

James Dickerson, AAS
Medical Assisting
Remington College, Dallas Campus
Garland, Texas

Gareth R. Dutton, PhD
Medical Humanities & Social Sciences
Florida State University College of Medicine
Tallahassee, Florida

Jasminka llich-Ernst, PhD, RD
Nutrition, Food, and Exercise Sciences
Florida State University
Tallahassee, Florida

Londa Ogden Haycock, RN, BSN, RMA
Medical Assisting Division
Keiser University
Fort Lauderdale, Florida

Marie A. Janes, Med, RHIA
Director, HIM & CHIA Program
The University of Toledo
Toledo, Ohio

Bonny Kehm, MSN, RN
Keiser University
Nursing, Medical Assisting
Fort Lauderdale, Florida

Alberto Leon, MD
Biology Department
Keiser University
Fort Lauderdale, Florida

Michelle McClatchey, BS, CHR
School of Healthcare
Westwood College
Calumet City, Illinois

Selinda McCumbers, BA
Director of Education
Brighton College
Hudson, Ohio

Norma Mercado, MAHS, BS, RHIA
Health Information Technology
Austin Community College
Austin, Texas

Dr. James Morley, BS, MA, PhD
Director of New Campus, Program and Online Development
Apollo College
Albuquerque, New Mexico

Janette Rodiguez, RN
Program Director Medical Assisting
Wood Tobe Coburn
New York, New York

Anita A. Rossell, BA
Medical Department
Pittsburgh Technical Institute
Oakdale, Pennsylvania

Pratima Sampat-Mar, M.Ed
Online Education Department
Pima Medical Institute
Mesa, Arizona

Janet R. Sesser, BS
Corporate Education
High-Tech Institute, Inc.
Phoenix, Arizona

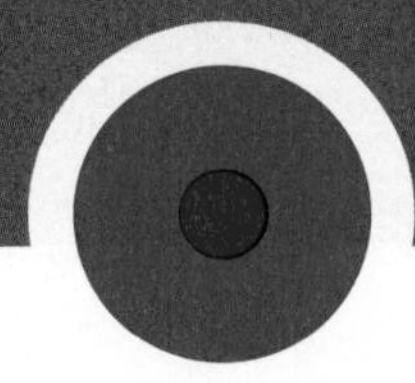

Walkthrough

Death and Dying

Learning Outcomes

After reading this chapter, you should be able to:

5.1 Describe the five Kübler-Ross stages of loss.
5.2 Understand denial.
5.3 Recognize anger in a patient and how to deal with it.
5.4 Discuss bargaining and how to work with the patient at this stage, including the use of empathy.
5.5 Identify depression and how to help patients cope with it.
5.6 Recognize when a patient has reached acceptance.
5.7 Discuss reactions and significance to changes in body image.
5.8 Describe the difference between positive and negative euthanasia and philosophies connected with right-to-die issues.
5.9 List five ways to help the dying patient and their family.

Key Terms

Acceptance
Anger
Bargaining
Body image
Defense mechanism
Denial
Depression
Hospice
Negative euthanasia
Positive euthanasia
Stages of loss
Thanatology

Chapter Openers

Every chapter opens with Learning Outcomes and a list of Key Terms that prepare the student for the chapter they are about to read.

Typically, jewelry should be modest in size and not detract from the health professional's message. Hairstyle and clothing should also fit the image of the professional. Many health facilities ask that piercing jewelry beyond a few modest earrings be removed when an individual is at work, although exceptions may be made if the clients being served are likely to be similarly adorned. Typically, it is also appropriate to keep tattoos hidden from view while at work. All these examples are subjective, and some health care employees choose to assert their individuality by persons of either gender keeping a nose stud or a male wearing a long ponytail, both of which may be a topic of negotiation within the workplace. However, one study found that patients want their health professionals to be dressed formally, not in blue jeans or sandals, as a carefully dressed provider may convey that he or she is meticulous and careful in practice.

Good hygiene—a clean body and neat, clean clothing—coupled with a pleasant or benign odor is ideal. Heavy perfumes or aftershaves are inap-

Key Point

Nonverbal message: communicating without using language. The most powerful way of communicating with patients. A relaxed yet steady gaze is generally ideal eye contact in the United States. Facial expression and professional appearance and adornment are key to sending the correct message. Adopt a relaxed posture with hands relaxed.

Key Points

Key Points boxes define and expand upon important terms or concepts.

CASE STUDY 5-1

For three years a daughter dutifully visited her mother in the nursing home. She came for two to five hours a day. She read to her mother, fed her, and helped to bathe her. Throughout these three years the mother was expected to die any time. Her condition, the result of a stroke, went from grave to critical. The health care providers involved made assumptions about the daughter's preparation for her mother's death. They believed the daughter was devoted to her mother, but they thought she would be tired of caring for her and worrying about her. Further, they reasoned that the daughter had come to accept death as the inevitable release for both. The nursing home staff was not prepared for the daughter's reaction the day her mother did die.

The daughter was called at her home at 7 a.m. She was told that her mother had died quietly during the night. When she heard these words, she began screaming hysterically, "She can't be dead, she can't be dead!" Fifteen minutes later, still wearing a nightgown, she arrived at the nursing home and dashed to her mother's door. There she flung on her mother's bed and sobbed and moaned. It was not until her own daughter was summoned from a nearby town that she was comforted.

Case Studies

Case studies illustrate common scenarios that the student might see in health care settings, and each case study has at least one question tied to it in order to encourage the student to think critically about communication and its implications.

Summary

Each chapter ends with a summary that emphasizes key information that was presented in the chapter.

Summary

Nonverbal communication skills serve the health professional well as you learn to observe and interpret the behavior of others. That which is non-neutral has some meaning. When nonverbal behavior contradicts verbal behavior, your attention must be focused there. Nonverbal interpretations also help you in establishing communication with those who cannot or will not talk. The nonverbal is often more revealing than the spoken word. The key elements of nonverbal language are kinesics, proxemics, haptics, oculesics, chronemics, olfactics, appearance and adornment, posture, locomotion, sound symbols, silence, and vocalics.

You must be aware of what specific physical positions, such as encountering a patient with arms crossed who is staring at the floor, might mean. You must always check your perceptions rather than assuming the meaning of nonverbal behavior, especially when cultural differences may exist. Good observational skills are an important component of the nonverbal process.

As health providers, you must cultivate the message you wish to send nonverbally. The right attire, good hygiene, and attention to body language are essential to success. You want to appear open, interested, and approachable. Facial expressions and proximity are significant, as is vocal usage. How you use your voice can significantly alter the way your message is received. Focusing on specific behaviors in a nonjudgmental way can be a primary communication tool for the health professional.

The ideal model for nonverbal communication is reviewed as follows along with suggestions of behaviors to avoid.

Ideal Communication Style

- Facing patient/client, holding gaze
- Arms at sides or gently folded
- Legs upright or gently crossed
- Posture erect but not rigid
- Distance of approximately one arm's length between professional and patient/client
- No barriers between health practitioner and patient/client

Chapter Review

The chapter review includes key term definitions, chapter review questions, critical thinking questions for every case study, references, and additional readings to reinforce the learning outcomes of each chapter.

Chapter Review

Key Term Review

Acceptance: Fifth Kübler-Ross stage of loss: resignation with fate, return to realistic existence

Anger: Second Kübler-Ross stage of loss: unreasonable anger directed at self or others.

Bargaining: Third Kübler-Ross stage of loss: delaying tactic to put off need for acceptance.

Body image: Mental picture of self including value judgments or psychological distortions.

Defense mechanism: Psychological means of avoiding conscious conflict.

Denial: First Kübler-Ross stage of loss: use of denial as defense mechanism by a bereaved client.

Depression: Fourth Kübler-Ross stage of loss: actual grief from loss.

Hospice: Supportive medical and home care focusing on dying with dignity; an organization that helps the dying and their families.

Negative euthanasia: The tacit noninterference with the process of death.

Positive euthanasia: *Directly* taking a life.

Stages of loss: Kübler-Ross' five stages of bereavement: denial, anger, bargaining, depression, and acceptance.

Thanatology: The study of death.

Chapter Review Questions

1. How is it possible for a patient to experience both anger and denial at the same time?
2. What counseling strategies will help you the most when dealing with dying patients?
3. What must you do to prepare yourself to work with dying patients?
4. What do you think the reason is for the statement "A big problem for the dying is to find someone who will listen to them?"
5. Why might a mastectomy patient suffer more emotional side effects than a patient who has just lost a kidney to cancer surgery (assume the same prognosis for each)?
6. What is it about body image that makes this a serious area of concern?

Case Study Critical Thinking Questions

1. Look at Case Study 5-1. How does bargaining differ from denial and how are they similar? What ideas have you about how to detect when a family member may be in denial?
2. Regarding Case Study 5-2, might you see a time when Dr. Kevorkian's ideas will be accepted as necessary? think society will deal with euthanasia if resources are plentiful?
3. Refer to Case Study 5-3. You are living through a period of history in which many American children regularly die of starvation and neglect. How do we, as a society, justify putting financial resources and

Therapeutic Communication for Health Professionals

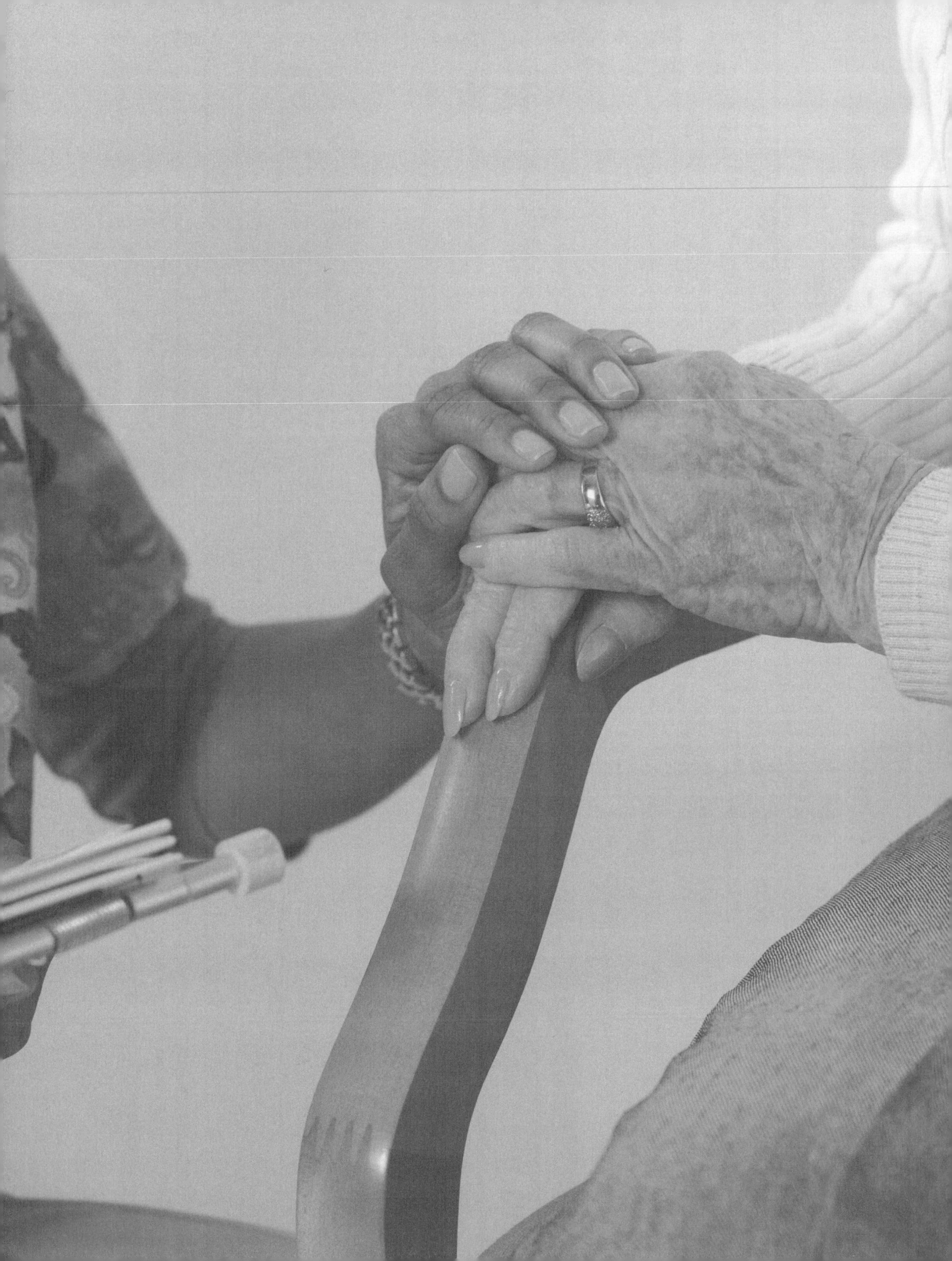

Body Language and Nonverbal Communication

Learning Outcomes

After reading this chapter, you should be able to:

1.1 Define nonverbal behaviors.

1.2 Recognize the effect on communication of using nonverbal language.

1.3 Illustrate several nonverbal behaviors and interpret a patient's nonverbal message.

1.4 Assess the message you are sending in nonverbal communication.

1.5 List the components of the ideal communication model.

1.6 Utilize the correct boundaries between patient and professional, especially where gender differences exist.

1.7 Explain sensitivity to cultural issues in communication.

Key Terms

Adornment
Atmosphere for communication
Behavioral observation
Boundaries
Chronemics
Cultural sensitivity
Haptics
Ideal communication model
Kinesics
Locomotion
Neutral position of behavior
Nonverbal behavior
Nonverbal language
Nonverbal message
Oculesics
Olfactics
Posture
Proxemics
Silence
Sound Symbols
Vocalics

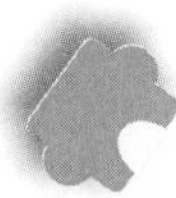

Introduction

What you know is important, but deciding what and how to share this knowledge is just as essential to your success as a health professional. The basic elements of communication are that there is a *message*, a *sender*, and a *receiver*. The *message* that needs to be sent (e.g., "You must get at least 30 minutes of aerobic exercise three times a week if you hope to prevent or delay cardiovascular disease") is an example of your professional knowledge. Your role as a health professional makes you the appropriate *sender* of that message (e.g., "I want to speak with you about an important matter as your [dietitian, nurse, physical therapist, sports medicine consultant, medical assistant, doctor] as there are preventive health strategies that will be very helpful to you." You then focus on the *receiver* to determine what may affect his or her ability to hear your message, such as cultural and age issues. Remember that messages may be sent in many ways, such as verbally, nonverbally, and in various written and electronic formats by the health care worker. Nonverbal skills are essential to being sensitive and effective and well received by the client.

This chapter helps you to focus on the nonverbal messages that augment those that are spoken or delivered face-to-face. Often nonverbal messages are made instinctively or unconsciously and deliver their own strong message. In the context of a professional setting, you must become aware of the messages you are sending nonverbally as well as those you are observing.

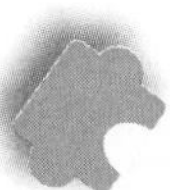

Nonverbal Behaviors

Throughout the day you witness many behaviors. But few people put their observations to use. Have you ever worked with someone who seemed so good at understanding others and predicting their behavior that you thought they might be psychic? Chances are they just use their observational skills more intensely than most people. Observing body language is a valuable skill, especially for those in the helping professions.

What is worn is also important in nonverbal communications because attire sends a message of its own. Have you ever noticed someone who wears a white lab coat all the time? What might be learned from this observation? When someone wears a lab coat, whether or not he or she is in the lab or treating a patient, it can safely be assumed that there is some meaning to this behavior. Perhaps the person has a busy schedule and no time to change out of the coat between jobs. Perhaps the person is self-conscious about his or her wardrobe and uses the coat to hide his or her clothing. Or perhaps the white lab coat has become a strong part of that individual's identity; that is, he or she wishes to be set apart from others and enjoy the visible recognition of being seen as a health professional.

This latter possibility has a definition as a defense mechanism called identification which will be studied in a later chapter. The important thing to note here is that you might easily misinterpret the meaning of the lab coat if you do not ask. But be sure, if someone is engaged in a non-neutral behavior such as constantly wearing a lab coat, then there is some meaning there.

What a person wears is just one example of **nonverbal behavior**. As health care providers you must be careful in your interpretations. You must learn to recognize universal neutral behaviors and to use this information to better understand your patients. A **neutral position of behavior** is the body's *natural* position. A neutral position is having your hands relaxed at your sides; other positions are purposeful and have some meaning. Dressing "as others do" is also neutral.

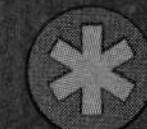

Key Points

Nonverbal behavior or kinesics using observational skills or reading body language to understand a patient's underlying feelings.

Neutral position of behavior the body's *natural* position. Hands relaxed at sides is a neutral position; other positions are purposeful and have some meaning.

Nonverbal language composite of eye contact, facial expressions, appearance, posture and proximity.

Components of Nonverbal Language

The main components of **nonverbal language** are listed as follows.

- **Kinesics:** Body motions such as shrugs, foot tapping, drumming fingers, clicking pens, winking, facial expressions, and gestures
- **Proxemics (proximity):** Use of space to make contact or to provide privacy
- **Haptics:** Touch
- **Oculesics:** Eye contact
- **Chronemics:** Use of time; pausing, waiting, speeding up
- **Olfactics:** Smell
- **Adornment:** Dress, cleanliness, jewelry, tattoos, piercings
- **Posture:** Body position, stance
- **Locomotion:** Walking, jumping, swaying, and moving with a wheelchair
- **Sound Symbols:** Grunting, ahs, pointed throat clearing
- **Silence:** Long pauses, withholding information, secrecy
- **Vocalics:** Tone, timbre, volume

Throughout this chapter, please refer back to this list as you learn to list examples of how nonverbal language is recognized and what effect it has on communication.

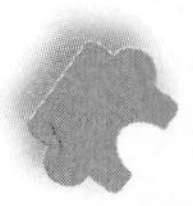

Nonverbal Language and Communication

In a classroom or hospital setting, you can learn a great deal about others simply by observing them. You will note that some people sit with their backs straight whereas others sit with their feet up on the chair in front of them; some sit close together while others seem to place themselves apart. Look around the classroom. Do you see students twisting hair or fidgeting with a pen or doodling? Perhaps you interpret these behaviors as reflections of what is going on inside these individuals.

Many people reveal more through their facial expressions (part of kinesics) than they may wish to convey. They may sit alone and frown at what appears to be nothing at all; others may exhibit a faint pleasant smile or offer a nearly vacant blank stare. Just by observations you can begin to formulate opinions about others and react according to your impressions.

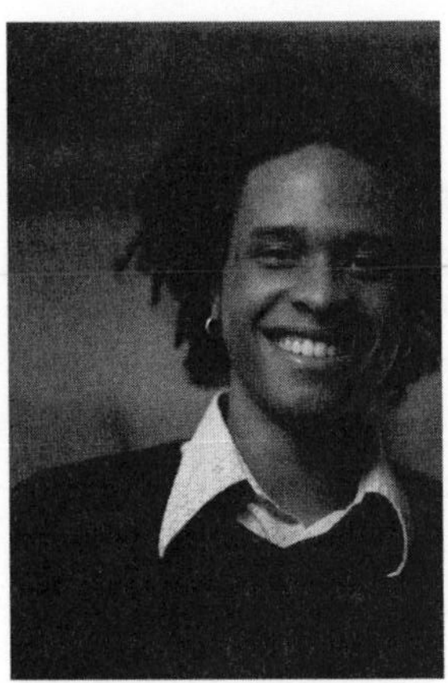

A warm and engaging smile appeals to those he approaches.

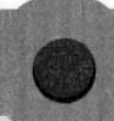

CASE STUDY 1-1

Two friends, a man and a woman, annually attended tournament games for which all attendees purchased tickets for two games on one night and one game on a subsequent day as a package. This meant that some fans at the end of the first game would know their team was out of the play and they would no longer be interested in staying around for the second or the final game. When their team was not playing in the first game, these friends would wait near the sections containing the preferred seats in which the losing team's fans were seated and approach them as they walked out, hoping to receive their seats for the remaining games. The woman always wore an expression of great sympathy and concern, but year after year she rarely received better seats. Her male friend, however, always upgraded his seat and usually had tickets to share with her and others they knew. Finally, the woman observed him in action and noticed that he approached each group with a kind smile on his face. Although some folks rebuffed him, most would stop and talk and invariably pass on their tickets. At the following tournament she approached the fans with a smile and her luck changed.

Observe two strangers from a distance. Jot down the behaviors you see. Guess at what may be communicated between or among them. Bring these notes to class for possible class discussion of what their behaviors may mean, describing one or more possible explanations or interpretations.

Once individuals begin to interact, verbal behaviors and mannerisms such as nail biting, pen flicking, and hair tossing enter the picture. For example, without examining content, what would you think of an individual whose speech was rapid and who twisted around in his or her seat throughout your interaction?

Vocalics and sound symbols refer to the pitch of a voice. Whereas a certain pitch may be pleasant to some ears, for others it will be difficult to detect. If you speak too rapidly or stumble with frequent "ahs," you may be hard to follow. When you think of the voices you enjoy in the broadcasting business, there are qualities and variations of tone. Certainly no one likes to hear a lecturer speak in a monotone unless he or she needs a nap! Training your voice to exude the feelings needed for the situation is part of a professional image. The sounds you make can convey confidence and warmth or frustration and fear. Discuss this response with your classmates:

CASE STUDY 1-2

Margie was a shy 14-year-old with a bad knee injury when she entered the physical therapy clinic. Her physical therapist was a hardworking and dedicated fellow about her dad's age named Jim. Jim was often anxious when faced with a new case because he wanted to do his best for every patient. His anxiety manifested itself in a chronic throat-clearing tic. When he first met Margie, he began clearing his throat and continued to do so every few minutes throughout their 30-minute session. Margie had her mother call the clinic the next day and ask for a different therapist. What do you think happened?

Margie, being shy, felt embarrassed every time Jim cleared his throat. She believed it called attention to her and to her problem. She couldn't bear having people look over every time Jim made that noise. They were not well-suited to working together.

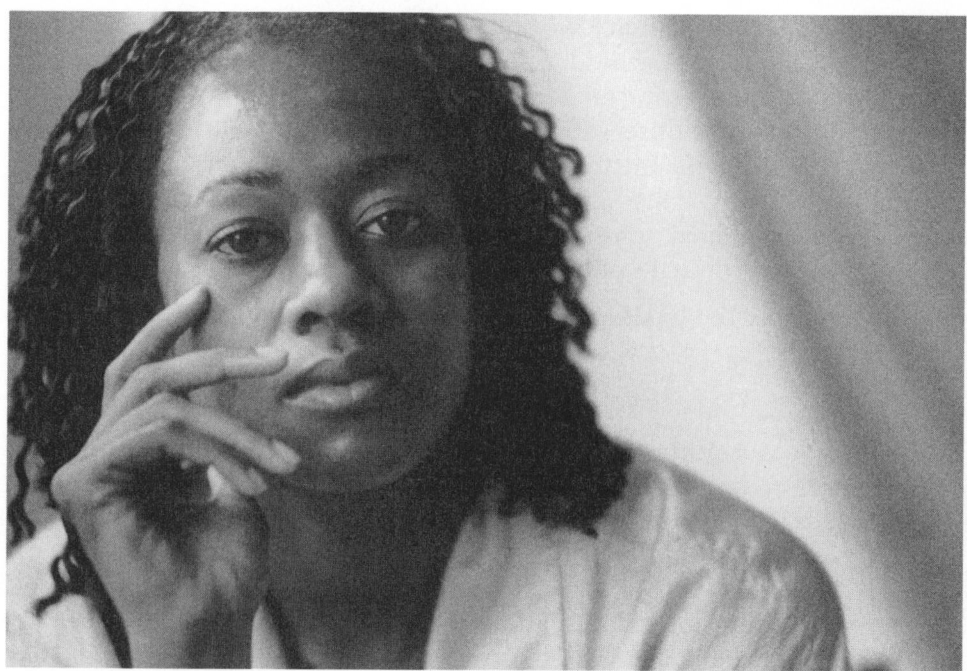

A relaxed, steady gaze

If you have a nervous condition, then you may need to work on it in order to avoid conflict for you in a professional setting. In most cases, however, vocalics simply refers to changeable habits or vocal qualities that skill and practice will allow you to correct.

The use of oculesics (eye contact) differs among cultures, but for the moment we will focus on what is typical for most Americans and later look more thoughtfully at cultural considerations. Certainly, all body cues need to be interpreted with a view toward the receiver's ethnic background. Typically, a relaxed yet steady gaze is ideal eye contact unless cultural information leads you to a different approach. Contrast a conversation with ideal eye contact with a conversation (same words) in which the speaker stares at the floor. Try this to exemplify the point: Client [staring at the floor] "I stopped taking my medication over the weekend." Now the same client states those words while making direct eye contact. In the first version you would instantly suspect a problem, but in the second your first thought might be that the client is feeling better.

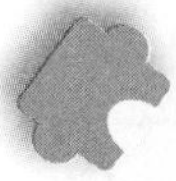

Nonverbal Behavior and Interpretation

Unfortunately, you cannot always be sure of what certain behaviors indicate. For example, if you observe patient X sitting with her arms folded across her chest, you must take care not to misinterpret her position. Perhaps she wants to protect herself from others, is hugging herself as a form of comfort, is self-conscious about her figure, or is simply cold and trying to warm up. Or, you might leave a party quickly because your beeper went off. The casual observer might guess you were bored or rude when neither was true.

What is your immediate response to the patient with her arms folded? Can you think of several other explanations?

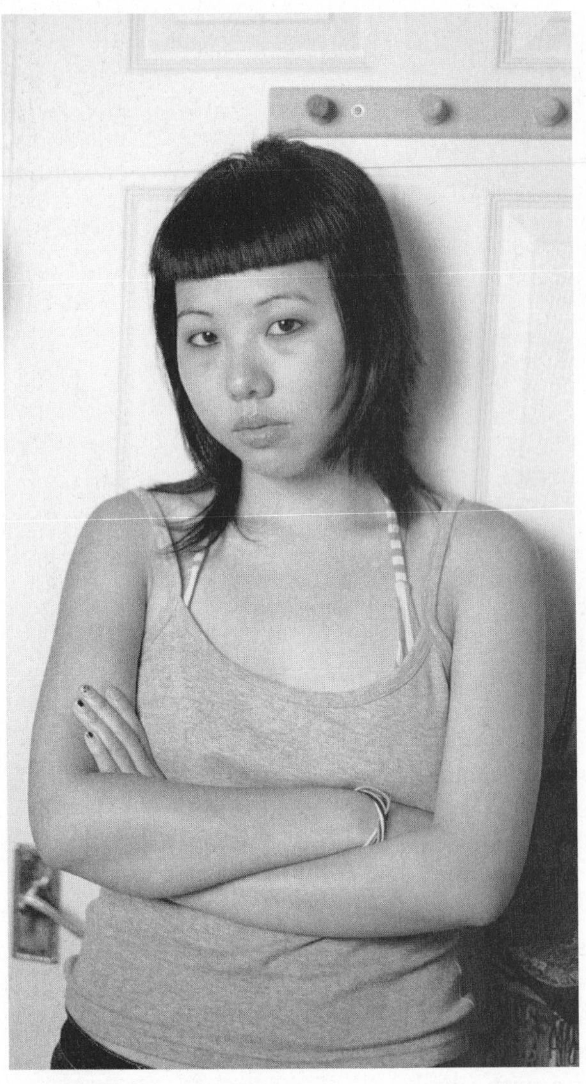
Hostile teen

If you are working with someone and wish to understand what they are communicating nonverbally, you must *first* take in the observation. *Then* you must follow your observation up with a question about what this behavior means to the individual. For example, you might say, "I see you've turned away from me and your arms are folded across your chest." You could follow that observation with one of the following comments:

"I'm wondering what that means to you."

or

"I guess you're feeling a little alone and frightened."

Either of these responses may be correct. The second, however, is recommended only if you have already established a rapport with the client. Otherwise you risk losing the client by labeling his or her feeling too quickly or inappropriately. Remember, first you make a strictly behavioral observation (nonjudgmental) such as "I see your arms are folded across your chest." Then you want to identify accurately what this non-neutral behavior means to the client. This type of reflection is very helpful in a clinical setting when you are first meeting a new patient.

Another benefit to making these observations in communication relates to conflicting messages. Often a patient will verbalize one message while indicating the opposite with his body. For example, a person may smile broadly while telling you how afraid he is of returning to work following a heart attack. By reflecting this obvious conflict back to the patient, you will be better able to appreciate what he is actually feeling.

"What does it mean to you when you are smiling while talking about your heart attack?"

"I wonder if you are smiling because that helps mask how frightened you really are."

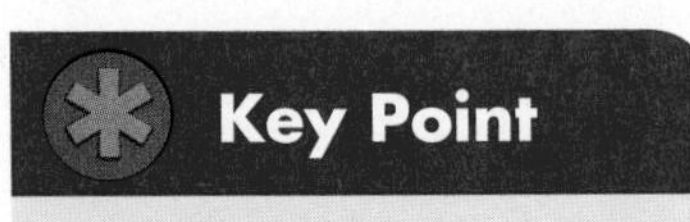

Behavioral observation studying the patient's kinesics, specifically, oculesics, facial expressions, appearance, posture, and proxemics.

Behavioral observation may also be the only tool you have for communicating with patients who are speech impaired or are unwilling to speak (silence). If the patient can hear and speaks a language you know, you may respond to them simply by reflecting what you see. For example, an adolescent may sit grimly and silently in the health professional's office after being dragged in by a parent. The health professional may find that the adolescent meets most verbal approaches with more silent resistance. But, if the following approach is used, the patient may decide to talk simply because someone has conveyed understanding.

"You've been sitting on my couch for nearly 20 minutes now without saying a word. You've kept your eyes on your hands, and your whole body is leaning forward. I'm getting the message that you don't want to speak with me."

or

"You haven't spoken in 20 minutes and you won't even look at me. Perhaps you are angry with your mother for bringing you here. If I were you, I'd probably feel the same way."

Again, the second approach involves some risk because it brings in more feelings. You should use feeling words with patients only when you are confident that you understand the emotional issues involved. How and when to use feelings is discussed in more detail in the section on empathy in Chapter 2.

Now that you have begun to see the value of body language in understanding others, you should also look at the messages you may be sending.

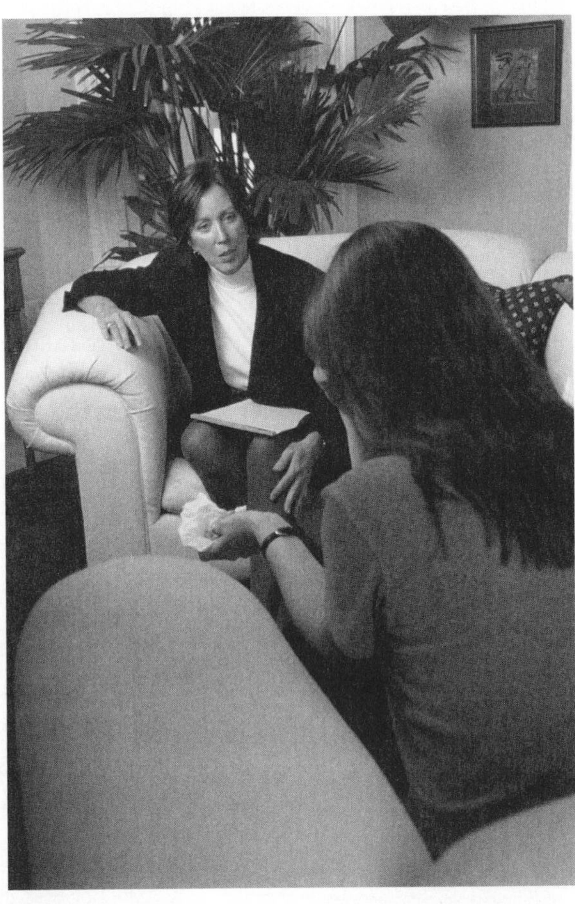

Woman listening

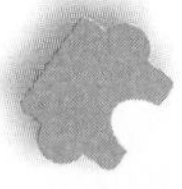

Assessing Nonverbal Communication

Perhaps the most obvious **nonverbal message** you send is your appearance, which includes adornment such as clothing, jewelry, tattoos, piercings, and hairstyles. To fit in as an entry-level health professional, you may want to begin by playing the role of the health professional complete with "costume." If professionals in your field generally wear white lab coats, uniforms, or tailored suits, you would do well to dress as they do, at least until you have established yourself professionally.

Typically, jewelry should be modest in size and not detract from the health professional's message. Hairstyle and clothing should also fit the image of the professional. Many health facilities ask that piercing jewelry beyond a few modest earrings be removed when an individual is at work, although exceptions may be made if the clients being served are likely to be similarly adorned. Typically, it is also appropriate to keep tattoos hidden from view while at work. All these examples are subjective, and some health care employees choose to assert their individuality by persons of either gender keeping a nose stud or a male wearing a long ponytail, both of which may be a topic of negotiation within the workplace. However, one study found that patients want their health professionals to be dressed formally, not in blue jeans or sandals, as a carefully dressed provider may convey that he or she is meticulous and careful in practice.

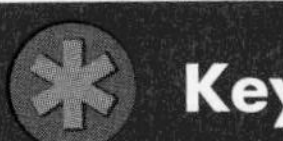

Key Point

Nonverbal message: communicating without using language. The most powerful way of communicating with patients. A relaxed yet steady gaze is generally ideal eye contact in the United States. Facial expression and professional appearance and adornment are key to sending the correct message. Adopt a relaxed posture with hands relaxed.

Good hygiene—a clean body and neat, clean clothing—coupled with a pleasant or benign odor is ideal. Heavy perfumes or aftershaves are inappropriate in a work setting. If oral disease or spicy foods make others back away from you, you will suffer for it professionally. These examples are grouped under the classification of olfactics, which relate to the way humans smell; in a professional setting, a neutral or nondetectable odor is recommended. Your sense of smell may also assist you clinically: If you smell sugary/fruity breath on a patient, he or she may be having trouble controlling their diabetes, or if you smell urine or alcohol, he or she may be homeless or exhibiting a drug problem. The nose gives health professionals another cue to focus in on with patients.

A less obvious consideration is your own facial expression. Just as you formulate a subliminal or unconscious opinion of another from his or her facial expression, others are responding to your facial expression as well. Few people realize how they look in random or candid moments. Generally, one prepares the face subconsciously for a moment before looking into a mirror. Shock may occur when viewing a photograph taken during an unexpected moment. Try to observe objectively what you see in such candid shots of yourself.

Sometimes, because of chronic pain or worry, an individual carries a sad or sour face into the world even long after those difficulties have been resolved. Others may look tough and unapproachable even though they are warm and friendly. Your colleagues and patients will observe you beyond the time you spend directly with them. They may form an opinion of you simply by observing how you walk down a hallway (locomotion). Try to get an objective analysis of your candid, off-guard expression, and train your face to change slightly if a problem is evident. Videotaping can be especially valuable, particularly if you record yourself interviewing another person.

Just as the man with the smiling face got the positive response in the earlier example, so will the health professional who smiles on the job, but instead of tickets, positive patient interactions will be the reward.

CASE STUDY 1-3

Two medical technologists (MTs) graduated from college together in a large midwestern city. Because they were friends, they applied to the same major metropolitan hospital for jobs, and both were hired with the same job title and salary. Both were young men of the same age and ethnic background. Both occasionally had a problem drawing blood from a patient. One man became quite agitated with himself when the draw did not go right, and this frequently resulted in a second missed attempt or in the patient refusing to let the MT try again. But the other MT would smile warmly at his patients, apologize for any inconvenience, and then calmly, and nearly always successfully, complete the second blood drawing. Obviously the effect demonstrated by the smile and warm response of the second MT made a difference to the patients observing him. After a year of work the second MT received a raise and promotion that his friend did not.

The kind of body language that makes you comfortable with others makes others comfortable with you. If you want to encourage your patients to talk openly, then you must offer open, approachable nonverbal as well as verbal cues. The rushed and tense health practitioner, an attitude perhaps conveyed through rapid speech (chronemics), does not stimulate dialogue nor does she or he escape detection. Recognizing the patient's nonverbal messages isn't enough; you must send the right nonverbal messages yourself.

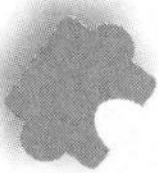

Ideal Communication Environment

To review, you will have noted that health care providers must take responsibility for sending out appropriate messages regarding their desire to interact with the patient. Through their behavior, they convey the following traits to patients:

- Friendliness
- Confidence
- Professionalism

Further, health professionals must develop highly attuned observational skills and learn by observing the patient. They use their observations to better establish rapport and to better understand patient problems and conflicts by appropriately reflecting them back to the patient.

The next aspect of nonverbal communication training entails creating the best **atmosphere for communication** to take place. A lot of this involves **proxemics**. Health practitioners and patients should not be separated by great distances or large barriers such as desks or machines. An arm's length apart is culturally acceptable in the United States. This distance is close enough for intimate conversations without making most Americans feel that their personal space is being violated. Reportedly, the "comfort zone" for standing is 30 inches apart for Americans.

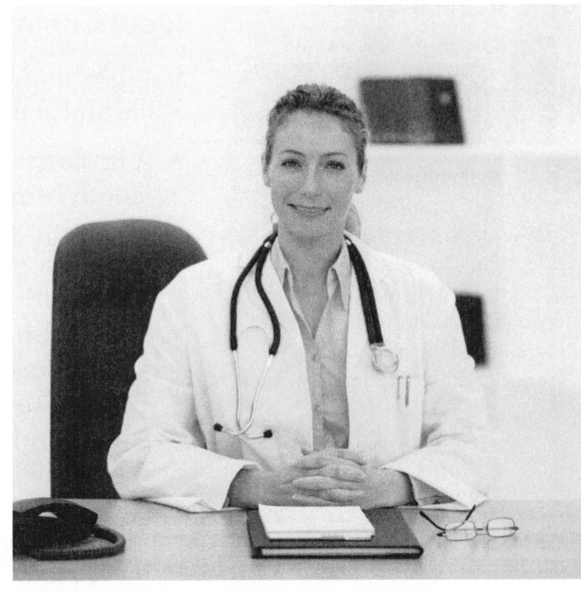

Is this woman too close?

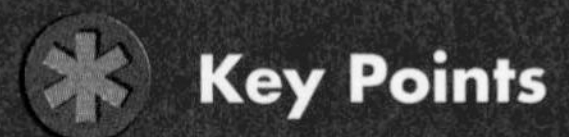

Key Points

Atmosphere for communication being at the correct distance from the patient, usually at arms length and without barriers.

Proxemics nearness, distance, or position from another.

Hospital settings can pose barriers or distractions that are less than ideal. The lack of privacy in most hospital rooms may necessitate some creative rearranging when professionals need to deal with sensitive questions. The patient's right and need for privacy can become a major stumbling block to communication progress if the health professional does not take it into account and will lead to problems with HIPAA and accreditation as discussed in Chapter 11. No matter what the barriers are, health professionals should strive for confidentiality by:

- Not holding discussions in hallways
- Closing doors when possible
- Gently suggesting that visitors wait outside when you must examine or treat
- Pulling drapes around inpatients when a roommate is present during a discussion

Patients may *need* to be touched (haptics). It was believed a few years back that there was an increased rate of healing in those who receive stroking or massaging as part of their treatment compared with those who are not intentionally touched. This may be especially true among elderly patients but also differs widely on the basis of ethnic variables (see the section Cultural Sensitivity in Nonverbal Communication in this chapter). Certainly you want to be close enough to your patients to hold a hand, pat a shoulder, or offer a tissue if emotions are strongly expressed. It is easy to believe that patients who may feel isolated and lonely will respond positively to the familiar yet missed sense of another person's touch on their arms. In times of psychological stress, a touch may be the only message that penetrates their pain; your hand on a patient's shoulder could feel like a lifeline. Yet, health professionals are wise to ask before touching a patient who is not well known to them to simply be certain that touching is okay with this person.

Ideal Communication Model

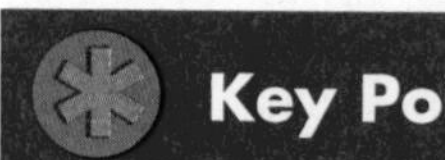

Key Point

Ideal communication model professionally attired; arm's length from the patient; private setting; relaxed, attentive posture; friendly expression and vocalics; holding patient's gaze; focusing on patient's body language and reflecting conflict.

Establishing the **ideal communication model** with respect to nonverbal skills and settings involves the following:

- A professionally attired health practitioner sits approximately an arm's length from the patient.
- The room is privately occupied for at least the duration of their interaction.
- The health professional is relaxed but in an attentive posture.
- The health professional's facial expressions and vocal tone are friendly and interested; eye contact is held throughout most of the interaction.
- The health professional focuses attention on the body language of the patient, reflecting out loud any aspects that may seem to contradict what is being said.

The health professional reflects back to the patient and interprets any body language that appears to carry a message of its own (such as tightly crossed legs or clenched fists).

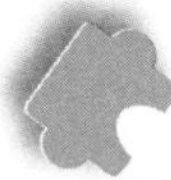

Correct Boundaries

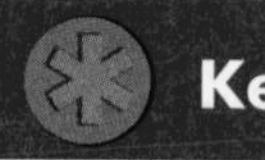

Key Point

Boundaries a mental or physical line delineating territories between two people that cannot be crossed, especially with gender or cultural differences.

Gender differences as well as cultural ones are a significant area of concern when you are practicing health care. Note the previous discussion of touching and proximity and the discussion in the section on cultural sensitivity. **Boundaries** are a concept essential to appropriate health care. Entry-level workers may need supervision to be certain they know the dangers of crossing boundaries. When men treat women or women treat men, it is especially necessary to be careful not to touch too often or perhaps not to touch when you are alone with the patient except as needed to strictly carry out your treatment. Certainly, male gynecologists have traditionally refused to treat their patients if a female assistant, usually a nurse, is not in the room. Not only does this custom add to the comfort of the patient, but it also helps protect the male practitioner from accusations of improprieties. Providers must also be alert that some patients are seductive, needy, or have mental health issues that may cause them all too easily to misinterpret a gesture. Therefore, it is the health care worker's responsibility to be certain all acts and comments are professional and not easily misunderstood.

A later chapter on ethics reviews the boundaries that must be maintained when dealing with any activities outside of the professional setting. It must be mentioned here that the chief concern is to be certain that no health professional becomes involved with a client outside of the professional setting and especially in a manner that could cloud or compromise the client–professional relationship. Certainly there should be no dating of a former patient until at least one year's time post-professional contact has elapsed or whatever guideline is established by the health provider's professional organization. Likewise, hiring of patients to provide any contractual service to the health care provider should also be avoided so that no conflicts can emerge.

If health care providers stay within their professional boundaries, studies indicate that patient responses to sensitive questions do NOT differ significantly, irrespective of gender differences between patient and provider. Remember good kinesics: Give positive, self-confident, professional, nonverbal messages to your clients, being especially sensitive to gender or cultural differences.

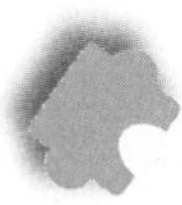

Cultural Sensitivity in Nonverbal Communication

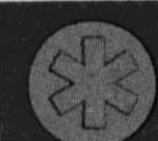

Key Point

Cultural sensitivity learning the differences among a culture's views of even haptics and oculesics. This will assist cross-cultural communication.

The world is frequently described as a "global village," indicating how much interdependence each country has. With today's technology and transportation, all but the most remote areas are quickly accessible. Naturally, the more overlap there is among peoples of the world, the more necessary it becomes to find ways of being **culturally sensitive** to and understanding each other. Not long ago, Americans tended to believe that people from different cultures must adopt American customs and were unwilling to learn anything of foreign peoples residing in the States. But the global marketplace and large increases in immigration have set the stage for Americans, and especially health care workers, to focus on learning about non-native peoples. A discussion of "body language" would not be complete without addressing the many nonverbal customs, signals, and gestures that are part of cross-cultural communication.

One caveat at the beginning of this discussion: It is not the authors' intentions to stereotype along ethnic or cultural lines; certainly there are exceptions to all that is stated. Further, customs and even food preferences are beginning to blur all over the world as markets collide and cross-pollinate. In this section, you will find behaviors that are considered "typical" of a group, and to the extent possible, these behaviors will be contrasted or compared with behaviors of people from different backgrounds. See also Table 1.1 that follows.

The following is a brief review of cultural preferences:

- *The current predominant culture in the U.S.*: Haptics—Americans may wish to be touched during difficult times or by close friends but generally stand 30 inches apart. Americans do shake hands. Young Americans do demonstrate affection publicly. Oculesics—Americans are taught to make eye contact. In terms of general kinesics, Americans use hand gestures to indicate "okay," give "a thumbs up" for a good job, and use head nodding to affirm a speaker's message.
- *African Americans:* Haptics—African Americans most commonly exhibit behaviors typical of all Americans, but this group tends to touch more, especially around other African Americans. Further, as a group, they stand closer to each other and display more emotion through laughter and touching than is typical of Euro-Americans. In the last chapter of this text the history of mistrust between whites and people of color in this country is reviewed. In this chapter on nonverbal communication, it is essential to mention that distrust is a major barrier to communications between patient and health professional. There are not enough health providers who are people of color, so health providers must find ways to bridge the trust gap, and nonverbal gestures can provide a good foundation.

Table 1.1 Generalized Nonverbal Behaviors by Ethnic/Cultural Background

	Nonverbal Behaviors						
Cultural Background	**Haptic** (Touch)	**Oculesics** (Eye contact)	**Kinesics** (Body motions, gestures)	**Vocalics** (Tone, volume)	**Posture** (Body position, Stance)	**Proxemics** (Use of space)	**Chronemics** (Time, speed, waiting)
Typical American	Generally like touch; shake hands; youth show affection in public	Eye contact expected	Used to signal; head nods affirm	Wide range varies by gender, age, social situation	Wide range; erect posture admired	30″ apart	Often in a hurry
African American* (Generally Fit as Typical American)	Touch more, especially with friends	———	———	More laughter and emotion in talking	———	Stand closer than Euro-Americans	Varies
Africans	More formal; expect respect	Quick eye contact	Nod heads to show listening	———	Erect	More formal distance until know others	Varies
Asians	Limited touch, both bowing and shaking hands; no public affection; do push in crowds	Avoid direct eye contact	Smiling covers many emotions	Never interrupt due to respect	Erect and balanced posture valued	———	———
Filipinos	Touch	Avoid long gaze	———	Laugh masks emotion	———	———	———
Hispanic	Enjoy touch	Avoid due to respect	Read others	Observe others	Observe others	Stand close	Anti-rushing

- *Africans* generally behave in a more formal manner, showing politeness with quick eye contact, erect posture, a nod of the head, and careful listening. They may be less interested in touching. When in the States they also expect to be treated with the same courtesy. This will differ somewhat by country and station in life; the more affluent and well-educated Africans tend to be more formal.
- *Asian cultures* (Chinese, Pacific Islanders, Japanese, and Koreans share much of the following): Haptics—Asians are generally not a touch-oriented society, although many cultures now use handshaking as well as bowing; public displays of affection are avoided, but pushing in crowds is common. Oculesics—Direct eye contact is typically avoided. Facial expression—Smiling covers a wide range of emotions, so be certain to reflect back what you see to clarify. Posture—Erect, balanced posture is highly valued. Silence while being spoken to is offered as a

sign of respect; great care is taken not to interrupt. People from Taiwan follow behaviors similar to these but are more likely to use handshaking than any other greeting.

- *Filipinos:* Haptics—The Philippines is generally a touch-oriented society, and people of the same sex often hold hands in public as a sign of friendship. Filipinos commonly shake hands irrespective of gender or may greet each other with a quickly raised eyebrow, the "eyebrow flash" (facial gesture). Oculesics—Prolonged eye contact is avoided as rude. Vocalics such as laughter may be used to mask embarrassment over another person's difficulties as well as to show joy.
- *Latino/Hispanic* cultures are extremely diverse; therefore, the following generalizations are made only in the interest of providing a guideline. Haptics—This is generally a culture that is comfortable with touching and closeness and requires far less personal space than do Euro-Americans. Men frequently greet each other with hugs and pats on the back. Oculesics—Avoiding eye contact may be a sign of respect. Children are often taught not to make direct eye contact with adults, and this can carry over to the patient-professional relationship. If a patient from a Hispanic culture does not wish to make eye contact with you, do not assume that there is a negative connotation as it may be a sign of respect. Vocalics and chronemics—Hispanics tend to read body language—vocal tone, speed of speech, gestures, and facial expressions plus posture—with great intensity. If you are impatient, for example, this can harm the patient-professional relationship as negative implications may be drawn from your nonverbal language that will indicate that you are rushing.

CASE STUDY 1-4

Provider (Anglo-male standing next to a Latina woman seated on an examination table): "Hello Mrs. Sanchez. What can I do for you today?"

Patient (spoken while staring at the floor): "I have a pain in my back."

Provider (stepping back from patient and speaking more loudly): "Well, where in your back, how bad is it, and how long have you had it?"

Patient (beginning to perspire): "I'm sorry to bother you, but I just bent over in the shower, and now it is hard to straighten up."

Provider (beginning to pace, looking at his watch, and reading some notes on his desk): "Well, let's have a look at the area."

Patient (shaking and eyes filling with tears): "No, that's okay; I have to go now."

The class should discuss what was happening here and describe alternative ways the health provider might have handled the situation.

The topic of cultural diversity is reviewed further in the last chapter of this text. Obviously, volumes can be written about the subject. In this chapter you should gain at least an insight into the necessity of making cultural sensitivity part of your arsenal as a health professional concerned with kinesics and peoples' health. Just to underscore the diversity of the world, this section closes with an additional cross-cultural gesture: The American signal for "okay" means zero in France; in Japan it means coins or money; and in Brazil, Germany, and the Commonwealth of Independent States it is an obscene gesture. Sensitivity and care will help improve our nonverbal communications with patients from different backgrounds and help avoid potentially dangerous miscommunications.

Summary

Nonverbal communication skills serve the health professional well as you learn to observe and interpret the behavior of others. That which is non-neutral has some meaning. When nonverbal behavior contradicts verbal behavior, your attention must be focused there. Nonverbal interpretations also help you in establishing communication with those who cannot or will not talk. The nonverbal is often more revealing than the spoken word. The key elements of nonverbal language are kinesics, proxemics, haptics, oculesics, chronemics, olfactics, appearance and adornment, posture, locomotion, sound symbols, silence, and vocalics.

You must be aware of what specific physical positions, such as encountering a patient with arms crossed who is staring at the floor, might mean. You must always check your perceptions rather than assuming the meaning of nonverbal behavior, especially when cultural differences may exist. Good observational skills are an important component of the nonverbal process.

As health providers, you must cultivate the message you wish to send nonverbally. The right attire, good hygiene, and attention to body language are essential to success. You want to appear open, interested, and approachable. Facial expressions and proximity are significant, as is vocal usage. How you use your voice can significantly alter the way your message is received. Focusing on specific behaviors in a nonjudgmental way can be a primary communication tool for the health professional.

The ideal model for nonverbal communication is reviewed as follows along with suggestions of behaviors to avoid.

Ideal Communication Style

- Facing patient/client, holding gaze
- Arms at sides or gently folded
- Legs upright or gently crossed
- Posture erect but not rigid
- Distance of approximately one arm's length between professional and patient/client
- No barriers between health practitioner and patient/client
- Professional attire
- Good hygiene
- Facial expression relaxed or matching that of patient/client
- Vocal tone moderate and clear
- Providing privacy whenever possible
- Demonstrating gender and cultural sensitivity

Communication Pitfalls

- Poor hygiene
- Inappropriate attire
- Too relaxed or rigid posture

- Failure to make eye contact or too intense contact
- Sitting too close or too far from patient/client
- Sitting behind a desk or large equipment when not necessary
- Creating a barrier with folded arms or legs
- Maintaining inappropriate behavior, such as hair twirling or gum snapping during an interview
- Lack of privacy
- Failing to take cultural differences into consideration

Health professionals should keep professional boundaries that do not allow for treating patients as casually as they treat friends. They must be sensitive to gender differences so that there is little or no confusion regarding their intent with a patient; sexual overtones, especially, must be avoided. Not treating a female patient behind closed doors without a female professional present is one example of a nonverbal message that will help keep the patient from feeling threatened and from misunderstanding the professional's intent. As we discuss in a later chapter, such a decision also will help the professional to avoid false accusations.

Care must be taken to avoid a tendency to stereotype diverse cultural populations. However, Asian populations are generally less comfortable with eye contact and touch than are some Euro-Americans and most Latino/Hispanics. It is also prudent to note that the friendly gesture of one culture may be an insult to another. Sensitivity to the body language of others will only improve the patient-professional relationship.

Chapter Review

Key Term Review

Adornment: Dress, appearing clean, jewelry, tattoos, piercings.

Atmosphere for communication: Being at the correct distance from the patient, usually at arm's length and without barriers.

Behavioral observation: Studying the patient's nonverbal behavior specifically, including eye contact, facial expressions, appearance, posture, and proximity.

Boundaries: A mental or physical line delineating territories between two people that cannot be crossed, especially with gender or cultural differences.

Chronemics: Use of time, pausing, waiting, speeding up.

Cultural sensitivity: Learning the differences among a culture's views of even haptics and oculesics. This will assist cross-cultural communication.

Haptics: Touch.

Ideal communication model: Professional attire; arm's length from the patient; private setting; relaxed, attentive posture; friendly expression and tone; holding patient's gaze; focusing on patient's body language, and reflecting conflict.

Kinesics: Body motions such as shrugs, foot tapping, drumming fingers, clicking pens, winking, facial expressions, and gestures.

Locomotion: Walking, jumping, swaying, and moving in a wheelchair.

Neutral position of behavior: The body's *natural* position. Hands relaxed at sides is a neutral position; other positions are purposeful and have some meaning.

Nonverbal behavior: Using observational skills or reading body language about a patient's underlying feelings.

Nonverbal language: Composite of eye contact, facial expressions, appearance, posture, and proximity.

Nonverbal message: Communicating without using language; the most powerful way of communicating with patients. A relaxed yet steady gaze is ideal eye contact. Facial expression and professional appearance are the key to sending the correct message. Adopt a relaxed posture with hands relaxed.

Oculesics: Eye contact.

Olfactics: Smell.

Posture: Body position, stance.

Proxemics: Nearness, distance, or position from another.

Silence: Long pauses, withholding information, secrecy.

Sound symbols: Grunting, ahs, pointed throat clearing.

Vocalics: Tone, timbre, volume.

Chapter Review Questions

1. How do behavioral observations differ from judgments?
2. What are the three basic elements of communication?
3. List six of the twelve components of nonverbal language.
4. Why is it dangerous to assume you know what someone is feeling on the basis of their kinesics alone?
5. What value may establishing rapport with a patient/client have for the client's physical well-being?
6. How might a careful observer of nonverbal behaviors know when they are *not* being told the truth?
7. What are the dangers when generalizing information across cultures?

Case Study Critical Thinking Questions

1. What does Case Study 1-1 tell us about "approachability"? Are you aware of what nonverbal impressions you may give out? What could you do to improve this or become more aware of the impressions you give off?
2. Reread Case Study 1-2. Do you feel more compassion for the physical therapist or the teenage patient? How could this be handled differently by the therapist without referring the patient to someone else?
3. Explain the meaning of "nonverbal behaviors may reveal more than spoken words do"? Take a look at Case Study 1-3. How might the "nonpromoted" medical technologist improve his work performance?
4. How may issues of proxemics be affected by gender? By culture? Look at Case Study 1-4. What message has the Anglo-provider sent to the Latina patient? How may health professionals manage a large number of patients and still treat each with patience and respect?

References

1. Carkhuff, R. R. *Helping and Human Relations* (2 volumes). Amherst, MA: Human Resource Development Press,* 1984.
2. Carkhuff, R. R. *The Art of Helping*, 6th ed.. Amherst, MA: Human Resource Development Press, 1987.
3. Danish, S., D'Augelli, A. R., Hauer, A. L. *Helping Skills: A Basic Training Program.* New York: Human Sciences Press, 1980.
4. Perls, Friedrich S. *The Gestalt Approach and Eye Witness to Therapy*. Lomond, CA: Science & Behavior Books, 1973.
5. Amin, H. "What are the Cultural Barriers for Native Americans and Hispanics Entering Science in our Educational System." *Socyberty*, March 2, 2009.
6. Axtell, Roger E. *Gestures: The Do's and Taboos of Body Language around the World.* Hoboken, NJ: John Wiley and Sons, 1991.
7. Bigelow, N., Paradiso, S., Andreasen, N. "Schizophrenia Impairs Body Language Comprehension." *Schizophr Res*: April 2006.
8. California State Polytechnic University Web Site for Asian Studies Summer Institute: *Gestures: Body Language and Nonverbal Communication*. Lecture by Gary Imai, 1997.
9. De Mente, Boye L. *Japanese Etiquette & Ethics in Business.* Chicago: NTC Business Books, 1994.
10. Eiser, A., Ellis, G. "Cultural Competence and the African American Experience with Health Care: The Case for Specific Content in Cross-Cultural Education." *Acad Med* 82(2):176–83; February 2007.
11. Ginige, S., Chen, M., Fairley, C. "Are patient responses to sensitive sexual health questions influenced by the sex of the practitioner?" *Sex Transm Infect* 82:321–322; 2006.

12. Kagawa-Singer, M., Blackhill, L. "You Got to Go Where He Lives." *JAMA* 286:2993–3001; 2001.
13. Preston, P. "Nonverbal Communication: Do You Really Say What You Mean?" *J Healthcare Manage* March 1, 2005.
14. Takahashi, et al. "Influence of Family on Acceptance of Influenza Vaccination among Japanese Patients." *Fam Pract* 20:162–166; 2003.
15. Ting-Toomey, S. *Communicating Across Cultures*. New York, NY: Guilford Press, 1999.
16. Yellow Bird, M., Snipp, C. American Indian Families. In Taylor, R. L. (Ed), *Minority Families in US: A Multicultural Perspective* (pp. 227–249). NJ: Prentice Hall: 2002.

Additional Readings

1. Betancourt, J. "Cultural Competency: Providing Quality Care to Diverse Populations." *Consult Pharm* 21(12):988–95; December 2006.
2. Biasco, Surbone. "Cultural Challenges in Caring for Our Patients in Advanced Stage Cancer." *JCO*: 27:157–158; 2009.
3. Kanzler, M., Gorsulowsky, D. "Patients' Attitudes Regarding Physical Characteristics of Medical Care Providers in Dermatological Practices." *Arch Dermatol*: 138:463–66; 2002.
4. Maguire, P., Pitceathly, C. "Key Communication Skills and How to Acquire Them." *Brit Med J* 325:697–700; September 28 2002.
5. Matsumura, S., et al. "Acculturation of Attitudes toward End-of-Life Care: A Cross-Cultural Survey of Japanese Americans and Japanese." *J Gen Intern Med* 17:531–9; 2002.

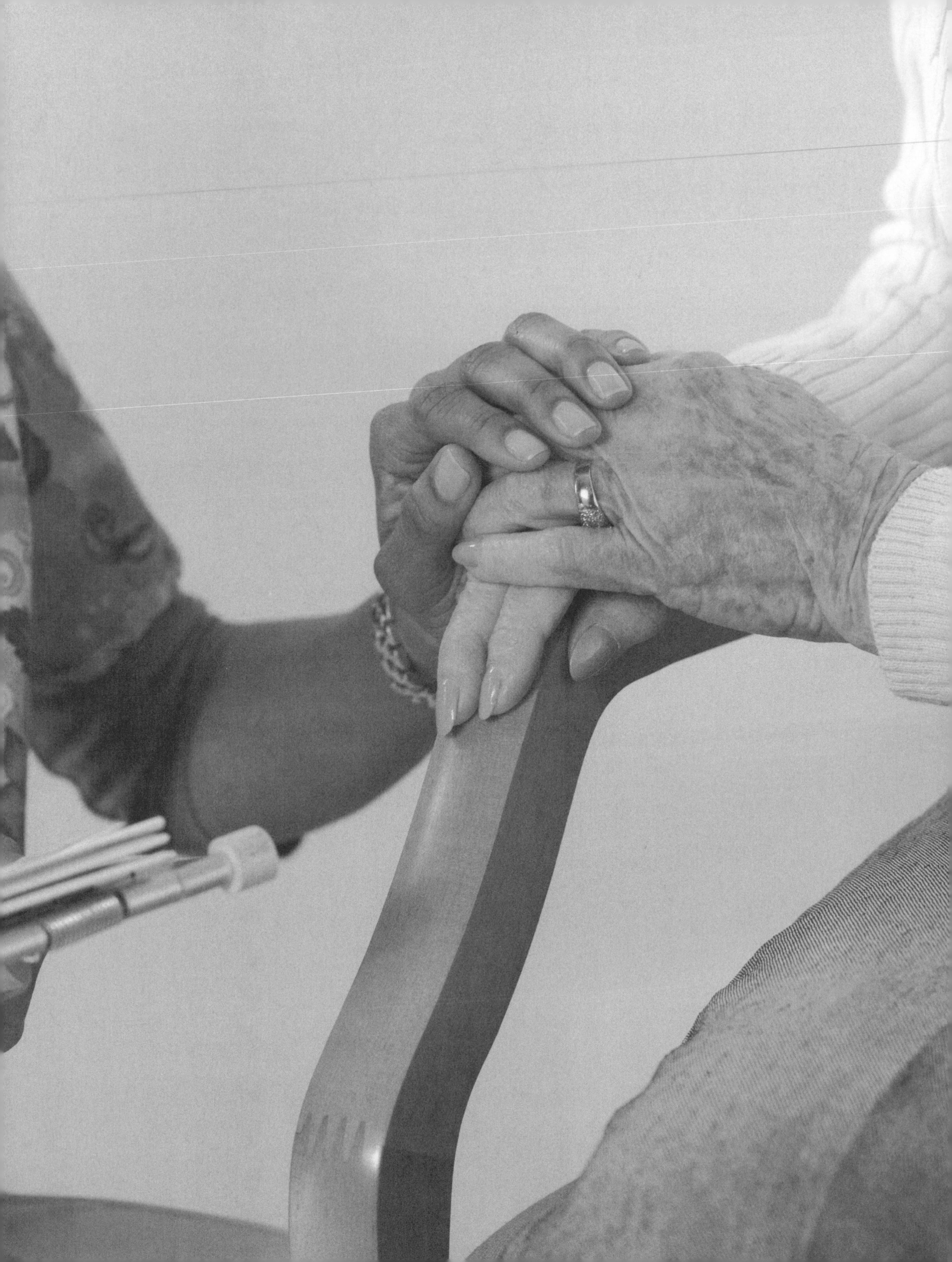

Basic Skills in Verbal Communication

Learning Outcomes

After reading this chapter, you should be able to:

2.1 Understand the value of good listening and paraphrasing skills.
2.2 Describe empathizing, the value of empathy versus sympathy, and being judgmental.
2.3 Identify feelings expressed verbally or nonverbally by clients.
2.4 Demonstrate open-ended questions appropriately.
2.5 Illustrate the limited role of closed questions.
2.6 Use nonverbal, paraphrasing, empathic, and questioning skills.
2.7 Evaluate the communication hazards common in social comment and with patient overinvolvement.
2.8 Demonstrate skill at giving and receiving feedback.

Key Terms

Boundaries
Closed-ended question
Cognitive
Communication sequence
Empathize
Feeling words
Giving feedback
Open-ended question
Paraphrase
Receiving feedback
Sympathy

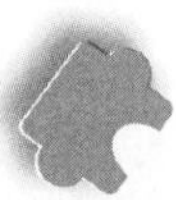

Recognize Listening and Paraphrasing

Naturally, you all want to be competent practitioners within your chosen fields. Competency is often equated with building professional skills based on new information. But, although knowledge may be the cornerstone of the health professional's repertoire, knowledge alone is not enough.

Not too many years ago, many medical schools chose their students purely on the basis of grades. These schools produced physicians who had a great deal of scientific knowledge but who often had weak interpersonal skills. They were excellent diagnosticians—when they could get a patient to come to them. Knowledge without the skill to impart or transfer it is like a fancy automobile without someone who knows how to drive: It looks good, but you aren't going to go very far.

Think about the patient contact you are likely to have. Although people see health professionals for a variety of reasons, fear or concern over their own health or the need for actual treatment is almost always involved. These feelings may be accompanied by pain, loss, and worry.

Many of you chose to become health care providers because you want to help people. Knowing how to take an X-ray may contribute a good deal to a patient's well-being, but you have to be prepared to hear a patient's fears and objections before you may be allowed to help.

Perhaps you can remember a situation in which you held back information because no one seemed to care or listen to you. This often happens during social conversation. You may begin to introduce a difficult or sensitive topic only to have the conversation abruptly turned to another topic. The person with whom you were talking did not really hear what you were saying. What you wanted was a good listener; what you got was a good talker. Thus an opportunity for sharing and intimacy was lost.

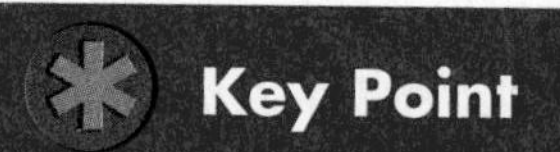

Key Point

Paraphrasing listening to speaker, then repeating what was said using different words.

Good listening skills require training and practice. You may occasionally be guilty of not hearing the true message in a conversation, but when you fail to hear your patient's true message, it affects your competency.

The foundation for developing listening skills is paraphrasing. To **paraphrase**, you simply listen to a speaker and then repeat what they have said. Although you can repeat exactly what they say, it is most helpful to rephrase the information in your own words, in other words, to paraphrase it.

EXAMPLE 1

Speaker: "I am so tired of working with Sandra. Every time I think she understands the importance of not skipping meals or taking laxatives she doesn't need, she turns around and gets herself into trouble."

Listener: "It sounds as though Sandra persistently ignores your helpful advice and therefore creates dangerous situations for herself."

EXAMPLE 2

Speaker: "I work so hard all year long. It doesn't seem that I'd be out of line to expect decent accommodations and good weather for two crummy weeks!"

Listener: "When you finally have a vacation you want things to go well!"

Of course, the listeners could have used other words as well. These examples are intended to convey the gist of paraphrasing—repeating concisely in your own words the relevant points you have heard, or finding another way of restating the topic.

Remember how easy it is not to hear what others are saying. What if you lived in a world where every speaker had to be paraphrased before the listener could make an original response? Your first thought might be that it would be a tedious world, but it would undoubtedly cut down on misunderstanding, hurt feelings, and errors. Certainly it is a necessary part of verbal communication training to begin each patient session (simulated or real) with paraphrasing.

There are five important reasons for paraphrasing:

- Paraphrasing is a check for the listener.
- Paraphrasing is a check for the speaker.
- Paraphrasing builds rapport.
- Paraphrasing focuses on the patient.
- Paraphrasing keeps the patient talking.

1. *Paraphrasing is a check for the listener.* Paraphrasing allows the listener to immediately check out his or her understanding of what has been said. Let us re-examine Example 2. What if the speaker had instead been trying to convey this thought: "I work so hard all year long I can't believe my only reward is a two-week vacation where anything could go wrong." By paraphrasing, the listener would then have been able to refocus on what the speaker really wanted to say: "Then what you are really saying is work takes so much out of you, you want more than two weeks off as compensation." The speaker's point would not have been lost or misunderstood.
2. *Paraphrasing is a check for the speaker.* Paraphrasing allows the speaker to hear what her or his words sound like. People often do not mean things exactly as they come out. Hearing your own words reflected back by a listener helps you to clarify what you really meant to say. Look at Example 1 again. A possible response to the listener's paraphrase might be, "It's not so much that I mind her ignoring my advice as it is that I can never relax and trust that she is safe." This change in focus may help both the speaker and the listener more quickly and accurately understand what is really troubling the speaker.
3. *Paraphrasing builds rapport.* Paraphrasing shows the speaker that he or she is actually being listened to, which effectively builds rapport. Remember how hard it can be to be heard. What a unique and warm experience it is to find someone who actually listens to you. What if the listener in Example 2 had said, "Your vacation couldn't have been as bad as mine. Not only did it rain every day, but my son called and he was upset that his cat had died." With such a response, the speaker would not have felt listened to.
4. *Paraphrasing focuses on the patient.* As we can see from the paragraph above, listeners can easily end up talking about themselves. (This type of response may be acceptable in a social setting, but it is usually unacceptable with our patients.) Listening and paraphrasing eliminates this danger. Sticking with what the patient wants to convey prevents the health practitioner from missing vital information or possibly offering impossible solutions. Until you have established firm rapport with your patient and followed his or her lead in exploring all the dimensions of

a problem, it is best to limit your responses to paraphrasing for the reason explained in Point 5.

5. *Paraphrasing keeps the patient talking.* Paraphrasing enhances a speaker's willingness to continue talking. If we are to get as much objective information as possible, we want the speaker to keep talking, at least in the first few encounters. Once we begin asking questions, we take the lead. See what happens with Example 2 if the listener starts asking questions right away.

Speaker: "I work so hard all year long it doesn't seem that I'd be out of line to expect decent accommodations and good weather for two crummy weeks!"

Listener: "Don't you enjoy any part of your work?"
"What kind of work do you do?"
"How long have you been living this way?"

Can you see how potentially distracting and off-center these questions may be? Although the speaker may eventually want to explore some of the issues these questions raise, the timing is clearly off. Asking questions too early in a session *prevents* rather than enhances good communication.

Listening and paraphrasing skills are the essential ingredients of good communication skills training. One cannot be overtrained: Take refresher training on these skills if it will help you to remain client/patient-focused. If, out of all the communication skills, a knowledgeable health care provider were to master only listening skills, she or he could be a successful practitioner. That is how valuable listening skills are.

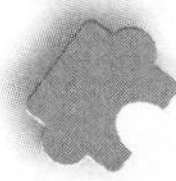

Empathizing

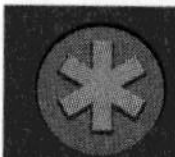

Key Point

Empathizing conveying understanding of another person's feelings.

To **empathize** is to convey understanding of another person's feelings. Empathizing is a skill you should learn only after you have mastered paraphrasing. It is a listening skill that relies on the proper use of paraphrasing before it can be introduced successfully. Whereas paraphrasing involves rewording a speaker's message, empathizing involves both the basic message and the emotion involved with the message. Thus the listener not only rewords the content of the message but also brings out and labels the speaker's underlying feelings. Empathizing is based on feelings rather than on thoughts. Empathizing may dramatically expand the meaning beyond paraphrasing while still keeping the focus on the patient. Consider two examples.

EXAMPLE 1

Speaker: "I am so tired of working with Sandra. Every time I think she understands the importance of not skipping meals or taking laxatives she doesn't need, she turns around and gets herself into trouble."

Paraphrasing Listener: "It sounds as though Sandra persistently ignores your helpful advice and therefore creates dangerous situations for herself."

Empathizing Listener: "It sounds as though you've tried very hard to help Sandra and you're feeling exhausted and frustrated."

EXAMPLE 2

Speaker: "I went in to draw blood from Mrs. Morgan this morning and she told me flat out to get out. She said she'd have nothing to do with anymore of us 'damn vampires.' Now what do I tell my supervisor when they can't run the tests?"

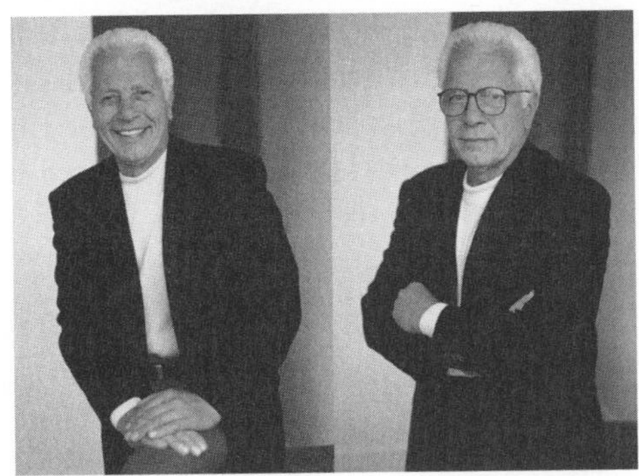

What kinesics do you imagine the man in this example would exhibit? Perhaps someone you know will volunteer to act out the speaker's role without using words. Empathizing in real life is easier than empathizing based on reading because in real life we have the advantage of nonverbal cues.

Paraphrasing Listener: "A patient stopped you from doing your job and you are on the spot to explain this to your supervisor."

Empathizing Listener: "I think what you are saying is you're feeling shaken by a patient's flat refusal to cooperate and afraid that you'll be seen as a failure by your supervisor."

What body language do you imagine the persons in these examples would exhibit?

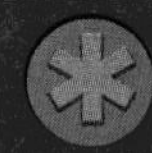

Key Point

Feeling words words that express emotional feelings rather than just cognitive thoughts.

Before reading any further, review the responses of the empathizing listener in Examples 1 and 2 above. List the **feeling words** contained within these responses. The use of feelings is the key difference between paraphrasing and empathizing. After you have identified these feeling words, try to make an empathic response to the speaker in the following example: "I worked so hard all year long it doesn't seem that I'd be out of line to expect decent accommodations and good weather for two crummy weeks." (One empathic response would be, "You seem to be angry about having a lousy vacation." Angry appears to be the essential feeling label for this example.)

What feeling words did you list when reviewing Examples 1 and 2 in this section? If you came up with *exhausted* and *frustrated* for Example 1 and *shaken* and *afraid* for Example 2, you are understanding empathy. If you are having trouble picking out feeling words or labeling and understanding human emotions, work on improving your skills as you continue.

Empathy–Sympathy–Judging

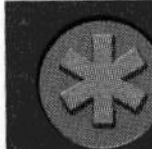

Key Point

Sympathy sharing pain with the sufferer; a nonprofessional situation.

Empathy is part of a professional set of skills used for good communications. It reflects the listener's understanding or comprehension of the speaker's feelings. The health professional "gets" what is troubling the client at a feeling level. Yet in the understanding, there remains some professional distance. There may be warmth and caring conveyed, but the health professional is NOT suffering along with/or overly involved with/ the patient's trouble.

Sympathy is best reserved for nonprofessional settings. **Sympathy** implies sharing pain with the sufferer in a way that is self-involving as though you actually experience the pain your patient is going through. This level of involvement could undermine your objectivity and your ability to work effectively.

Judging: Health professionals need to be objective when treating patients. To empathize and understand what they are going through, you must suspend judgments that place your values in opposition to the patient's. That is, you need to meet the patient "where they are." If needed, referrals can always be made to assist patients in dealing with behavioral issues.

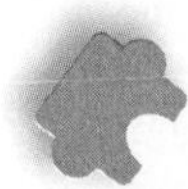

Comprehending Feelings

Key Point

Cognitive of thought, factual knowledge, thinking skills

We live in a world biased toward the **cognitive** (what can be reduced to factual knowledge). Being a thinking person is thought of as superior to being an emotional person. Although we may find some merit in this view, it also has limitations. Many individuals fail to develop their emotional antenna as they seek to feel less and think more. Males especially may believe it is unbecoming or unmanly to show emotions. Even in the face of acute sorrow, there are those who will not shed a tear.

Many of you have been raised in this "big boys and girls don't cry" culture and then have to learn how to get in touch with your feelings. As an introduction, turn to the accompanying list of feelings. Table 2.1 contains the words most commonly used to describe feelings. Becoming familiar with these words will make it easier for you to recognize them when you are listening to others. But familiarity with this list alone is not sufficient.

Just as you may have difficulty picking up on feelings, your patients often have trouble clearly conveying what they feel. Even the feeling words listed can be used in such a way that they are not truly feelings. For example: a patient can "feel down," and you understand a sense of depression or despair; that is a feeling use of a feeling word. But what does the speaker *feel* who says, "I feel that he was putting me down."

The use of *that* after the word *feel* tells you that you are about to hear a thought, not a feeling. If you rewrite the above message to read, "I *think* that he was putting me down," it makes more sense. The word *feel* is often used instead of the word *think* when the speaker is confused about or blocking her or his feelings. Probably the speaker in this example was feeling angry that someone was insulting him.

Besides the difficulty you may have in recognizing and expressing feelings, you may also be reluctant to deal with certain feelings. You may even consider some feelings taboo. The group of feelings that people may consider taboo encompasses emotions that can be seen as harsh or negative. Of these, anger is probably the most significant. Every human being experiences varying levels of anger on a relatively frequent basis. Those who are constantly angry, hostile, and negative are certainly not well and are not pleasant to be around. But human beings who never express anger have their own set of emotional problems. Obviously, there are degrees of difficulty between these two extremes. A typical patient may feel angry but not know how to show it appropriately. When you are the empathic listener, keep in mind that many people have difficulty expressing their anger and may need your help to focus. Otherwise, that anger comes out in less direct but often damaging ways, especially when it is turned inward. Also be certain to look for a deeper, perhaps hidden, feeling when the speaker starts with "I feel that ..."

Table 2.1 Partial List of Feeling Words to Help Improve Your Empathic Responses

Feeling Words				
Abandoned	Daring	Grief stricken	Maligned	Stable
Adequate	Delighted	Grouchy	Mean	Strong
Affectionate	Desperate	Happy	Miserable	Stupid
Agreeable	Dirty	Hardy	Misunderstood	Sweet
Amused	Discouraged	Hated	Mocked	Tender
Angry	Disgusted	Helpless	Moody	Terrible
Annoyed	Dissatisfied	High	Nervous	Thrilled
Anxious	Disturbed	Hopeful	Nice	Tight
Apprehensive	Doomed	Hostile	Numb	Tired
Badgered	Dreadful	Humiliated	Obsessed	Torn
Baffled	Eager	Hurt	Offended	Tremendous
Beaten	Ecstatic	Ignored	Open	Triumphant
Betrayed	Elated	Impatient	Optimistic	Uncomfortable
Bitter	Embarrassed	Inadequate	Panicky	Unhappy
Bored	Empty	Inept	Patient	Unloved
Brotherly	Enraged	Inferior	Peaceful	Unsatisfied
Bruised	Enthusiastic	Insecure	Powerful	Unstable
Calm	Exasperated	Insulted	Proud	Unsure
Carefree	Excluded	Intimidated	Puzzled	Valuable
Caring	Fantastic	Irate	Quiet	Virile
Cast off	Fearless	Jealous	Rejected	Vivacious
Cautious	Flattered	Joyful	Relaxed	Vulnerable
Cheated	Foolish	Jumpy	Resentful	Warm
Cheerful	Fortunate	Justified	Responsible	Weak
Cold	Friendly	Kind	Ridiculed	Well
Comfortable	Frightened	Lame	Rotten	Withdrawn
Confident	Frustrated	Lonely	Sad	Witty
Confused	Furious	Lost	Satisfied	Worried
Content	Generous	Loving	Savage	Wounded
Cranky	Giddy	Lucky	Secure	Zonked
Crushed	Glad	Mad	Selfish	
Curious	Good	Majestic	Sensitive	
Cut	Greedy	Malicious	Sick	

Timing and Power of Empathy

What do you think would happen if your first words to a client focused on feelings? Although your response might be well-received, chances are that it would be too threatening for your client to accept. It is important that you listen first and analyze later. You must establish rapport before you shift the focus to your patient's feelings. Remember that labeling feelings accurately is not an easy task.

One of the key values of paraphrasing is that it allows the patient to realize that you are with him or her. You must build trust through paraphrasing before you attempt to label feelings. If you mislabel a feeling without first developing rapport, your patient might well feel hurt, misunderstood, and angry—a reaction that will make it difficult for you to establish trust. Patients will often retreat with their feelings if they are frustrated by an early mistake on the part of the health care provider.

Another advantage to timing empathy correctly is that you reduce your chances for making errors. Remember that an essential purpose of paraphrasing is to find out if you actually understand what the patient is saying. If you label feelings without being certain that you have clarified the message, the outcome is likely to be disastrous.

An example of how you might reach the wrong conclusion follows:

Patient: "My daughter cannot make up her mind whether she wants to live with me or her father."

Health Care Worker: "Sounds like you are feeling rejected by your daughter's ambivalence."

Patient: "I'm not worried about rejection—I'm scared to death she'll ruin my life by moving back in. Don't you see how destructive that would be?"

A well-labeled empathic response can be a powerful tool. It can further establish you as a caring, understanding health care provider and can assist in rapidly helping your patient. Poorly timed, however, an attempt at empathy can frighten your patient into putting up a defensive roadblock. The key to success is *timing*. An empathic response is well-timed if you established rapport and clarified your interpretation of the patient's issues. Both are accomplished through paraphrasing.

One further caution about making judgments: Be careful not to use judgmental comments when responding to patients. If your response indicates criticism or a negative value for the patient's position, you will shut off communication. How would you react if you were the patient in the following situation?

Patient: "I hate my brother. He has everything: good looks, good grades, and he is a great athlete. Meantime, I'm an ugly duckling crippled kid."

Response: "Now you don't mean that about your brother. You're just having a bad day and feeling sorry for yourself. That doesn't give you the right to hate anybody else."

Can you see how insensitive such a response would be? Even though the patient is exhibiting some self-pity, reflecting his words back to him with such judgments is not going to help him work out these feelings. Remind yourself that you are on the patient's side. Your job is to assist him in understanding himself and helping you to help him. It is not your job to judge what you hear, at least not in the sense of this example. Strong judgments on the part of the health practitioner only inhibit true understanding.

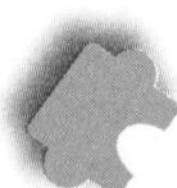

The Role of Open-Ended Questions

Once you have established rapport and a clear understanding of the patient's issues through paraphrasing, you can proceed to empathic responses. These responses permit you to communicate your understanding of the patient's feelings and to expand on the content of what the patient has said. While you remain focused on the patient, you want to expand the patient's understanding of the issues in which she or he is involved. The only kind of question that lends itself to paraphrasing and empathizing is the **open-ended question** (a question that can't be answered simply but encourages further discussion). It is the only kind of question you should use during the beginning of your interactions with a patient. Perhaps you have been using open-ended questions already in your practice work. Such a question sounds something like the response in the following example.

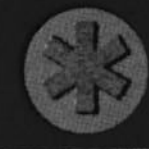

Key Point

Open-ended question a question that cannot be answered simply but encourages further discussion.

Speaker: "If you ask me to do any more of those leg-lifting exercises, I'm never coming back."

Response: "So you're pretty bothered by the leg lifts and you want me to understand how hard they are for you?"

Such a response relates directly to what the patient has said. It does not lead the patient away from discussing his or her needs or problems. Once you have established rapport and understand the patient's issues, you may have to ask a limited number of questions. Again, you begin asking only after you are certain that you understand the patient's needs and are not leading the patient away from further explaining those needs.

Even at this stage, you should ask only open-ended questions. Remember that open-ended questions encourage the patient to discuss issues further. Can you distinguish between the open-ended questions and the **closed-ended questions** in the list on the next page?

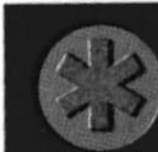

Key Point

Closed-ended question a question that can be answered simply and that does not encourage further discussion.

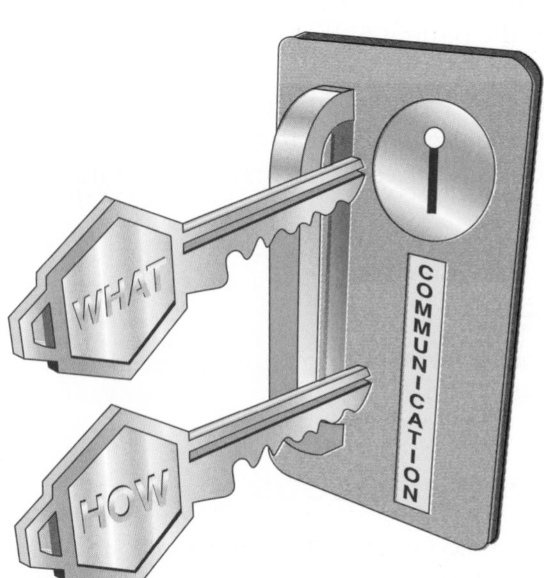

Keys to communication

1. Can you tell me how you feel?
2. How did it feel to be on a strict diet when you were only nine years old?
3. What can you describe as contributing to your problem?
4. Have your parents been divorced long?
5. Did anyone else in your family have high blood pressure?

If you said 2 and 3 were open-ended you were correct. The other questions could be answered with a single word (especially yes or no). Closed questions do not allow us to learn any substantiating information. Also, the way we ask closed questions can determine the answers we receive. Remember that many people, especially when ill, feel emotionally frail and overwhelmed by the health care system. They may respond to questions as they believe they are expected to respond. If you ask questions that threaten them in any way, you will get the easiest answers they can come up with. Something as simple as "Did you eat breakfast this morning?" may cause a patient to feel defensive and cover the truth.

A key to enhancing your ability with open-ended questions is to remember two little words: *how* and *what*. Ninety-five percent of all how and what questions are open-ended. Use these two words whenever you are struggling to ask an open-ended question. But your questions must be carefully thought out to avoid closing off discussion. Here is an example:

1. Would you describe the situations in which you begin to experience pain?
2. Can you tell me how often you feel pain?

Sentence 1 might elicit an open-ended response because the word *describe* opens the question. Sentence 2 might elicit a response with some depth, but note that it could be answered with a word or two, leaving an information gap. What do you think about using one of the following two questions?

1. How would you describe your pain?
2. What can you tell me about this pain?

These sentences flow easily and invite the patient to share information. It is important to keep in mind that there are times when you may need to get very specific information from the patient and closed questions may be more appropriate.

In general, you shouldn't ask *why* questions. Gestalt therapy (see Chapter 3) teaches us that in truth there may be no real answer to a why question. Further, many why questions come across as threatening and confrontational:

"Why did you do that?"

"Why didn't you call for help?"

"Why don't you take your medicine?"

Questions that sound threatening generally go unanswered or are answered dishonestly.

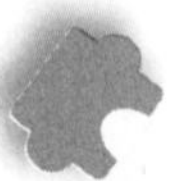

The Role of Closed Questions

As a health professional, much of your contact with patients will still consist of closed questions. A closed question is one that is designed to elicit a short, focused answer like "yes," "no," "5 years," "20 pounds," "I quit in 2002," or "sometimes."

It is important that you can judge when to ask open-ended and when to ask closed questions. For example, a nurse could start a patient history with questions such as "Tell me about yourself" or "What brings you here?" But, if the nurse has a four-page questionnaire to fill out in 15 minutes, she or he will not have much time for such open-ended questions.

As a general rule, health practitioners ask too many closed and not enough open-ended questions. Interestingly, more information can often be elicited faster by using open-ended questions, perhaps because patients feel less on the spot. On first meeting a patient, even if you have only 15 minutes with him or her, it is often advisable to allow the patient to ramble for at least a couple of minutes. It has been reported that most health professionals will interrupt the patient within 15 seconds. Yet, this rambling may contain the seeds of the person's problems, which two hours of direct questioning may not elicit. According to one old rule, if you listen, the patient will tell you the diagnosis.

Of course, some questions—"Which knee is it?" or "Are you single or married?" for example—have to be closed questions. The point is that it is more productive to start with general questions before zeroing in on specifics. For instance, "What can I do to help you?" would be better than "What are your symptoms?", and "What is bothering you?" is better than "Which tooth hurts?"

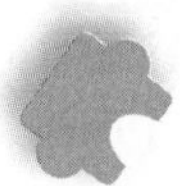

Nonverbal, Paraphrasing, Empathic, and Questioning Skills

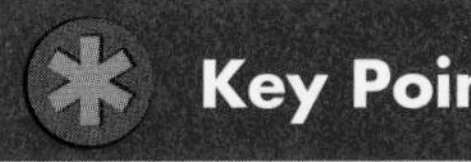

Communication sequence paraphrasing (with use of nonverbal language), then empathizing, then asking open-ended questions.

You begin a session with a new patient by offering paraphrasing responses until you fully understand the individual's situation and have established rapport. Recall from the previous chapter that this involves observation and checking of nonverbal skills. You may then focus in on the underlying feelings related to the message you are hearing by using empathic responses. When the patient begins to flounder or needs help in continuing the discussion of her or his situation, you can ask open-ended questions. These questions should be well thought out and should be based on an understanding of the patient's problems. This is called the **communication sequence.** As a health care provider, never ask a question simply to satisfy your own curiosity. A question you may wish to ask yourself is, What question does the patient want me to ask?

Paraphrasing ⟶ empathic responses ⟶ open-ended questions (Using nonverbal)

Such a line of questioning will often help the patient to come up with solutions for his or her own problems. For example, if a patient says to you, "I only experience this pain after a fight with my husband," she is clearly asking whether she can talk about her husband, and you must respond. She may well begin to see what really needs to be worked on further. Solutions always work better if they come from the patient.

Learning the art of helping patients to help themselves is the purpose of acquiring the skills described thus far in this chapter. When you stick to the patient's issues long enough and develop an understanding of his or her feelings, you may be able to assist in focusing on meaningful discovery. Just remember that questions asked without an empathic understanding are likely to be wasted.

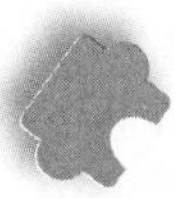

Communication Issues

If you have ever felt inadequate or insecure about your skills, you are not alone. Beginners in every field experience the fear that they will not be good enough to perform the work for which they are training. Feeling confident about developing communication skills is no exception. Repeated practice and experience are the keys to security and success. The issues addressed in this section are included as preventive medicine in the hope that they will help you avoid some of the most common mistakes new professionals make. When you do make errors, it is important that you recognize them and then continue your practice work.

Social Comments

The most common communication errors entail what is called *social comments:* giving advice, talking about yourself, and saying, in effect, that you know what the other person feels. Each of these responses has its own drawbacks.

Giving advice

Listen to someone explaining their problems to a friend. Usually the friend has begun to "solve" the problem before the speaker has even stopped talking. Offering such rapid advice generally serves to close off discussion before the listener really even hears what is being said. Remember that it takes concentration on paraphrasing to actively understand most problems. By giving advice, you offer solutions that might work for you but are rarely helpful to the speaker. Your goal is to clarify the problem. When you help someone to better understand their own problem, solutions often emerge. The natural emergence of a solution without the need for outside advice is ideal; giving advice may be totally unnecessary.

Talking about yourself

Students often ask whether they should say they have had the same problem when that is so. Ask yourself what would be gained? The paramedic on the scene of an accident is best advised to listen and *not* to report the circumstances surrounding her own auto crash.

Although wanting your patient to feel at ease is kind and admirable, telling her or him something about yourself may not be the best way to do it. If you respond to a patient by describing trouble in your own life, what have you done? You've switched the focus from the patient to you. An occasional patient may be interested in your common experiences, but generally patients are not interested. They want to be heard! They want to be listened to. Remember that a therapeutic dialogue should generally be one-sided. Your job is to focus on the patient and understand his or her problem. Discuss yourself with your friends. Keeping the focus on the patient also helps you to avoid the boundary issues that we discussed in Chapter 1 and will discuss further on in this chapter.

Saying you know how the other person feels

This common mistake overlaps talking about yourself. By saying "I know how you feel," you may be hoping to empathize, but most likely you will be talking about yourself. You then lose the patient focus. In general, you should avoid self-disclosure. The few occasions on which it may be appropriate are discussed later in this chapter.

You also are making a false claim when you say you know how someone else feels, for you have no way of knowing if you truly know how someone else is feeling. Even when you have had the same experience as another, your innermost reactions may not mesh with theirs. A very good and caring counselor we know once had the following experience. The counselor was working with a man who had ceased to function at his high-level job following the sudden death of his son. Years before, the counselor had tragically lost a 10-year-old daughter. When her patient began to review the agony of his grieving, she replied, "I know how you feel; I lost a daughter."

His response was totally unexpected as he exclaimed, "How could you know how I feel—I lost a son!"

His response was not an arrogant or sexist comment; it was a reflection of inappropriate timing and empathizing on the part of the counselor. This patient was unable to hear that his pain was like anyone else's. Grief is lonely and private. It often dissolves the world around the griever. The counselor wanted to break through this barrier of grief and show that she too had been there and survived, but her client was not ready. His pain was greater, more exquisite than anything he could imagine sharing with another human being.

Although it may become appropriate for the counselor to mention her own loss to this patient, this was not the time. She should have empathized without self-disclosure. If she had realized how angry he was, she might have timed her disclosure better. We will study the emotional stages of grieving in a later chapter.

When you understand a patient's problems well, it may be okay to reveal something about yourself if the disclosure is worded to be supportive. Never use yourself to show the patient how to be, however. Holding yourself up as an example usually invites a hostile reaction or a sense of dependency. You don't want the patient to feel that she or he can only do well by doing it your way. The patient will then depend on you for all major decisions.

Occasionally a troubled patient may ask for your help by saying something such as, "What would you do if it were your mother?" You might wish to answer this question cautiously in a way that supports the speaker. It is best for everyone, however, if the answer does not come from you. Some honest sharing may be appropriate in situations where a stigma may be involved, for example, for an ostomy therapist or for someone working with a woman postmastectomy.

Overinvolvement

The subject of dependency opens another major topic: overinvolvement. Involvement and identification with the patient are important, but overinvolvement drains you and leaves you ineffective. When you are too entwined with the patient's issues, you have crossed a boundary that must separate you. Your goal is independence for the patient, not making a friend or possibly feeding your ego by how much your patients need you.

You have invested time, money, and energy in becoming a health practitioner. Chances are you are very committed to the goal of helping others.

Until now, you have probably not been in a position to assist people in need. Now that you are entering the health field, you may be filled with energy and enthusiasm. Such zeal is welcome in any setting provided that it is well-directed.

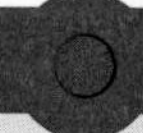

CASE STUDY 2-1

A young social worker wanted to help every kid he came into contact with. If a client needed shoes or a place to stay for a few days or couldn't deal with a parent, this social worker tried to meet the need. His caring was boundless. He worked day and night for his clients. He lost sleep over them as well. The sadness in their lives touched him deeply. Instead of assisting a child's parents to develop resources for a needed pair of shoes, for example, this social worker bought the shoes himself. But what is going to happen next year when the child again needs shoes? And how many feet can the salary of one social worker cover?

Overinvolvement means that you are doing more for your patients than is necessary or really helpful in the long run. Much as with "sympathy," you lose effectiveness when you become overinvolved. Further, when you become too important to a patient, you may well disappoint him or her by setting up unrealistic expectations. Once a patient feels disappointed, the rapport you have built and the work developed between you will be lost.

Although our social worker friend had the best intentions—helping his clients to have better lives—his actions actually prevented them from finding their own solutions. Not only did he foster their dependency on him by being the sole source of their solutions, but he also overworked himself. If your job has no limits, then you have no breaks, no places to rest, and no joy outside the work.

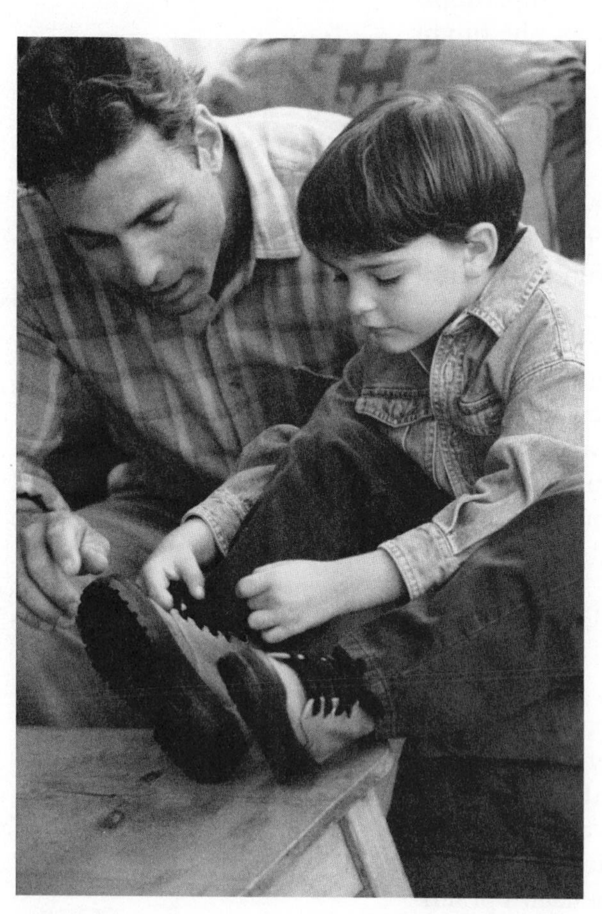

Overinvolvement

Health care providers who become too involved with their patients usually burn out early and leave their profession. The work becomes too sad, too demanding, too overwhelming. A balance between personal life and professional obligations is essential. Depression and anxiety are often signals that burnout has begun.

Yet you want to help people and the idea of being cold and objective in the face of human suffering is abhorrent to you. So how do you strike a balance between being too involved and too callous? Practice and experience will be your best teachers.

If you see an abused child about whom you cannot stop thinking, you could be heading for trouble. Talk about your feelings to a trusted colleague when you first sense that they may not be appropriate. Often we must become conditioned to the troubles we see. Few people feel relaxed when they first view surgery or a cadaver, but a few repeated exposures generally take the mystery and horror away. Anatomy students often eat lunch while studying in the morgue.

You must live through your first experiences with difficult patient problems in order to build up your stamina and understanding. Be quick to recognize your own inner warnings of trouble. Then talk to a more experienced person for help in dealing with your feelings. Someone who has recently been a student may be of great help to you. Chances are that he or she also went through a similar time.

Occasionally, we come upon a patient problem that overwhelms us because it strikes too close to home. For instance, if you were a battered child, you might react too strongly to an abused child's situation. Yet, if people in your field are to work repeatedly with battered children, you must do something about your reaction. Health care providers sometimes need help themselves. If your personal problems affect your work, you must resolve those issues in a manner that will permit you to function with all your patients. Otherwise, the patient you are overinvolved with may get a disproportionate amount of your time and your other patients may pay a price for your unresolved problems. Or you may be so upset in the presence of a certain patient that you cannot practice what you are hired for. As discussed, all the sympathy in the world will not compensate for deprivation of treatment.

To avoid problems of overinvolvement, ask yourself these questions: What is my role here? What are the possible consequences (to me/to my patient) if I overinvolve myself? Will this affect my ability to function with other patients? Is there a better way to serve this patient?

Could you become overinvolved with a patient? With what type of patient might it be difficult for you to work? With what type of problem or patient might you overidentify? It is important to think about these situations before you must cope with them.

Self-preparation, early recognition of problems, talking with a colleague or a professional, and balance at home are keys to beating overinvolvement. In a few rare instances it might be best simply to remove yourself from a case. Doing so could be appropriate in an isolated incident, but if several cases are too much for you, you have work of your own to do.

Taking Things Personally

Becoming personally involved may overlap slightly with another area of concern: taking things personally or becoming defensive on the job. We are focusing here primarily on practitioner–patient interactions. Personalizing issues with colleagues is another issue.

The health care provider who is trying too hard to make the world a better place or to win love from patients is very vulnerable. Patients often take their own frustrations and pain out on whoever is available. Although the nurse entering Mrs. Brown's room may be the kindest nurse in the world, Mrs. Brown may hate *anyone* who is up and about while she is bedridden with pain. Our kind nurse will likely be attacked for no reason. If she is an experienced practitioner, the attack will simply key her in on how unhappy Mrs. Brown is. But, if she is overly sensitive, unsure of herself, or emotionally needy, Mrs. Brown's attack may be very damaging.

As a health care provider, you cannot allow yourself to require praise and appreciation from your patients. If you do, you will often be hurt and disappointed. When you learn more about the needs of patients and the

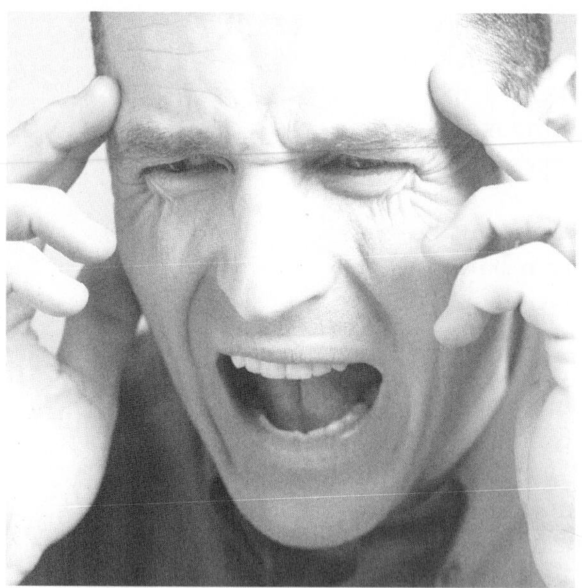

When patients attack, don't take it personally, paraphrase their anger.

losses they are suffering, you can distance yourself from attacks. Attacks are usually a call for help and require attention and understanding. Defensiveness and arguments are not appropriate responses.

What do you do if you walk into a patient's room and are yelled at for no understandable reason? Well, you could cry or run or shout back, but we hope you won't. So, what do you do? How about paraphrasing? Reflect back to the patient, in nonjudgmental tones, the complaint you are hearing. Don't panic. Chances are this approach will serve to soothe the patient and allow you to perform your job. Remember that patients are not really upset with you as an individual; they are angry with their own situations. Consider this example:

> **Patient:** "Why can't you damn nurses do anything for this pain?!
>
> **Nurse:** "It must be overwhelming always to be in pain. I will check with your doctor about more medication. While I'm doing that is there anything else I can do for you?"

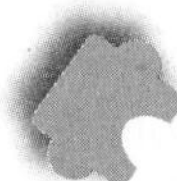

Receiving and Giving Feedback

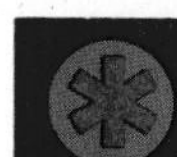

Key Point

Receiving feedback thanking the giver, paraphrasing the giver, seeking clarification, and discussing how you can change.

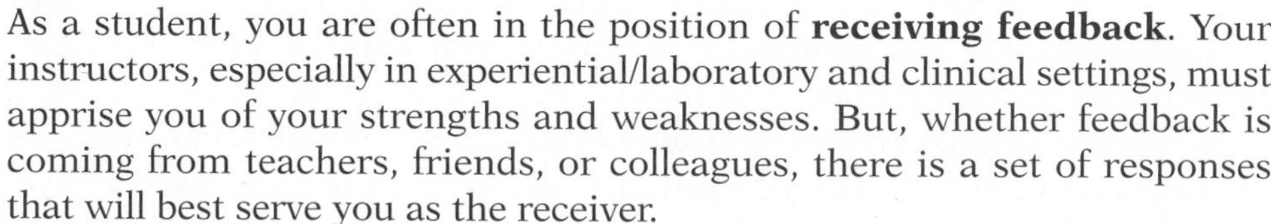

As a student, you are often in the position of **receiving feedback**. Your instructors, especially in experiential/laboratory and clinical settings, must apprise you of your strengths and weaknesses. But, whether feedback is coming from teachers, friends, or colleagues, there is a set of responses that will best serve you as the receiver.

You may recall our discussion about defensiveness in the previous section. A defensive response means you are blocking out the value of any feedback that is directed toward you. Besides preventing you from developing your skills, a defensive response is like waving a red flag that reads "I am insecure."

There are four steps to follow in receiving feedback. Note how they guard against defensiveness.

1. **Thanking the giver.** By thanking the person who gives you feedback, you immediately set a receptive tone. You are saying, in essence, "I am glad to have your input so I can profit from what you see." An automatic thank-you gives you time and prevents you from making a short or defensive opening remark.
2. **Paraphrasing.** In the context of receiving feedback, paraphrasing will do two things for you. First, it will allow you to be sure you have heard the feedback correctly. Even the best communicators can be ambiguous at times. And, when you're dealing with any form of criticism, oversensitivity can easily distort your hearing. You want to be certain that your understanding of the message is what the speaker intended.

   Second, paraphrasing gives the speaker a second chance. Hearing his or her own words of evaluation repeated may allow him or her to see that it sounds too strong or too all-encompassing. Feedback will seem more appropriate following paraphrasing.

3. **Seeking further clarification.** Once paraphrasing has occurred and you fully understand the issues, you may still need to clarify certain points. Consider this example:

Evaluator: You are spending too much time with your patients.

Student: Do you mean I am working too late?

Evaluator: No, I mean you should limit the time you spend with each patient so you can see all patients by noon. If there is a special needs case, you can return to it once you've reviewed the needs of all the patients.

By seeking clarification, you are demonstrating a desire to fully understand what you might need to change. You are asking specifically what it is that the evaluator is suggesting you do. If feedback is not specified and behavioral, it may be impossible to follow, as described in Case Studies 2-3 and 2-4. Seeking to clarify feedback shows that you are willing to work on change if the evaluator can be clear about what you need to work on.

4. **Discussing how to correct weaknesses** Once you understand precisely what needs work, you can discuss how to make the necessary change.

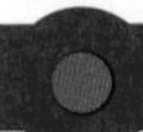

CASE STUDY 2-2

Evaluator: I wonder whether I might speak to you in private. I have been getting complaints about your notes in the charts.

Student: *(Thank you)* Thank you for bringing this to my attention. *(Paraphrase)* It sounds like my notes aren't up to hospital standards. *(Seeking clarification)* What do I need to change?

Evaluator: You need to give more details when reporting your conclusions. Otherwise, no one knows why you are picking up various patient problems the rest of us have not seen.

Student: *(Discussion of what can be corrected.)* If I take just a few extra minutes with each patient, I should be able to describe the patient comments or behavior with which I am concerned. Would that take care of it?

Evaluator: Yes, that sounds very helpful.

Contrast Case Study 2-2 with the two that follow.

CASE STUDY 2-3

Evaluator: I wonder whether I might speak to you in private. I have been getting complaints about your notes in the charts.

Student: Oh no! I've been writing down everything you taught us to. Who has been criticizing me?

Evaluator: Now please calm down. We are all trying to help you learn. But several people have questioned your conclusions on patient problems. They especially want to know why you think Mr. London is upset by his daughter's visits.

CASE STUDY 2-4

Evaluator: I wonder whether I might speak to you in private. I have been getting complaints about your notes in the charts.

Student: Oh dear! I'm so sorry. I knew I couldn't handle all this. Does this mean I am out of the program?

Evaluator: Heavens no. This is probably not at all serious, but we do need more information when you make a statement about a patient problem.

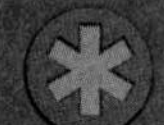

Key Point

Giving feedback starting with the positive, being specific, focusing on behavior, knowing your motives, being immediate, and being private.

Which of these three responses would you most likely have made? Discuss. (Hopefully you picked Case Study 2-2.)

We have made several assumptions in the preceding discussion regarding the receiving of feedback. One is that the evaluator is acting for the good of the receiver. Another is that the problems can be corrected. These two assumptions are essential to **giving feedback**.

Whether you are giving feedback to a patient, a colleague, or a friend, you need to be aware of certain basic guidelines. The first is that you must examine your reasons for giving the feedback. Feedback that is not intended to help the receiver is bound to be received negatively. If you are angry with or want to hurt or punish the receiver, you can count on not being well heard.

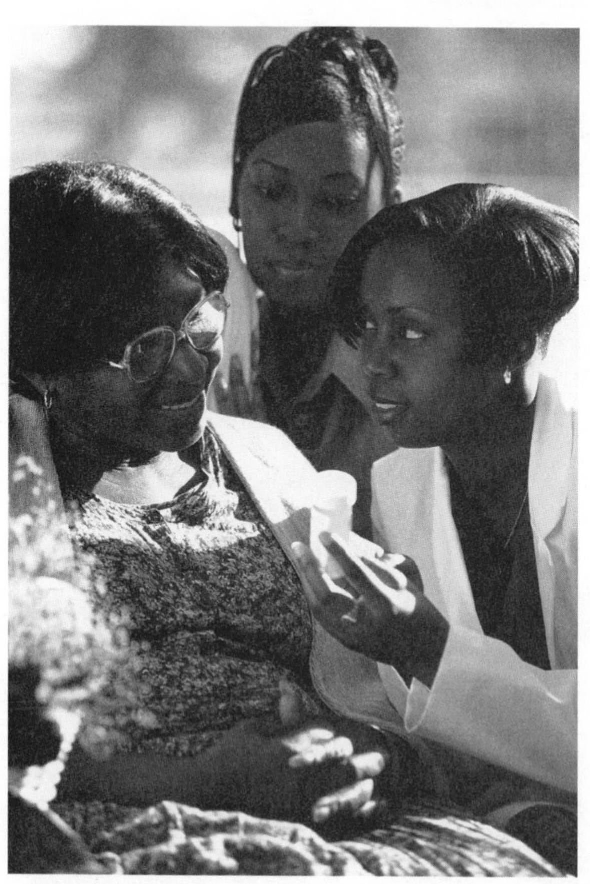

A home care nurse explains medications to a patient and asks for feedback.

One way to guard against giving punitive (aimed at punishment) feedback is to keep feedback specific and behavioral. Never suggest that someone change an intangible. Consider this example: "Why don't you just grow up? Your immature attitude is hurting the whole department!" What is the receiver to do? Wait five years and try the job again? Note, however, that if the criticism relates to specific behavior, there is hope for change: "It is difficult for the staff to work around your irregular hours. If you will give us an updated copy of your schedule from week to week, I am sure things will go smoothly."

The first giver, who sounds hurt and angry, made negative character judgments based on hidden behavioral issues. When the behavioral issues themselves (irregular hours) become the focus, the giver makes more sense and the receiver knows what is bothering the staff. It is much easier to change a schedule than to try to "grow up."

Well-intentioned behavioral feedback is productive feedback; it is advice given expressly to help the receiver become aware of and change her or his behavior.

Knowing when and where to offer feedback so that it will be best received is essential. Generally speaking, feedback should be given immediately so that it is clearly connected to the event under discussion. Further, the receiver is less likely to be embarrassed that the situation has been allowed to go on with him or her being seen in a critical light.

There are a few exceptions, however. Most individuals prefer to receive feedback in a private setting. Although some classroom and clinical situations may offer the opportunity for everyone to learn from the errors of one, most feedback is best given in private. The impact of delayed feedback may not be weakened if the delay is for the sake of discretion. Giving immediate feedback in front of others at the risk of embarrassing the receiver is not productive.

Finally, remember to look for the positive. Begin a feedback session by reviewing the receiver's strengths. No one wants to feel that he or she can do nothing right. Tell the receiver what you like before mentioning what you do not like. Doing so will increase the receiver's receptivity. To summarize, the rules for giving feedback are:

1. Begin with something positive.
2. Be specific.
3. Focus on behavior.
4. Be certain your motive is to be helpful.
5. Be immediate.
6. Be private.

What do you do if you follow these rules and the receiver becomes defensive anyway? First, remember that anyone can have a bad day. You may be giving feedback to a person who is undergoing a personal crisis. Or you may be offering well-intentioned feedback to someone who is too insecure to deal with it.

How should you respond when the receiver is clearly in distress? Your first reaction might be to clarify what you are trying to say to be sure there is no misunderstanding. Beyond this, you could choose either to back off and perhaps try again another time or to stick with the issues and pursue the receiver's difficulties in hearing it.

Either of these responses may be appropriate. Who the receiver is with respect to you and your role may dictate how you proceed. If you are responsible for the training or well-being of the receiver, the second approach may be more beneficial. Ideally, feedback is being given upon request; that is, it has been solicited or is expected by role definition. Keep professional **boundaries** in mind.

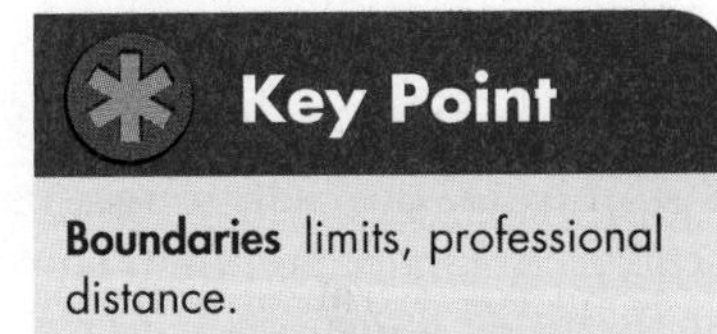

Summary

This chapter emphasized the value of learning and applying good listening skill synthesizing the use of nonverbal skills, paraphrasing, empathizing and using questions appropriately while remaining client focused. Paraphrasing is restating the client's problems in your own words.

Paraphrasing is used for several reasons. It helps the health provider to verify what he or she has heard, it allows the speaker to hear what his or her words have conveyed, it helps to build rapport, it keeps the focus on the client, and it keeps the client engaged in talking.

To be most effective, you must go beyond the actual words a patient uses and connect these words with the underlying feelings to give an empathic response. This should only be attempted once rapport has been established. Empathy is understanding how another feels and differs from sympathy as sympathy is a connection to personal and mutually shared feelings and is not recommended in the professional setting. Suspension of value judgments is an essential component of developing these empathic responses. A list of words which convey feelings was provided.

This chapter also taught the skill of using open-ended questions. Open-ended questions keep the focus on the client and allow the health professional to learn more about the client without leading the conversation in the health professional's direction. The timing and use of closed-ended questions was also reviewed as such questions are necessary to quickly assess basic facts and items of the patient's health history.

Evaluating possible communication hazards was also discussed, with a review of common issues such as those found in social comment: giving advice, talking about yourself, and claiming to know how another person feels. Also, the dangers of overinvolvement and taking client comments personally were reviewed.

Finally, the chapter discussed the important skills of receiving feedback with steps that involve: thanking the giver, paraphrasing what the giver has said, clarifying if necessary, and accepting what may need correcting. Similarly the steps of giving feedback were also outlined: Begin with something positive; be specific; focus on behavior; know that your own motive is to be helpful; be immediate; and when possible, be private.

Chapter Review

Key Term Review

Boundaries: Limits, professional distance.

Closed-ended question: A question that can be answered simply and that does not encourage further discussion.

Cognitive: Of thought, factual knowledge, thinking skills.

Communication sequence: Paraphrasing (with use of nonverbal language), then empathizing, then asking open-ended questions.

Empathize: Convey understanding of another person's feelings.

Feeling Words: Words that express emotional feelings rather than just cognitive thoughts.

Giving feedback: Start with the positive, be specific, focus on behavior, know your motives, and be immediate and private.

Open-ended question: A question that cannot be answered simply but encourages further discussion.

Paraphrase: Repeat message in different words.

Receiving feedback: Thank the giver, paraphrase the giver, seek clarification, and discuss how you can change.

Sympathy: Shared feelings of pain over a loss best used in a social context.

Chapter Review Questions

1. List five reasons for paraphrasing.
2. What effect might it have on the world if every speaker had to be paraphrased before the listener could make an original response?
3. It is easier to empathize with a real-live person, face-to-face, than it is to empathize with most problems as described in a text. Please explain this statement.
4. What is the difference between empathy and sympathy?
5. Discuss the pros and cons of overinvolvement for the patient and for the health care provider. What is the importance of appropriate boundaries?
6. What types of patients or human problems are most likely to lend themselves to "overinvolvement"?

Case Study Critical Thinking Questions

1. After rereading Case Study 2-1, comment about overinvolvement. Have you felt a similar feeling? How did you deal with the feeling? Is professional distance just another word for coldness?
2. Look at Case Studies 2-2, 2-3, and 2-4. Describe your personal problems with giving feedback and receiving feedback. How might you overcome them? There are members of the health care team who are always working their own agenda, such as how to make themselves look better than others or how to do less work. What impact do their goals have on the team—on communication and on feedback?

References

1. Aring, C. "Sympathy and Empathy." *JAMA* 167(4):448–52; May 24, 1958.
2. Baile, W., et al. "Breaking Bad News, More than Just Guidelines." *J Clin Oncol* 24:3217; 2006.
3. Barrier, P., Li, J., Jensen, N. "Two Words to Improve Physician-Patient Communication: What Else?" *Mayo Clin Proc* 78(2):211–4; February 2003.
4. Bellet, P., Maloney, M. "The Importance of Empathy as an Interviewing Skill in Medicine." *JAMA* 266(13):1831–2; October 2, 1991.
5. Coulehan J., et al. "Let Me See if I Have This Right ... Words that Help Build Empathy." *Ann Intern Med* 135(3):221–7; August 7, 2001.
6. Hardee, J. An Overview of Empathy. *The Permanente J*. 2004.
7. Suchman, A. et al. "A Model of Empathic Communication in the Medical Interview." *JAMA* 277(8): 678–82; February 26, 1997.
8. Freeman, P. *Verbal Communication* Shrewsbury, U.K.: Axis Education, February 2007.

Additional Readings

1. Audrey, S., et al. "What Oncologists Tell Patients about Survival Benefits of Palliative Chemotherapy and Implications for Informed Consent: Qualitative Study." *Brit Med J* 337:a752; 2008.
2. Back et al. "Efficacy of Communication Skills Training for Giving Bad News Discussing Transitions to Palliative Care." *Arch Intern Med* 167:453–460; 2007.
3. Leaper, Ayres. "A Meta-analytic Review of Gender Variations in Adults' Language Use: Talkativeness, Affiliative speech, and Assertive speech." *Pers Soc Psychol Rev* 11:328–363; 2007.
4. Maguire, P. Pitceathly, C. "Key Communication Skills and How to Acquire Them." *Brit Med J* 325:697–700; September 28, 2002.

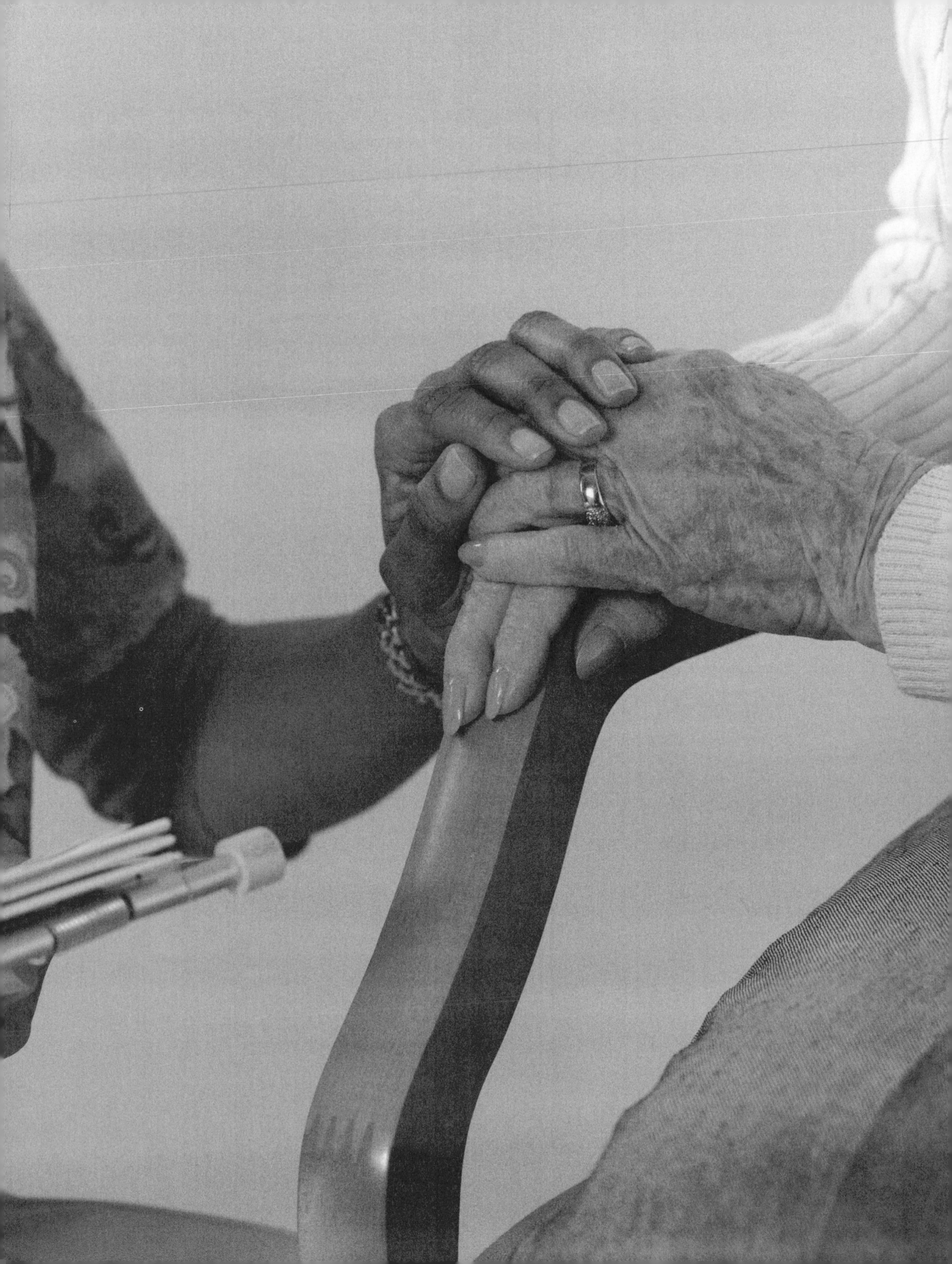

Basic Psychology

Learning Outcomes

After reading this chapter, you should be able to:

- **3.1** Summarize the historical perspective of basic psychology.
- **3.2** Describe Maslow's hierarchy of human needs.
- **3.3** Explain Pavlov's conditioned reflex.
- **3.4** Understand Freud's concept of the unconscious mind.
- **3.5** Identify Freud's life and death instincts.
- **3.6** Discuss Adler and the inferiority complex.
- **3.7** Explain Jung's theory of the collective unconscious.
- **3.8** Apply eclectic decision making.
- **3.9** Define Gestalt therapy.
- **3.10** Analyze games people play.
- **3.11** Describe nondirective or client-centered therapy.
- **3.12** Illustrate examples of psychological defense mechanisms.

Key Terms

Anima
Behaviorism
Collective unconscious
Compensation
Complex
Conditioned reflex
Countertransference
Defense mechanism
Denial
Displacement
Ego
Eros
Eclectic
Electra complex
Extrovert
Gestalt
Hierarchy of basic human needs
Id
Identification
Inferiority complex
Introvert
Inversion
Libido
Life instincts
Masculine protest
Oedipus complex
Persona
Positive regard
Rationalization
Repression
Regression
Resistance
Rogerian approach
Sublimation
Superego
Suppression
Symbolism
Thanatos
Transactional analysis
Transference

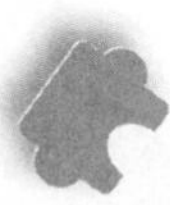

Historical Perspective of Basic Psychology

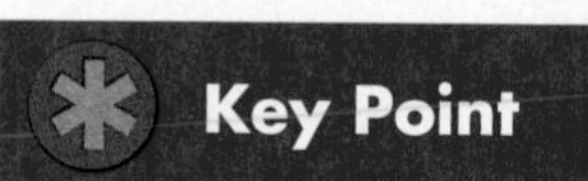

Rogerian approach nondirective or client-centered counseling.

Human behavior can be analyzed in several ways. Much of this book uses the **Rogerian approach**. The Rogerian approach is client-centered, as described in Chapter 2. By contrast, the older psychoanalytic approaches are more of a theoretic explanation of client behavior. Combining both kinds of approaches will be most helpful to the aspiring health care worker. This chapter covers many of the psychoanalytic explanations, which form a framework for thinking about client behavior.

Effective communication demands at least some knowledge of psychology. A basic understanding of psychology will add a conceptual framework to the skills the reader has been developing. This chapter condenses an enormous field into the basic essentials for understanding human behavior. Also contained within this chapter are the definitions of many terms related to the field of psychology.

People's belief systems vary, and rather than judge them as old-fashioned, different, or alternative, we need to understand their belief systems to communicate with them. Look at different psychological theories and apply them to human beings and illness behavior. There is no one-size-fits-all theory. Rather, traditional psychological theories offer metaphors that give insight into human behavior. For example when counseling a patient to stop smoking, you can look at smoking at several levels: a Freudian level (satisfaction of libidinous instincts at the oral level), a Pavlovian level (light up after each meal), an addictive level (to nicotine), or a Jungian level (a persona projected by smoking fine cigars). Without this historical background, your understanding will be limited.

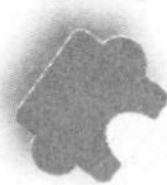

Psychoanalytic Theory

Maslow and the Hierarchy of Human Needs

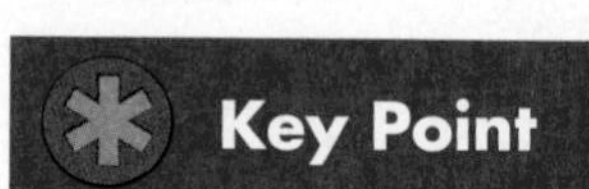

Maslow's hierarchy of human needs physiological, security, affiliation, esteem, and self-actualization.

Abraham Maslow (1908–1970) linked together existential philosophies (ideas relating to existence) and human psychology. He began by acknowledging a **hierarchy of basic human needs** common to all individuals. These needs, in order of priority, are:

1. *Physiological needs*—food, water, and shelter
2. *Security needs*—safety and security, freedom from illness or threats
3. *Affiliation needs*—sex, affection, relationships, a feeling of belonging to something
4. *Esteem needs*—feelings of self-worth and achievement
5. *Self-actualization needs*—self-fulfillment, finding meaning to life, transcendental change

In simple terms, Maslow said that, to understand a patient's motivation, one must first see at what level of human need the patient is being threatened. For example, a patient who is facing a grim diagnosis or extraordinary surgery may withdraw to varying degrees from friends or family. Further, such a patient may regress to a childlike state, with no interest in affiliation or self-esteem needs. These emotional and behavioral changes can be understood by determining at what level the patient is being threatened. If this patient believes that her life is at risk or her security is totally jeopardized, then her inability to relate to higher level needs is understandable.

Only those rare individuals who have become self-actualized can transcend disruption at lower levels. Such remarkable individuals live life always in search of more, taking every turn of events for its peak value. The self-actualized cannot, therefore, be threatened.

Self-actualization was a goal for which even Maslow himself continued to thirst. However, Maslow described a state of homeostatis that many persons who do not reach the level of self-actualization experience during their lifetime. Homeostasis is not a zero point, which might indicate low motivation, boredom, or lack of challenge, but rather a sense of optimal functioning.

Finally, you must acknowledge something in human beings that goes beyond basic human needs. This is the autonomous (able to do for or exist on one's own) self or pure psyche—the unique essence of the individual. Awareness of this essence can free up the definition of an authentic or healthy person, making one able to better value human beings and better understand motivation as defined by the individual's own right or uniqueness. Perhaps it is the individual's karma.

Pavlov and the Conditioned Reflex

Ivan Pavlov (1849–1936) is famous for his work on conditioned reflexes. He measured salivation in dogs in response to food. He then found that salivation occurred as soon as the dogs saw food coming. He then paired ringing a bell with presenting food. When he finally stopped bringing food, the dogs still salivated in response to the ringing bell, an unrelated stimulus. This was called a **conditioned reflex** (that is, a learned response to the stimulus). Consider this example:

Key Point

Pavlov's conditioned reflex learned response to stimulus.

CASE STUDY 3-1

The medical assistant is drawing blood from Mrs. Benson, who is sitting in the exam room with her daughter. Her daughter tells the assistant that she used to drive her mother to a local restaurant for dinner every Sunday. But Mrs. Benson always felt sick in the car and eventually had to stop going out. Subsequently, Mrs. Benson developed severe nausea every time her daughter visited. She did not become nauseated at any other time.

The car made Mrs. Benson sick. But when the stimulus was withdrawn, the unrelated stimulus (her daughter's company) still evoked the same response.

This case illustrates a conditioned reflex. It helps the health professional to understand illness behavior as discussed later in this text. Some patients become conditioned to avoiding treatments if they associate all health professionals with pain or loss. Knowledge of conditioned reflex may need to be applied to solve a variety of patient concerns.

Behaviorism is a school of psychology founded by John B. Watson and William James. It holds that you should be concerned primarily with an individual's behavior. Behavioral therapy involves using conditioning to change a person's behavior.

Psychoanalytic theory might suggest that Mrs. Benson secretly disliked her daughter. Behavioral theory would say that you should accept Mrs. Benson's symptoms more at face value. Therapy might consist, for example, of a simple explanation of conditioned reflexes or counterconditioning (associating her daughter with another stronger cue to oppose the nausea such as the daughter always bringing a present or ice cream).

Freud and the Unconscious Mind

Key Point

Freudian psychology the belief that the conscious mind represses thoughts that are painful into the unconscious mind.

Sigmund Freud was the founder of modern psychoanalytic theory. In *The Psychology of Everyday Life*, he explained unconscious motivation. Some events may be pure chance; others may be subconsciously motivated. Obviously, he said, it is not your fault if a brick falls on your head. But spending a day in bed with a splitting headache is an excellent way of missing work and gaining the family's attention. Note how well this description dovetails with the discussion in Chapter 4 of "secondary gains" of illness. Freud could predict this type of behavior.

Freud also explained the concepts of **repression** and **resistance**. Repression means the conscious mind will not allow unconscious thoughts to enter. Emotions that are undesirable conflict with the conscious mind. They are repressed or pushed back into the unconscious. Once there, they cannot reenter the conscious mind because of resistance (the mind holds off the painful reality).

CASE STUDY 3-2

Mr. Green was told that his wife would be dead in a matter of weeks. She had advanced cancer that was no longer responding to any drugs. Knowing that she had always wanted to travel around the world, he bought tickets for the two of them to go on such a trip six months later. The painful thought was that his wife would die. He repressed this thought to the unconscious. It is obvious that he repressed the thought because he bought a ticket for her that she could clearly not use. His conscious mind resisted the painful thought because he paid a lot of money for those tickets.

This kind of situation comes up frequently in psychology because it is conflict that is painful. This example helps to establish further understanding of death and dying, which is the subject of Chapter 5 of this text. In psychological treatment, this example helps to explain mental health issues when patients have a pattern of abnormal behaviors that all began around the same date. For instance, a girl's drinking, doing poorly in

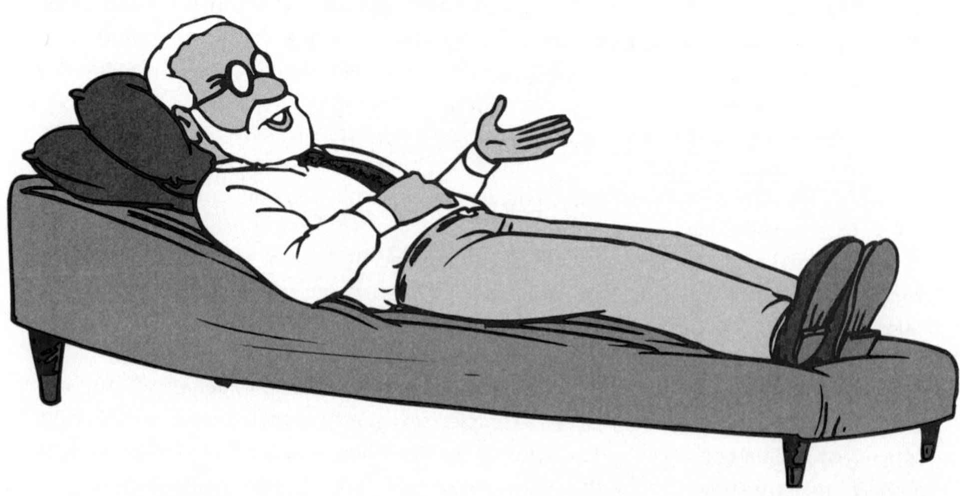

Freud's theories may be down played today but his concepts are actively used in patient care.

school, and getting arrested may all have occurred when she was 16 and was raped. The rape was a precipitating event, and the patient will require extensive psychotherapy to unlock the trauma.

Freud's Life and Death Instincts

Another of Freud's theories involved the **life instincts**—sexuality and self-preservation. His theory of infantile sexuality became of profound importance to later psychologists. He believed that two drives were innate in a young infant: the drive for self-preservation and the drive to procreate (which he claimed was thwarted till later).

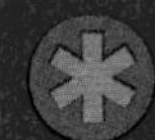

Key Point

Freud's life instincts or Eros sexual drive or libido (three phases: oral, anal and genital) and self-preservation.

He noticed frequent reference by patients to three erogenous areas. On the basis of these references, Freud formulated his theory of **libido** or sexual drive. The child's interest in each of the erogenous zones follows a set chronological sequence. Until the end of the first year, interest is centered on the mouth. Eating and smoking therefore represent, according to this theory, a persistence of infantile libidinous (or lustful) instincts at the oral level. This, according to Freudian theory, is why people who give up smoking tend to eat more.

From the end of the first year, until the end of the third year, the child's interest is centered on the anus. The bowel habits of the young infant are said to bear a direct relationship to later traits such as possessiveness or stubbornness. Feces become associated with belongings and especially with money. ("He's got pots of money," "He's stinking rich," "She's rolling in the stuff.") Constipation represents the child's desire to hold onto possessions and indicates that the child is trying to assert control over the parent doing the toilet training.

From the end of the third year to the fifth year, interest is on the genital area. At this time Freud's renowned **Oedipus complex** arises. The boy is sexually attracted to his mother and sexually jealous of his father. The situation usually resolves itself through the castration complex, in which the boy fears that his illicit desire will be punished by his father through castration. Freud seems to have been rather uncertain about girls. He explained the situation in terms of penis envy, which causes the girl to be sexually attracted to her father. Freud called this the **Electra complex**. This complex resolves itself more easily than the Oedipal complex because the girl feels that she *has been* punished, whereas the boy feels that he *may be* punished.

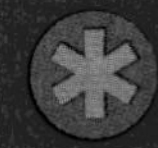

Key Point

Freud's death instincts or Thanatos innate destructiveness and aggression.

Freud later called his sexual phases and instincts **Eros**, or self-preservation instincts, the feeling that you do not wish to die, to be the underdog, or to be controlled or defeated by others; you choose instead self-determination.

In contrast to the life instincts, the death instinct, or **Thanatos**, represents the individual's innate destructiveness and aggression either toward himself or toward others. Thanatos plus libido produces sadomasochism (sadists enjoy inflicting pain; masochists enjoy pain). In Freud's theory, examples of self-aggressive behavior include addiction, accident proneness, and recurrent failures.

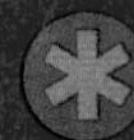

Key Point

Id, ego and superego *id* is based on the pleasure principle and is the demand part of our personalities that strives from infancy to get our basic needs met; *ego* is largely an unconscious part of the personality that mediates the demands of the id, the superego and reality; *superego* begins to develop around age 5 as our moral or ethical side, which tells right from wrong.

Another of Freud's theories involves the **id**, the **ego**, and **superego**. The *id* is the inherent instincts in a newborn child and remains in our unconscious, influencing our personalities as we strive to get our basic needs met throughout life. The *ego* represents the realization that the child is a unique person. The ego develops just after the id and is largely unconscious.

The ego acts as a sort of arbitrator between the subconscious id, the morals of the superego, and the reality of the outside world. When moral prohibitions of society are imposed, the superego emerges from the ego. Much of the superego is preconscious and is responsible for an adult's character. The *superego* knows right from wrong and is our ethical side, but it begins forming in the young child.

Adler and the Inferiority Complex

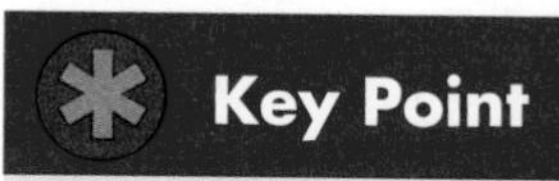

Key Point

Adler inferiority complex and masculine protest.

Alfred Adler (1870–1937) introduced the concept of the inferiority feeling that results from a real or imagined defect. This inferiority feeling determines what stance in life a person takes. A strong feeling of inferiority with undue pessimism is termed an **inferiority complex**. The conscious or subconscious overcompensation for feeling inferior leads to a superiority feeling or complex: Thus people with superiority complexes act the opposite of how they actually feel.

Another corollary of feeling inferior is the natural tendency for people to move from a passive, or feminine, role to an aggressive, or masculine, role. This is called **masculine protest**. The yin and yang of masculine protest (that is, the passive conflicting with the aggressive) was to Adler a major cause of anxiety.

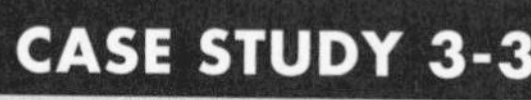

CASE STUDY 3-3

Carlos, aged nine, injured his knee playing football with some friends in the street. When he saw the physical therapist, he was pessimistic. Rather than do the exercises the physical therapist prescribed, Carlos chose to sit around. He spent much of his time indoors. Despite a seemingly mild injury, he seemed convinced that he would never again be able to play football. This in turn would stop him from being able to get back with his new gang of friends. He said he didn't mind that so much because he liked to spend time with his rabbit.

Clearly, Carlos has an inferiority complex. It is affecting his motivation to cooperate with physical therapy. The comment about his rabbit can be viewed several ways. It may be his **rationalization** of why his most important striving (to be with the gang) did not matter. It may be simple **displacement** activity for something else that he would have rather done (playing with the gang). It may be a cry for help. "If I say something so pathetic, perhaps she will help me to do what I really want to do."

The physical therapist's mandate here is to attend to more than Carlos's knee. It is to use his knee to help him with his inferiority feelings. The physical therapist can accomplish this by first accepting the patient's problem. Although the patient may be exaggerating the knee injury, he may be using it as a symptom to legitimize his relationship with the therapist.

By accepting the symptom, the health professional can use the patient's agenda and help him to achieve his goals. Additional questioning may allow the patient to maintain his control without undue threat: "How's the knee doing this week?" "How is it improving?" "When do you think you'll be able to manage to get back on the football field?" "When did you last see your friends?"

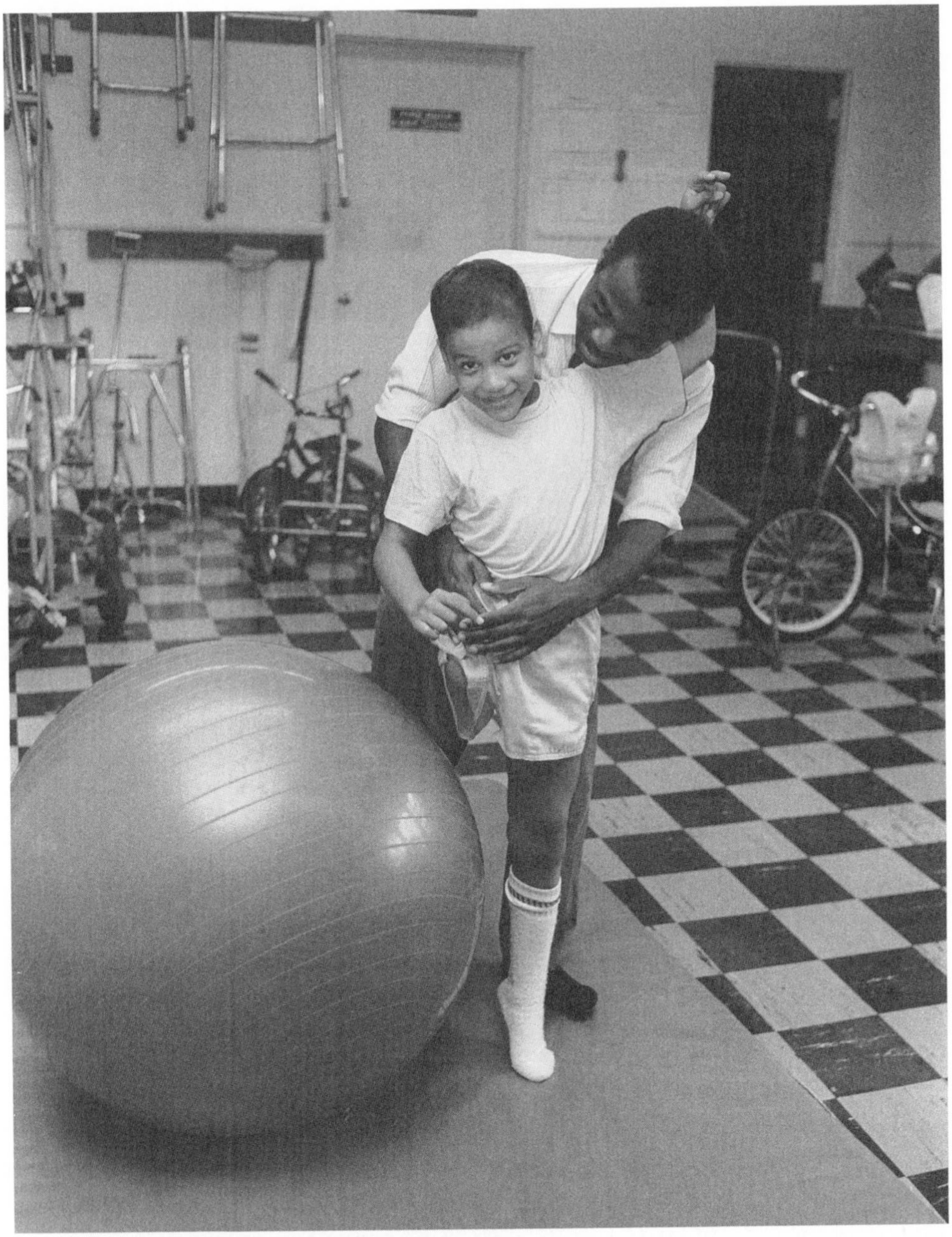

Injuries may reveal more than is physical. What should your role be?

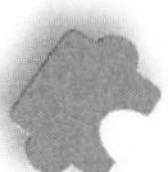

Jung and the Collective Unconscious

Carl Jung (1875–1961) believed that all humans are born with a genetically preprogrammed unconscious. He called this the **collective unconscious**. He also introduced the idea of a **complex,** a group of ideas with a common feeling or tone. Jung described the inner self as the **anima** and the front a person puts on for the world as the **persona**. He also described the now well-known personality types called the **introvert** and the **extrovert**. An introvert is shy and introspective. An extrovert is sociable and outgoing.

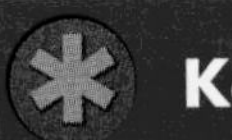

Key Point

Jung anima and persona; introvert and extrovert.

These personality types have become common references within our culture. A basic understanding of the introvert and extrovert may help not only with understanding how to be sensitive to our patients but also how to work better with members of the health care team as discussed in Chapter 10.

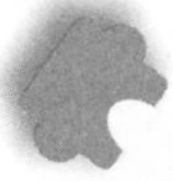

Other Theories of Human Behavior

Key Point

Eclecticism the use of many different theories to input decision making

It is obvious from this historical perspective that there is no one "correct" explanation for human behavior. Some old philosophies are simply viewed as inappropriate or sexist in today's world. There are many systems of psychological explanation to choose from. Each health practitioner will chose different items from the menu and will use them in individual ways. That is appropriate and is referred to as **eclectic**. What works for one health care provider may not work for another. What works with one patient may not work with another.

Thus far, this chapter has reviewed schools of psychoanalytic thought that seek to explain what makes the personality of one person unique. Some other important theories are **Gestalt** therapy, **transactional analysis**, and Rogerian counseling.

Gestalt Theory

Key Point

Gestalt therapy treating the patient as a whole, focusing on current feelings.

Fritz Perls (1893–1970) developed Gestalt therapy. Or, as he might have said, he *worked on developing* Gestalt therapy, for Perls never considered Gestalt a finished product, just as he viewed all of development as a confirming process. The word *gestalt* is German for a pattern or whole that is more than the sum of its parts. Gestalt therapy treats the patient as a whole. It concentrates on finishing the patient's unfinished business by focusing on current feelings. Role-playing techniques may be used to bring old unfinished situations into the present. Gestalt therapy can be used if a patient has unfinished business with a deceased parent, for example. As role play is used to deal with the parent, the patient may complete or get closure on something critical from the past. Completion may result in the patient's changing a destructive behavioral pattern.

Transactional Analysis

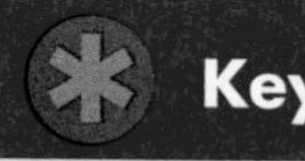

Key Point

Transactional analysis the belief that, in their transactions, people assume different roles at different times

In *Games People Play*, Eric Berne (1910–1970) developed transactional analysis. In their transactions, he said, people assume different roles at different times. He labeled each of these roles as a different ego state: parent (dominant), adult (equal), or child (submissive or immature). Any series of interchanges can be written as a diagram showing which ego states are involved (sometimes two are involved if the exchange has an ulterior meaning).

Therapeutic relationships usually call for a patient to assume a dependent role. Take the example of a female nurse giving a male patient a backrub. An appropriate response for him afterwards might be, "Thank you, nurse." Such a response establishes him in the child role and her in the adult role. If during the backrub he said, "That feels good, don't stop," he would be reversing the roles. Or he might say afterwards, "Thank you, that felt good. Will you be in tomorrow?" This could be taken both ways: child to parent and parent to child.

People, Berne said, need "stroking," physically or socially. They structure their time to receive strokes through four activities—pastimes, games, intimacy, and nonsocial activity.

Pastimes are semiritualistic, simple transactions used commonly at parties or during waiting periods. Games differ from pastimes in that ulterior transactions are involved or because there is a psychological payoff. The following exchange is a simple pastime: "Have you seen the latest hybrid Toyota has developed?" "Yes, the Ford has that too. It saves a lot of gas." But, if the response to the question is, "Of course we ordinary mortals can't afford that—maybe I should raise my prices like you pharmacists," it is a game. Games can be very complex and can be played without the participants being aware. Games can involve a simple transaction, a life situation, a marriage, or a professional situation. Intimacy involves lovemaking, and nonsocial activity includes cycling, collecting coins, and watching DVDs.

Rogerian Counseling

Carl Rogers (1902–1987) has been a major influence in the areas of behavioral prediction and control. Rogerian counseling initially was called *nondirective* or *client-centered therapy*. Patients have their own way of understanding themselves and getting better. A supportive, nonjudgmental, deeply caring therapist can activate this understanding and bring about change.

Rogerians focus on what the client is saying and then paraphrase and empathize. A key concept is **positive regard**. The therapist is careful to make the patient feel special. The patient is then free to trust that someone cares and understands. This judgment-free positive regard is thought to be especially helpful to those who have suffered from lack of parental support. Rogers also believed that psychotic patients should receive reassurances and warmth.

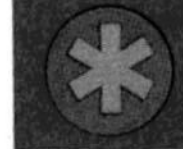

Key Point

Rogerian non-directive or client-centered counseling that uses positive regard

Rogers' theory, like any of the others, can be criticized, but it has been used extensively. Much of today's therapy and inpatient mental hospital treatment has a Rogerian base. It has also led to the encounter group movement. Do you see any similarities between Rogerian counseling and the paraphrasing, listening, and empathizing discussed in Chapter 2?

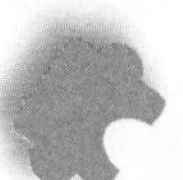

Defense Mechanisms

Psychoanalysis has long theorized the existence of the subconscious mind and that two conflicting stimuli produce either psychic pain or resolution of the conflict. The psychic pain can manifest as anxiety or some other pathology. The conflict can be resolved through various mental mechanisms—also called **defense mechanisms**, ego defenses, or dynamisms.

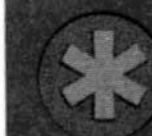

Key Point

Defense mechanisms subconscious ways for the mind to avoid painful conflicts.

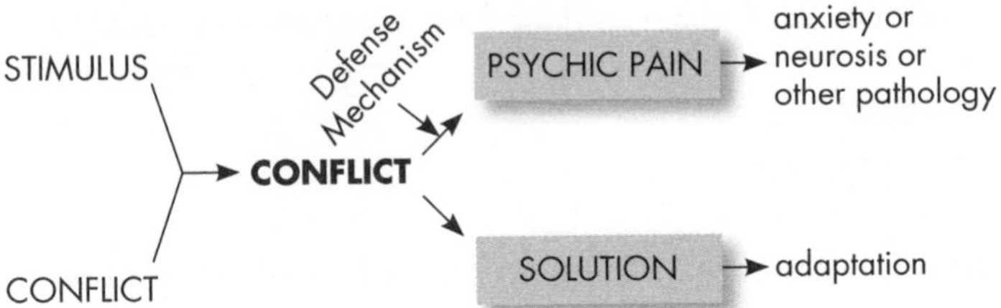

Theory of conflict resolution

The simplest defense mechanisms are repression and **suppression**. Repression is an involuntary relegation of consciously intolerable ideas into the unconscious mind. Suppression is the conscious equivalent of this.

CASE STUDY 3-4

Mr. Cage, aged 85, is normally a model patient. But one night he developed a fever, became confused, and struck his nurse. A few days later, after his fever and confusion were gone, he was told that he had struck his nurse. When the incident was mentioned to him a week later, however, he had no recollection of being told. To Mr. Cage, the idea of striking his nurse was in conflict with his normal character. Rather than leave such conflicts in his conscious mind, he repressed the painful thought into his unconscious. He was not forgetting or lying. He was not being malicious. He found the memory too painful to bear; repression was the way he dealt with it.

Sublimation is finding a socially acceptable outlet for a socially loaded problem. For example, a normal devoted husband finds that his wife has lost all interest in intimacy. So he devotes his evenings to committee meetings of various charitable organizations. Another example is an avid athlete who develops multiple sclerosis and becomes a jazz fan instead.

Identification is the unconscious transfer of outside character traits into one's own mind. Identification is what makes you cry at the movies. Group identification is of major importance in the armed forces (for example, "I am a Marine. Marines are the best"). Parents often live vicariously through their children's lives. Fathers may, for instance, identify with the sporting achievements of their children. Mothers may push daughters to be popular in ways that they were not.

CASE STUDY 3-5

The medical office assistant thought Mrs. Gefarb lived a boring existence. Meals on Wheels came once a day. Once a week her daughter brought some groceries and talked briefly about her children. Mrs. Gefarb had no television or radio and took no papers. Yet she didn't seem to be depressed. In fact, she always seemed very happy. Much of her conversation revolved around the achievements of her two grandsons, who were both at Princeton. The assistant thought of trying to increase Mrs. Gefarb's socializing, and she suggested getting a television set. She could not understand why her patient wasn't interested. However, Mrs. Gefarb was living a vicarious existence. By identifying with her two grandsons, she perceived fulfillment through their achievements. She didn't need any other fulfillment. Her daughter's 15-minute conversations about her children were Mrs. Gefarb's weekly "soap opera." Remarkably, a short conversation kept her going all week long.

Transference is when a patient identifies the health professional with someone else. Commonly the health professional is viewed as a parent. Feelings the patient has toward his or her parent are transferred to the health professional. **Countertransference** is when the health professional has personal (nonprofessional) feelings toward the patient.

A health provider can analyze his or her own feelings toward a patient and find there are two parts. The first part is a reaction toward the patient that is similar to other people's reactions. A patient, for instance, may have a habit that is annoying. The annoyance the health professional feels will also demonstrate how others may react to the patient. The second part of a health professional's feelings may be a response that goes beyond objectivity: The health professional might recognize feelings of love or hate. These feelings are countertransference and can be a problem. This is when a health professional must be on guard to follow the boundaries of a professional, rather than to develop a personal role with the patient.

Health care providers must strive for a subtle balance between overidentification and insufficient identification. This comes through experience and learning. To learn, be objective; to be objective, examine your own feelings: Am I reacting to the patient objectively or for some need of my own? Am I feeling anger or prejudice?

Excessive identification makes the health professional too involved, and he or she loses objectivity; insufficient identification makes it difficult to understand the patient's point of view—to empathize. Establishing professional distance does not mean you are being impersonal. It means treating the patient as you yourself would like to be treated. Objectivity is most commonly lost when you step out of your professional role into the role of friend. This can happen, for instance, if you overidentify or become a friend with a patient outside of the professional setting. You must retain your boundaries.

CASE STUDY 3-6

Irene, a middle aged nurse, worked on the pediatric oncology ward. She chose this area because her six-year-old son had died from leukemia 10 years previously. Unfortunately, all her patients became her substitute children. She was unable to switch from one patient to the next, became too involved, and soon had to transfer to a general pediatric floor. Once moved, she worked much more effectively. Overidentification had caused her to lose her objectivity and her effectiveness.

Inversion is when a person does the opposite of what he or she wants. For example, if you are rejected by someone you love, you may be able to deal with this more easily by hating that person instead. (The word inversion was used by Freud differently to refer to homosexuality.)

Denial is another defense mechanism in which painful truths are denied. Denial is the verbal equivalent of suppression. It is described in more depth in Chapter 5 on Death and Dying.

CASE STUDY 3-7

A girl who loved her father very much often came home from school to find him drunk. He often assaulted her physically. She found this so unpleasant that she simply did not think about it and so appeared to be quite contented. This is suppression. When a nurse asked her if her father ever beat her she said, "No, he loves me." This is denial.

Other common defense mechanisms include:

- **Displacement:** Shifting feelings, especially negative ones, onto someone or something other than the direct cause of those feeling, for example, yelling at your mother because you were embarrassed by your teacher.
- **Compensation:** Making up for a shortcoming by achieving in another area, for example, the person with an amputation who goes into professional athletics.
- **Regression:** Assuming childlike behavior.
- **Symbolism:** When one idea comes to stand for another, for example, money for love.
- **Rationalization:** When unacceptable events are made acceptable through a pseudo-logical argument, for example "I beat her because she talks back" or "I don't have enough time to do those exercises."

Summary

Historically, many different schools of psychological theory have described human behavior. They all offer insight, but no single theory is necessarily correct. Maslow's hierarchy of human needs describes successive layers of need to be satisfied: physiological security, affiliation, esteem and self-actualization. Pavlov described the conditioned reflex, and this led to the early behaviorists. Freud, the founder of modern psychoanalytic theory, had an elaborate system of yins and yangs: conscious/subconscious, Thanatos/eros, and id/ego/superego. Adler described the inferiority complex. Jung described anima versus persona, and introvert versus extrovert. Gestalt therapy uses role playing to bring up unfinished business. Transactional analysis views human interactions as time structuring to receive "stroking" through pastimes, games, or intimacy. Rogers focused on paraphrasing, empathizing, and positive regard. Defense mechanisms stem from Freud's idea that two conflicting stimuli produce psychic pain that can be resolved by a long list of subconscious mechanisms.

Most people use a "mix and match" menu from all of these theories called eclecticism.

Chapter Review

Key Term Review

Anima: Inner self theorized by Jung.

Behaviorism: School of psychology focusing on patient behavior.

Collective unconscious: The preprogrammed unconscious that all humans are born with.

Compensation: Addressing a problem by excelling in another area.

Complex: Group of ideas with a common feeling or tone (e.g., inferiority complex).

Conditioned reflex: A learned response to a stimulus.

Countertransference: Nonprofessional feelings of a health professional toward the patient.

Defense mechanism: A psychological method of reducing psychic pain from mental conflict.

Denial: A defense mechanism in which painful truths are denied.

Displacement: Putting (usually) negative feelings on someone or something other than the cause.

Ego: The realization of a person's conscious mind as a unique individual.

Eros: Life instincts.

Eclectic: The use of many different theories to make decisions.

Electra complex: A theory by Freud that penis envy causes a girl to be sexually attracted to her father.

Extrovert: A person who is sociable and outgoing.

Gestalt: A form of therapy that treats the patient as a whole, focusing on current feelings.

Hierarchy of basic human needs: Human needs in order of priority as theorized by Maslow.

Id: The mass of undifferentiated instincts in newborn child.

Identification: The unconscious transfer of outside character traits into one's own mind.

Inferiority complex: Strong feeling of inferiority with undue pessimism.

Introvert: A person who is shy and introspective.

Inversion: When a person does the opposite of what they want.

Libido: Sexual instinct.

Life instincts: Sexuality and self-preservation instincts as theorized by Freud.

Masculine protest: The natural tendency of people to move from the passive or feminine role to the aggressive or masculine role.

Oedipus complex: The sexual attraction of a boy to his mother and his sexual jealousy toward his father, as theorized by Freud.

Persona: The front a person puts on for the world.

Positive regard: Deeply caring, nonjudgmental, supportive behavior that makes a patient feel special.

Rationalization: A defense mechanism in which unacceptable events are made acceptable through psychological argument.

Repression: Pushing painful thoughts into the unconscious mind.

Regression: Assuming childlike behavior.

Resistance: The holding off of painful reality by the mind.

Rogerian approach: Nondirective or client-centered counseling.

Sublimation: Finding a socially acceptable outlet for a socially loaded problem.

Superego: The conscious mind responsible for the adult mind.

Suppression: The conscious rather than unconscious pushing away of painful thoughts.

Symbolism: One idea standing for another; for example, money for love.

Thanatos: Death instincts.

Transactional analysis: The theory that people assume different roles and play games in their interactions.

Transference: The identification of the health professional with someone else by the patient.

Chapter Review Questions

1. Give three examples of overcompensating.
2. Discuss how the gender of the health professional may influence transference.
3. How could money become a symbol for love?
4. How does Rogerian Counseling fit with Chapter 2 (Basic Skills in Verbal Communication)?
5. It has been observed that many introverts appear to be outgoing. In light of this chapter how would you explain this?

Case Study Critical Thinking Questions

1. In Case Study 3-1, what strategies could you suggest to avoid Mrs. Benson's nausea?
2. In Case Study 3-2, give some other examples of denial that Mr. Green might have exhibited in a similar situation.
3. In Case Study 3-3, please explain how the rabbit could be either Carlos' rationalization or his displacement. What makes the authors say Carlos has an inferiority complex?
4. In Case Study 3-4, please describe the underlying feelings that have led to Mr. Cage's repressing the incident where he struck the nurse.
5. In Case Study 3-5, how would you as a health professional use the information about Mrs. Gefarb's vicarious existence?

6. Reread Case Study 3-6. Do you have any personal reasons why you entered the health care field? Will those reasons be helpful to you and your patients?
7. Review Case Study 3-7. This is a question for only the most advanced students, or you may wish to review with your instructor. Look up the term *dissociative disorder* online. If the girl in this case is so traumatized by her dad's abuse, how might her lack of awareness or acknowledgment of it be explained by this new term?

References

1. American Psychiatric Association. www.psych.org
2. American Psychological Association. www.apa.org
3. Berne, F. *Games People Play*. New York: Ballantine Books, 1973.
4. Cramer, P. *Protecting the Self: Defense Mechanisms in Action*. New York: Guilford Press, 2006.
5. Kahn, M., *Basic Freud: Psychoanalytic Thought for the 21st Century*. New York: Basic Books, 2002.
6. Masters, W., Johnson, V. *Sex and Human Loving*. New York: Little, Brown and Company, 1988.
7. National Institute of Mental Health. www.nimh.gov
8. Maslow, A. H. *Toward a Psychology of Being*, 3rd ed. New York: John Wiley and Sons, 1999.
9. Rogers, C. R. *Client-Centered Therapy: Its Current Practice, Implication, and Theory*. London: Constable and Robinson, 2003.

Additional Readings

1. Hothersall, D. *History of Psychology*, 4th ed. New York: McGraw-Hill, 2004.
2. King, D. B., Viney, W., Woody, W. D. *A History of Psychology: Ideas and Context*, 4th ed. London: Allyn and Bacon, 2008.

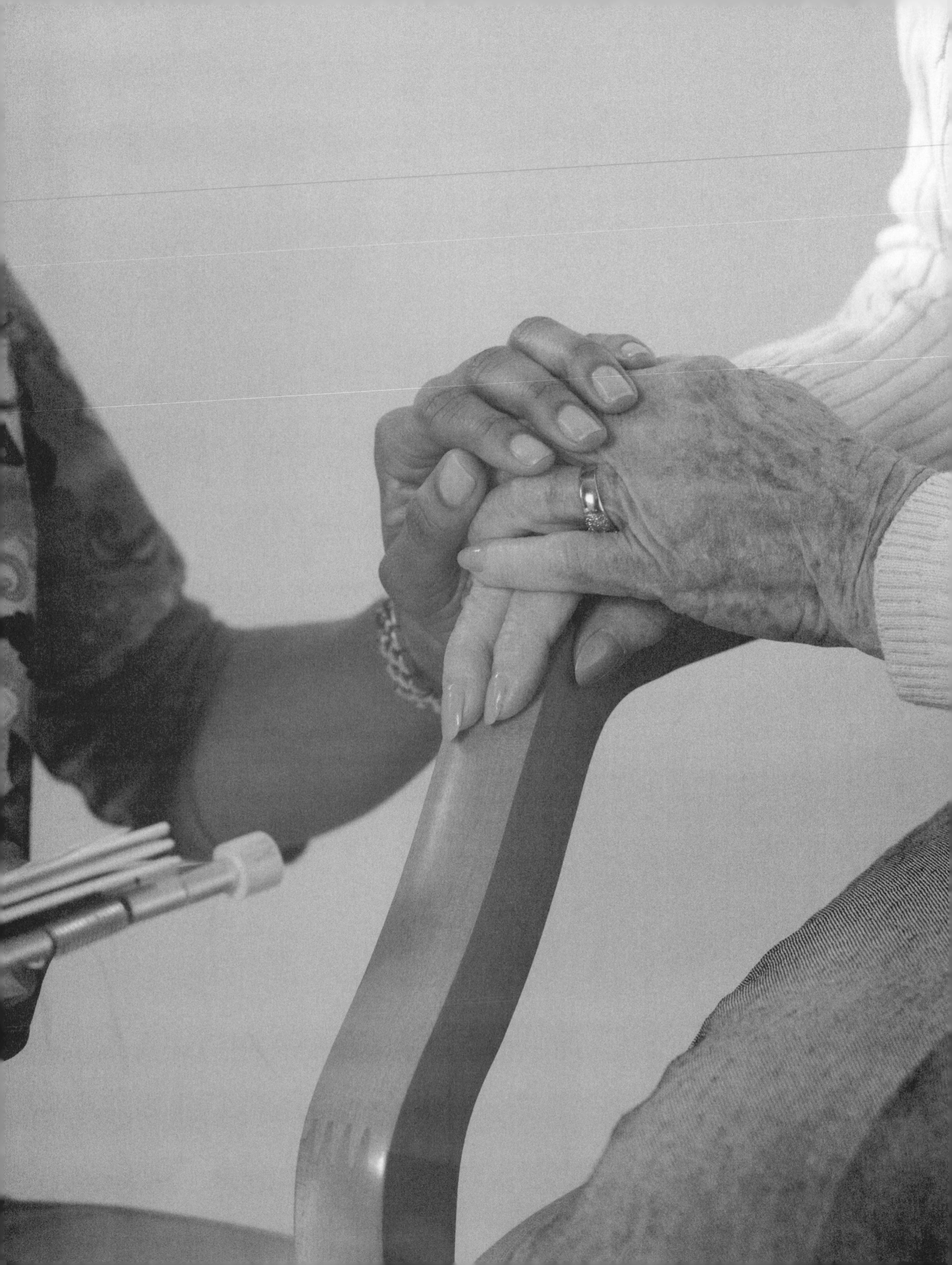

Mental Health and Adaptive Disorders

Learning Outcomes

After reading this chapter, you should be able to:

4.1 Explain what DSM IV TR is.
4.2 List and classify some clinical syndromes and personality disorders.
4.3 Understand illness behavior.
4.4 Describe some major psychosocial stressors.
4.5 Discuss family myths and traditions.
4.6 Discuss sickness roles.
4.7 Illustrate examples of primary and secondary gain.
4.8 Summarize how to determine who the patient is and what the disease is.
4.9 Identify illness behavior related to work.
4.10 Discuss bridging the gap between psychological and physical.
4.11 Evaluate how personality types, intellectual capacity, and illness itself affect patient behavior.
4.12 Identify a patient's primary relationship.

Key Terms

Adaptive regression
Cartesian dualism
Distant relative syndrome
DSM-IV-TR
Illness behavior
Lonely immigrant syndrome
Primary gain
Primary relationship
Psychosocial stress
Secondary gain
Sickness role
Type A personality
Type B personality

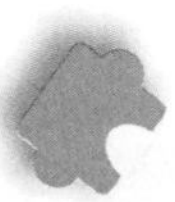

Mental Health and Adaptive Disorders

One of the reasons health professionals ask for consultations from a social worker, counselor, or psychologist is to get an encapsulation of the patient's problems and lifestyle in a revealing and easily understandable way. Health professionals may say "there is something about Mrs. Smith that is just not right, but I cannot put my finger on it; unless I can really understand the patient I don't know how to react to her or whether I can help her." This chapter seeks to answer this question.

Early classifications of psychological disease centered on mental retardation, dementia, and neurosyphilis (a venereal disease that sometimes affects the brain in its later stages). Later classifications broke mental diseases into retardation, neuroses, psychoses, and psychopathology. The neurotic lived in the real world but worried about it. By contrast, the psychotic lived in an unreal world, detached from reality. One old aphorism was that neurotics knew 2 + 2 = 4 but were worried about it, whereas psychotics knew 2 + 2 = 5 and were not worried about it. Another aphorism was that neurotics built castles in the air, psychotics lived in them, and in both cases the therapist collected the rent! The psychopath was simply unable to get along with others, was later called a sociopath, and most recently is said to have an antisocial personality disorder.

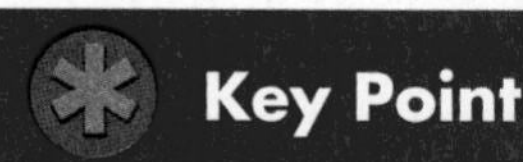

Key Point

DSM IV TR Classification of psychological diseases into five axes: Axis I, clinical syndrome; Axis II, personality disorder; Axis III, physical disease; Axis IV, severity of stress; Axis V, level of functioning.

In 1994 the American Psychiatric Association rewrote a diagnostic and statistical manual of mental disorders (DSM-IV). The text was revised in 2000 as **DSM-IV-TR** (TR means text revision). (In 2012 a DSM-V is planned.) In it, mental disorders are classified in five different "axes," a practice that many find pedantic. These axes are as follows:

Axis I Clinical syndrome (e.g., neurosis)

Axis II Personality disorder (e.g., compulsive)

Axis III Physical disorder (e.g., dry skin from excessive washing)

Axis IV Severity of stress (e.g., severe)

Axis V Highest level of functioning in past year (e.g., cannot work because of bleeding hands)

Obviously, Axes I and II are what would commonly be called mental illnesses. The first is the clinical syndrome presenting itself, and the second is the underlying personality disorder (see Table 4.2 for descriptions and definitions).

Although most of you will not be making DSM diagnoses on patients, as a health professional you need to understand diagnosis, which is the shorthand of mental health. It is often helpful to create for yourself a picture, or vignette, of a particular patient's problems, such as nervousness, self-destructiveness, alcoholism, or paranoid dementia, which makes a patient likely to be violent. This technique is intended only to provide a loose framework upon which to build patient understanding. You can work to treat or change problems on Axis I whereas those on Axis II are believed to be far less likely to change.

Table 4.1 Clinical Syndromes (Axis 1)

Cognitive Disorders

- Delirium (acute confusion caused by medical illness)
- Dementia (most commonly caused by Alzheimer's disease)

Substance-related Disorders—substance dependence, abuse, intoxication, and withdrawal

Psychosis—most commonly schizophrenia, characterized by delusions (false belief with no basis in reality) and hallucinations (false perception with no basis in reality)

Depression—major depression, dysthymia (chronic inability to enjoy life), or bipolar disorder (formerly called manic depression)

Anxiety Disorders

- **Panic Disorder**—repeated attacks of physical symptoms associated with a feeling of panic
- **Agoraphobia**—fear associated with open spaces, causing panic attacks; patient may become house-bound
- **Social Phobia**—constant fear of social situations
- **Obsessive-Compulsive**—repeated thoughts and behaviors that the patient knows are unreasonable but cannot suppress
- **Posttraumatic Stress Disorder**—chronic anxiety precipitated by an acute trauma like war
- **Generalized Anxiety Disorder**—chronic worry. The patient is often characterized as a "worry wart."

Somatoform Disorders—physical symptoms substituted for psychological disease, for example, a somatization disorder in which numerous different symptoms plague the patient though no physical cause is ever found for these symptoms. Somatoform disorders include hypochondriasis, hysterical paralysis, and chronic pain syndrome.

Factitious Disorders—made-up symptoms that allow the patient to assume a sick role without material gain in mind. This is different from malingering, in which the patient invents symptoms to obtain money or drugs or to avoid work or punishment.

Dissociative Disorders—disturbances in awareness, identity, or memory that result in altered states of consciousness, for example, split personality disorder in which two or more identities intermittently seize control of the patient's behavior

Sexual Disorders—problems with sexual identity or performance, for example, hypoactive sexual desire, erectile dysfunction, or inability to achieve orgasm. Paraphilias are disorders in which the patient is attracted to substitutes for sex, for example, sadomasochism, fetishes.

Eating Disorders—anorexia nervosa, bulimia nervosa, binge eating disorder

Sleep Disorders—insomnia, hypersomnia, narcolepsy

Impulsive Disorders—kleptomania, pathological gambling, pyromania, intermittent explosive disorder (severe temper)

Adjustment Disorders—impaired functioning in response to stress

Personality Disorders—traits that are bad enough to impair functioning and disrupt underlying psychological makeup (see Table 4.2 for more details)

Childhood Disorders—a disorder of childhood, for example, mental retardation, learning disability

Table 4.2 Some Examples of Personality Disorders (Axis II)

- **Paranoid Personality Disorder**—Patient seems to be unjustifiably suspicious, tending to suggest that others have ulterior motives.
- **Schizoid Personality Disorder**—Patient is socially withdrawn, has peculiar ideas, is unable to integrate into society, may be described as eccentric or bizarre.
- **Histrionic Personality Disorder**—Patient is overactive and dramatic and engages in attention-seeking behavior.
- **Dependent Personality Disorder**—Patient has poor self-esteem, seeks approval, and gets others to be responsible for important things in life.
- **Passive-Aggressive Personality Disorder**—Patient displays aggressive behavior in passive ways, for example, forgetting intentionally or being obsequious and stubborn.
- **Borderline Personality Disorders**—Patient acts impulsively in ways that are detrimental to himself or herself, has unstable but intense interpersonal relationships, is temperamental, makes suicidal gestures, has many surgeries and frequent accidents, has an unstable mood.

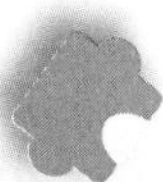

Illness Behavior

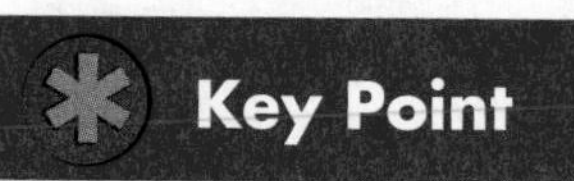

Key Point

Illness behavior ways different people respond when suffering the same symptoms.

The key to understanding illness behavior is to remember that each patient is an individual. A common misconception is that people simply have or do not have diseases. Studies have shown that groups of people who see their physician frequently (more than five times a year) suffer in fact the same frequency of commonly reported symptoms like colds, backaches, hemorrhoids, and headaches as do those who see their physician infrequently (less than once every five years). **Illness behavior** describes ways that different people respond when suffering the same symptoms.

You must think of a patient as a complex gestalt: in their relationships within the family and to authority; within work and society; and developmentally within their culture, traditions, myths, and sickness beliefs. You must also take into account emotional and intellectual makeup as it affects illness behavior.

Each time you see a person, and particularly when things do not seem to be going as they should, think about this gestalt. Realizing this gestalt can make brief encounters with patients much more productive, as you will not always have the time for an in-depth analysis. Lack of time will occasionally put you in the position of taking shortcuts. And, of course, you bring to each patient your knowledge from other patients you have seen. In a sense, this is using a preconceived notion about the characteristics and needs of the individual. It is still important to spend time on paraphrasing, empathizing, and asking open-ended questions. But awareness about the patient as a whole can enable you to zero in on things more effectively. The pitfall, of course, is that patients are unique and our assumptions can backfire if we are not paying attention.

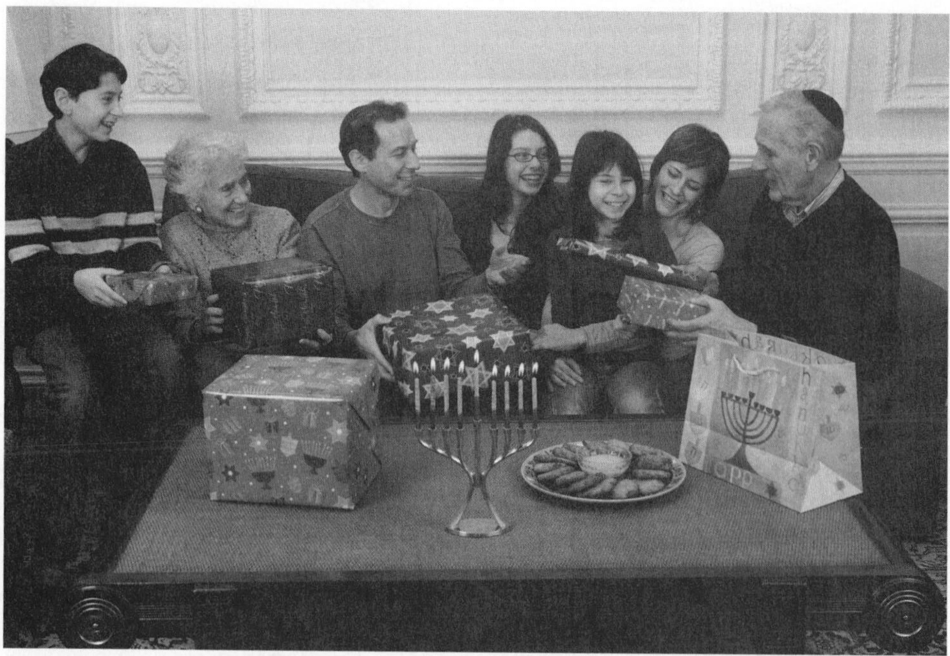

Illness behavior is shaped by many relationships and factors. Can you think of any influences from your culture, traditions, myths, and sickness beliefs that have helped form your illness behavior?

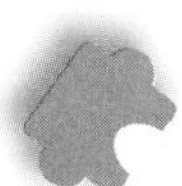

Psychosocial Stress Level

Epidemiological work suggests that illnesses within a patient tend to occur in clusters. There is also evidence to show that these clusters occur at times of **psychosocial stress**. Illness at such a time can be seen as maladaption to stress. All people experience stress, but the level alters during life. We must be attuned to likely stressors.

Recent bereavement is the most obvious major stressor; others include a recent geographical move when social support systems have to be remade, a change of job, a pregnancy, or taking on a mortgage (see Table 4.3).

It is a fairly good bet, for instance, that most illnesses presented in the context of recent bereavement could be regarded as symbols of stress. Generally speaking, the best way to deal with such illness seems to be on a symbolic basis. A patient, for instance, who wants physical therapy on a knee in such a situation should be given the therapy (as long as it will not harm the patient) even if nothing abnormal is found. It takes a lot of courage for such a patient to present themselves to you in the way he or she feels is most appropriate, which is to come to you in your area of expertise. To deny that communication is to reject the patient. To accept it makes the pain a little easier to bear and can open up more significant underlying problems.

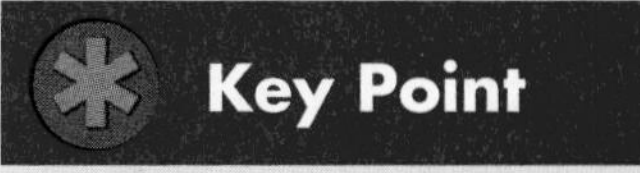

Psychosocial stress stress most commonly caused by death of loved one, divorce or separation, jail, and illness.

Table 4.3 Major Stressors According to Holmes and Rahe*

1. Death of spouse
2. Divorce
3. Marital separation
4. Jail term
5. Death of close family member
6. Personal injury or illness
7. Marriage
8. Being fired at work
9. Marital reconciliation
10. Retirement
11. Change in health of family member
12. Pregnancy
13. Sex difficulties
14. Gain of new family member
15. Business readjustment
16. Change in financial state
17. Death of close friend
18. Change to different line of work
19. Change in number of arguments with spouse
20. Mortgage or loan for a major purpose
21. Foreclosure of mortgage or loan
22. Change in responsibilities at work
23. Son or daughter leaving home
24. Trouble with in-laws
25. Outstanding personal achievement
26. Spouse beginning or stopping work
27. Beginning or ending school
28. Change in living conditions
29. Revision of personal habits
30. Trouble with boss
31. Change in work hours or conditions
32. Change in residence
33. Change in schools
34. Change in recreation
35. Change in church activities
36. Change in social activities
37. Mortgage or loan for a lesser purpose
38. Change in sleeping habits
39. Change in number of family get-togethers
40. Change in eating habits
41. Vacation
42. Christmas
43. Minor violations of the law

**Institute for Stress Research*

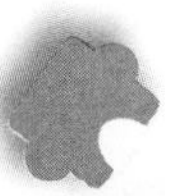

Family Myths and Traditions

CASE STUDY 4-1

Mrs. Gelineau says, "My daughter has always been very delicate." One day Mrs. Gelineau and her husband argue about this issue. Mrs. Gelineau then takes the daughter to the school nurse to complain of a cough. (This is an example of a defense mechanism, in this case displacement activity—the threat of conflict with her husband is switched to a concern about her daughter's health.)

The school nurse examines the child and agrees that she has a cold. All it takes is a little pressure from Mrs. Gelineau to obtain permission to keep her daughter out of school the next day. Mrs. Gelineau comes home to dad and recounts the day's goings on, adding, "I told you she was very delicate."

Mr. Gelineau loses this game and so learns that it is best not to argue. If he has any frustrations, he will have to figure out some other way of dealing with them. He agrees that his daughter is delicate. To deny it would start a game that he knows he would lose again. Thus, a family myth has been perpetrated. The daughter will be raised in the *family myth* that she is a medically delicate person.

This behavior spills over into *family traditions of illness*. A mother may not take her daughter to the school nurse each time she gets a cold because of any game. It may be simply a tradition. "When I sin, I must confess to the priest, so when my daughter has a cold, I must seek medical attention." The mother feels she may be seen as negligent if she does not check with the nurse. Health education—telling her it isn't necessary to seek medical attention for every cold—may not work. Her tradition is part of her ego system, which, if undermined, may increase rather than decrease her stress level. Both myths and traditions are reinforced when the health professional agrees to participate in them.

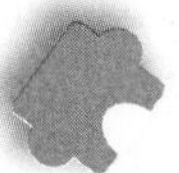

Sickness Roles

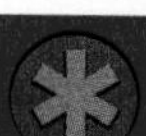

Key Points

Sickness role adaptive regression by significantly ill patient to accept treatment.

Adaptive regression ability to take on the child role when ill as a patient.

Normal illness confers roles on the patient and the health provider. The most usual role in terms of Berne's transactional analysis is for the patient to be child and the health provider to be adult. This is called the **sickness role**. The patient's role has been labeled dependent as opposed to independent.

CASE STUDY 4-2

A hard-driving businessman suffers a heart attack, is admitted to the coronary care unit of a hospital, and gives the nurse a difficult time. He pulls out his intravenous lines, refuses to take medication, and insists on having his cell phone and laptop by his bedside so he can continue to run his business.

This patient, who is used to playing an adult role, now finds he must regress into a dependent, childlike role. Although this would be good for him under the circumstances, his lack of **adaptive regression** puts his life at risk.

A normal healthy person can drop the dependent role as she or he recovers. Some people, however, demonstrate excessive regression, which is a defense mechanism caused by anxiety. It can be difficult to loosen the patient's clinging grip. Although health professionals may feel flattered by such dependency, it usually becomes emotionally draining very quickly.

Another way of looking at the sick role is to consider the advantages (or secondary gains) that might be accrued outside the health professional–patient relationship. For example, a patient is unable to work at home or at his job, although he is needed there. If he cooperates with what the health professional says, he gains the privileges of the sick role. This allows him to be off work or to avoid duties at home.

These roles are difficult to apply to all illnesses; they apply best to acute illness. Consider, for example, the difference between chronic disability and a health risk. A patient with a chronic disability may play any role from chronic dependency (child/parent) to mutual cooperation (adult/adult) to excessive assertiveness (parent/child). A patient with high blood pressure has a health risk rather than a sickness.

CASE STUDY 4-3

Irene went to a screening clinic, and the nurse told her that she had high blood pressure. Her doctor prescribed medication and a low salt diet. A nurse practitioner was asked to see her because she would not take her pills or follow the diet. The nurse explained to Irene that she was not sick. Further, she would not become a sick or disabled person if she took care of herself. After a while, Irene came to understand that taking pills was acceptable and that it did not signify that she was an ill person.

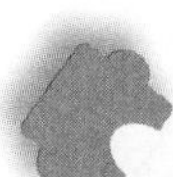

Primary and Secondary Gain

CASE STUDY 4-4

Mrs. Sanger, a middle-aged housewife, tells the medical assistant that she is ill. She says the doctor diagnosed a prolonged viral infection. She does not seem particularly upset by the idea. Indeed, she seems somewhat pleased. What has she got to gain from being ill?

First, she has the illness itself. It has become a new center of attention. The doctor listens to her. The medical assistant listens to her. She does not usually have such an audience. She can be egocentric and talk about her illness and nothing else. This is called **primary gain**. It is the advantage the illness itself creates.

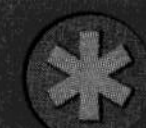

Key Points

Primary gain the advantage an illness itself produces.

Secondary gain the bonus gained from being ill.

But there are more advantages. Mrs. Sanger can tell her husband that she has been advised by her doctor to avoid housework and rest in bed for the weekend. This is called **secondary gain**. It is a consequence of the illness that has a bonus aspect for the patient.

The worst case of secondary gain is maintaining or producing illness only because of its advantages. One patient suddenly developed paralysis of his legs and was unable to go to work. No physical cause could be found. He had a little electric repair shop in his back room where he sat in his wheelchair and enjoyed his lifelong hobby of electronics. This released him from his boring factory work and gave him a disability pension. These were the secondary gains of his hysterical paralysis (or conversion reaction). Behaviors are maintained when they are rewarded. We discuss this further in Chapter 9.

Another patient was a passenger in a car crash. He suffered a whiplash injury that gave him neck pain and headaches. He talked with an attorney and found that he might get a lot more than his medical bills paid. Soon he was unable to work. He won an out-of-court settlement of $280,000 and decided to apply for disability. This is another example of secondary gain.

The rewards of sickness to children can be just as real. They get to stay home from school, watch television in bed, have favorite foods brought to them, and get more attention from mother. They do not have to worry about schoolwork, teachers, or peer criticism. Sometimes the thought of returning to the real world can be downright threatening. The onset of some illnesses in children may actually reflect a psychological problem within the family. For example eating disorders in children often arise when the parent's marriage is in trouble. The focus is removed from the parents and everyone rallies to help the child. The children often believe that their being unwell holds the family together and they may be right.

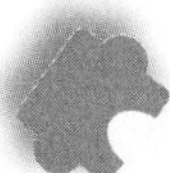

Who Is the Patient and What Is the Disease

Perception of Who Is the Patient

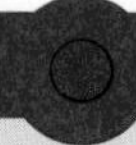

CASE STUDY 4.5

Mrs. Smith is an aging lady with dementia who has lived for many years with her daughter, who cares for her devotedly. Mrs. Smith's urinary incontinence means that her daughter must wash bedclothes constantly. The house looks like a laundry. The caregiver daughter, the doctor, and the visiting nurse are all aware of a gradual overall deterioration in Mrs. Smith. From time to time, Mrs. Smith's second daughter from California comes to see her mother. She has not seen her mother for several years when she arrives on her latest visit. Although she has certainly heard stories from her sister, she is expecting to find her mother not much different from when she last visited. What she finds shocks her. She immediately calls the visiting nurse agency that provided the home health aide. The visiting daughter reports that Mrs. Smith has fallen, is covered with bruises, and needs to be admitted to the hospital immediately.

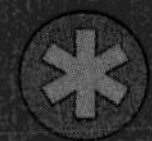

Key Point

Distant relative syndrome the whirlwind of criticism about a previously stable patient's care created by the visit of a distant relative because she or he does not understand the gestalt.

Who is the patient? Certainly you can all see that the first daughter, who regularly cares for her mother, is likely to be severely stressed. But she is not the patient. She and all the other caregivers have acknowledged the deterioration. They also acknowledge that, given the circumstances, the mother would like to continue to be cared for at home. But is the mother really the patient? No. This is the **distant relative syndrome**, not uncommon in geriatric care. The situation, previously stable, is a surprise for the guilty absent relative, who is shocked. The visiting sister from California has not seen her mother for several years. By precipitating a crisis, she has assuaged her guilt that she has not cared for her mother. If she did not feel guilty, she would have grasped the fact that multiple caregivers have already acknowledged the situation, decided what was best, and given their best. The true patient is the visiting sister. It is she to whom the health professional must talk. In this case the skilled visiting nurse meets with her in person to listen, paraphrase, and empathize. A harmful hospital and nursing home admission is prevented.

A stressed mother brings her children to the nurse practitioner approximately monthly for colds. The children are not necessarily the patients; the mother needs more help than they do.

What Is Perceived as Disease

Health is defined as a state of complete mental, social, and physical well-being, not simply as the absence of disease. Some may see a cold as an illness requiring treatment. Others may ignore a cold unless there is extreme suffering.

A problem viewed as an illness by the patient may not be seen as one by the health professional. An example would be the onset of normal menstruation in an unprepared pubescent girl.

The wife of an Iranian engineering student constantly visits the student health clinic. The nurse practitioner can never figure out what is the matter with her. This may be an example of the **lonely immigrant syndrome**. Is the Iranian woman or the society she lives in really the patient? The problem is that she needs to socialize, but she has no one who shares her culture and language.

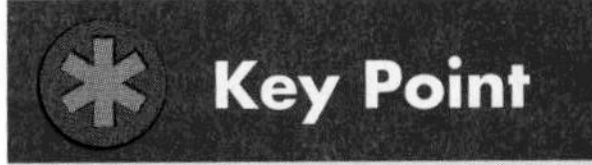

Lonely immigrant syndrome the substitution by an immigrant of medical care for lack of socialization.

A couple who have sexual difficulties to the point of contemplating divorce may see the pharmacist to ask for sexual stimulants especially for erectile dysfunction. The pharmacist may be infinitely more helpful if she or he refers them to a counselor if the problem is emotional rather than physical. Although low sexual drive could be seen as an illness (and treated with medication), such a perception might limit or restrict actual help.

Sickness beliefs may depend on a patient's upbringing. A patient may choose a medical model, see a physician, accept treatment, and present physical symptoms. Or a patient may have a psychoanalytical model and expect the illness to be treated through psychological insights. Or a patient may have a primitive model of illness—for example that suffering is a retribution for sin. Is mental illness an illness? Is drug addiction an illness? Is gambling an illness? It depends not only on the health professional, but also on the patient and on the society in which it is occurring. Mental illness and addictions are currently seen as related biological behavior.

Cultural Determinants of Illness Behavior

Certain cultures may have styles for expressing sickness. Pain, for example, is often expressed differently in different cultures. Specific groups may have their own health beliefs that persist in a different country. Any minority group may cling to early beliefs of their country of origin—a sort of medical expatriate syndrome, passed through several generations.

The DSM-IV-TR offers a section on Cultural Formulation and a Glossary of Culture-Bound Syndromes. This appendix is meant to assist health professionals in understanding and evaluating the impact of the patient's cultural context on presenting problems. This will be discussed more in the chapter on Multiculturalism and Health.

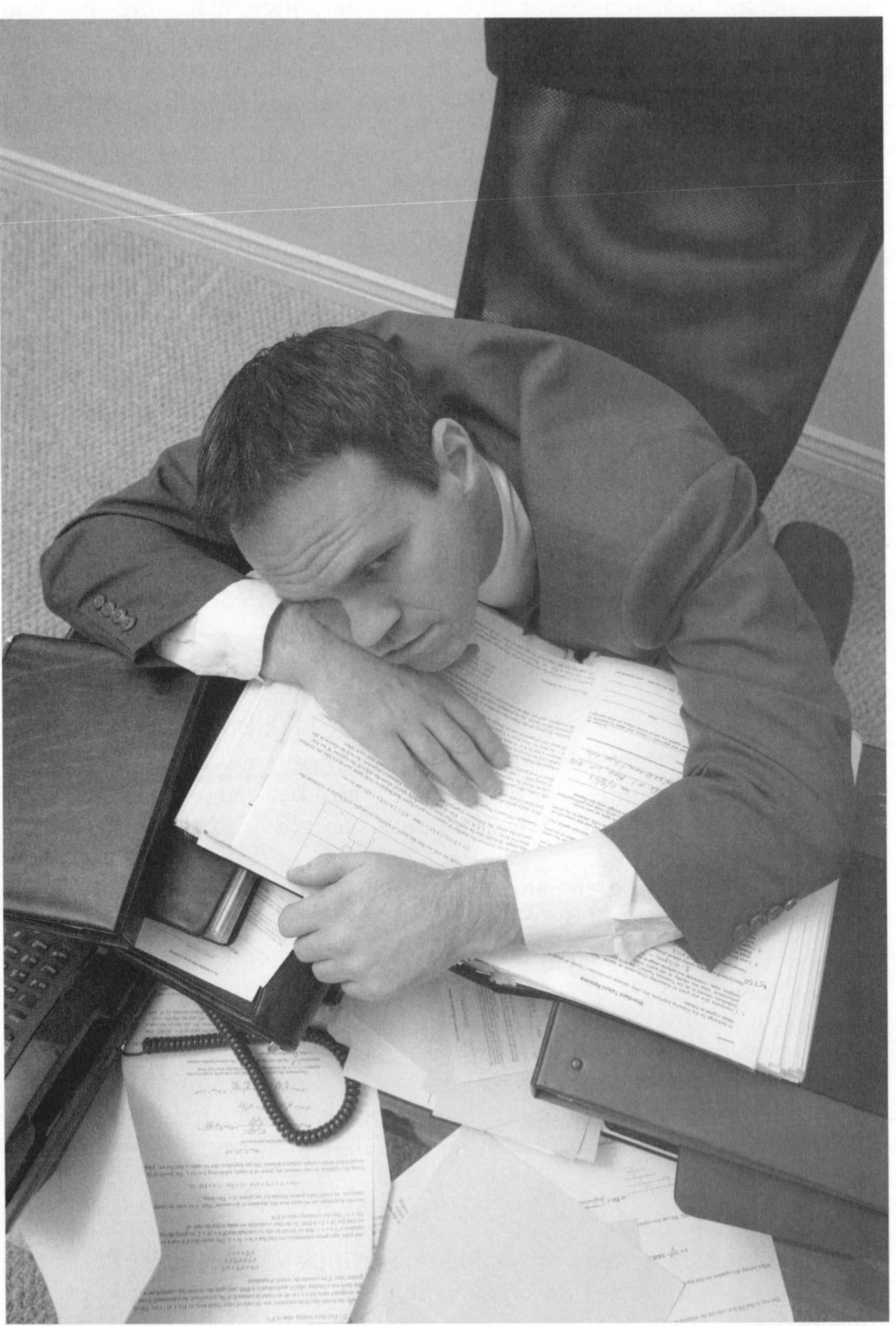

How would you react to a spouse who kept on taking time off work for illnesses that you never took time off for?

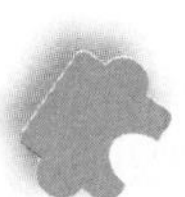

Illness Behavior Related to Work

As already described, the sick role involves permission to stop work or school and get better. The housewife with the flu who goes to bed can reasonably expect some help looking after the children. A person who is the dominant figure at her or his place of work may find it difficult to accept a dependent role in sickness. Recall the businessman in the intensive care unit.

Many people have learned that physically demanding work is hard and that looking busy makes life a little easier. Likewise, time off makes life a little easier. If you are allowed to take two weeks of sick time per year, you soon learn that a cold, previously not much of a problem, will give you a welcome break from work (another example of secondary gain).

Others have a very strong work ethic. One hospital dietitian took only two days off in her entire life—on each occasion to have a baby! Some types of work have traditions or what appear to be occupational diseases. Physicians, for instance, are likely to take little time off. Psychiatrists and dentists have a higher addiction rate than most professions. Military personnel have high rates of alcoholism.

Work stress in the modern workplace often leads to psychological disease, for example, panic disorder from conflict, or physical disease, for example, carpal tunnel syndrome from excessive computer use.

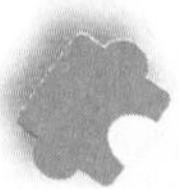

Cartesian Dualism

Rene Descartes (1596–1650) first postulated a philosophical difference between the body and the mind. Ever since, it has been difficult to bridge the gap between the psychological and the physical. **Cartesian dualism** says that the body and mind are two separate though parallel entities. The body is physical, and the mind is nonphysical.

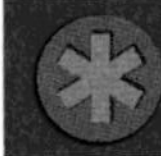

Key Point

Cartesian dualism the belief that the body and mind are two separate entities.

In particular, patients have a difficult time relating anxiety to sickness. A patient can suffer a purely physical problem such as pneumonia or can present with pure anxiety to the health practitioner. Some symptoms of anxiety are tremors, sweating, palpitations, jitteriness, insomnia, or feeling physically exhausted. Some anxious people find specific symptoms more bothersome during periods of anxiety, for example, diarrhea, loss of appetite, headaches, or frequent urination. Because pure mental illness is still taboo or is looked down upon in American society, a patient may come to the health professional with these physical symptoms, thinking they are more acceptable. Often, however, a patient understands how close such symptoms are to simple anxiety, is afraid of rejection, and therefore believes that he or she must present the correct ticket to the health care provider. This has been called the "symptom on the plate."

Rather than say, "I grind my teeth," a patient may prefer to present with a toothache to the dentist. Perhaps he is already aware that tooth grinding is a symptom of anxiety. Presenting with a toothache will at least prevent the dentist from telling him that the problem is anxiety. The patient may simply want reassurance or fixing so that his teeth will not fall out.

The dentist can still treat the patient, but a new sensitivity can make him or her more receptive to the patient's world and symptoms. If the dentist can probe (psychologically!) in the right way, even the slightest hint from the patient may enable the dentist to respond more appropriately and learn what is really bothering the patient.

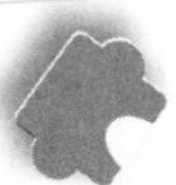

Behavior and Illness

Each illness has its own story; illnesses do not have the same psychological effect. A patient with chronic renal failure on dialysis has needs that are different from those of a patient with paraplegia, diabetes, chronic pain, or stage IV cancer. Multiple sclerosis patients often seem to be inappropriately euphoric, despite a seemingly disastrous future, although underlying depression is common. Alcoholics frequently use denial—a part of the illness itself—as a defense.

It is important that you, as a health care provider, not be sidetracked by behaviors that may be part of the illness itself. For example, you cannot assume that every multiple sclerosis patient who seems to be happy is happy.

Secondary depression in illness is also common. Such depression can be regarded as a grief reaction to learning the diagnosis of some chronic problem. If the patient can adapt, life will become enjoyable again. If not, the patient will suffer from chronic grief, a surprisingly common and hidden reaction in chronic sickness.

Behavior affects illness in several ways:

- personality types
- intellectual capacity
- negotiating appointments
- manipulative patients

Personality Types in Illness Behavior

The histrionic personality (a person who displays emotions for effect) is apt to play out in the health professional's office as much as in the outside world. Symptoms are exaggerated, dramatic, sudden, and presented in an alarming fashion. Understanding a person's style is likely to help the health professional see such symptoms in their true perspective.

Dependent personalities may quickly reveal themselves to caregivers through their desire to please ("Yes, nurse," "Whatever you say, nurse"). Of course, the way a patient comes across to you also tells you how he or she may deal with other people. Perhaps the patient is also dependent on his or her spouse or peers. If a patient's problems are psychological, excessive dependency on a health professional may block the patient's ability to stand on his or her own two feet again. The aim of psychological treatment is to promote independent functioning.

Obsessive-compulsive personalities may dwell excessively on particular symptoms, especially their bowel habits. However, there are effective psychotropic medications available that do well in helping obsessive-compulsive disorders.

A lot of interest has been paid to **Type A personalities** and **Type B personalities**. Type A behavior entails a sense of time urgency, striving for perfection, and difficulty in accepting things if they are not the way the person wants them. Most successful business people are Type A. Type Bs

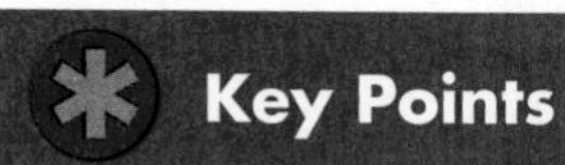

Key Points

Type A personality a personality characterized by sense of time urgency, striving for perfection, and difficulty in accepting things if they are not the way the person wants them.

Type B personality a personality that is easygoing and accepting of people and events because the person is without frustration and feels no compulsion to compete.

are not bothered by lateness, accept people and events as they are without frustration, and feel no compulsion to compete. Type As are thought to be more prone to heart attacks than Type Bs, possibly because Type As produce more adrenaline as a result of the hostile part of their personality. A chronic high adrenaline level may stress the heart.

Intellectual Capacity

As a health care provider, it is important for you to be particularly sensitive about a patient's literacy level. Illiterate patients seldom announce the fact. An illiterate person will accept written information graciously. When asked to fill out forms, the person will have a friend or family member do it for them, offering an excuse such as forgetting their glasses that day. It is difficult to detect that a patient is illiterate, but you must learn how to do it so you can provide effective treatment. Literature or schedules for pills are, of course, inappropriate for an illiterate person. Pill tables can be constructed by taping each pill to the left of a table that has check marks indicating when pills should be taken. Even for many literate patients, graphs are often difficult but pictures work very well.

Whether patients can read or not, communication is of vital importance. A study of discussions with patients about informed consent for operations showed patients remembered or understood virtually nothing at a later date. Patients remember best what is said first. Older and more intelligent patients remember about the same as younger or less intelligent patients. Most patients can consistently and easily recall only two statements or ideas.

More educated patients tend to visit multiple health care specialists for various problems. By contrast, the less educated may take their financial, moral, psychological, and legal problems all to their primary caregiver, whether that be the parent figure in a dependent relationship, their landlord, a grandmother, a nurse, or a physician.

Appointment Negotiating

No discussion of illness behavior would be complete without an examination of how patients handle the making and keeping of appointments in the outpatient world. Many patients, regardless of the diagnosis, take a distant appointment to mean that they are doing well. They may resist having appointments close together because they see this as a symbol of how ill they are. Never mind that they need the appointment!

Other patients may wish to have frequent appointments regardless of actual need. They may be frightened and want extra support from the health professional, or they may be using their health problems to get attention. Frequent appointments mean that they get attention from the health professional, or they may get sympathy from their family and friends for having to see a health practitioner so often.

Other patients use the breaking of appointments to manipulate the health care provider. Providers may be

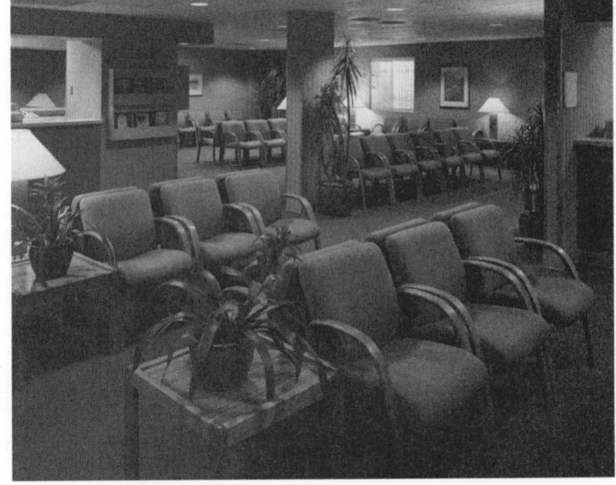

People need to keep appointments when possible.

wise to refuse service to patients who break appointments frequently. The symbolic implications around the scheduling of appointments make negotiating them a phase of treatment to which you and all health care practitioners must be alert.

Manipulative Patients

Manipulative patients cancel their appointments or are "no shows." They may switch from one health professional to another as though they were shopping for tuna fish. They may seek multiple consultations for no apparent reason without proper communication. If, for instance, they are seeing you as a physical therapist, you may be unaware that they are seeing two other physical therapists at the same time.

Manipulative patients do not get better in ways that health professionals devise, desire, or control. They may do some or all of what they do because they cannot tolerate the dependent role, because they deny illness, or because they wish to manipulate their own treatment. They need to be in control.

The reason for being manipulative can be analyzed on several levels:

1. It may be an expression of a passive-aggressive behavior or of a borderline personality disorder.
2. It may be, in the terms of transactional analysis, that the patient cannot accept the sick role; that is, he or she cannot assume a dependent role because of an ego disorder (like the businessman in the coronary care unit example).
3. It may be a defense mechanism. The patient is being dictated to, and he or she does not want to be. This conflict either produces anxiety or can be resolved through defense mechanisms such as:
   - Denial—"I forgot my appointment."
   - Rationalization—"My sister told me the physical therapist down the street specialized in back pain."
   - Substitution—"The pills you suggested I try didn't work, so I decided to try acupuncture."
4. It may be a social phenomenon. Some patients may use manipulation as a style. It is the only way to assert themselves, especially when they know they may spend the rest of their lives with little power. Manipulative behavior is a common difficulty for the health professional (think of the cost in time lost when patients repeatedly fail to show up for appointments). The following somewhat detailed example illustrates this.

CASE STUDY 4-6

George, aged 61, frequently worked at the hospital as a volunteer. He sometimes had epileptic seizures and had been hospitalized many times, though usually not for epilepsy. Chest pain frequently brought him to the hospital, although cardiologists said there was nothing wrong with his heart.

(continued)

CASE STUDY 4-6 *(continued)*

When he first saw the nurse practitioner at the health center, George was charming. His medical story was extremely complex. Soon letters started arriving from a cardiologist, two neurologists, and a gastroenterologist. None of these referrals had been made by the health center.

The nurse practitioner called his previous family practitioner and discovered that he switched primary care specialists about every two or three years. The family practitioner also revealed that he had learned not to criticize George. He had heard through the grapevine that George would tell the nurses and the patients at the hospital negative things about all his caregivers. George had already had a run-in with an x-ray technician at the local hospital and so refused to have anymore x-rays there. He had also said that Oprah gave better advice on her show than the hospital's chief dietitian.

The nurse saw George's pattern of behavior as a problem. One day George cancelled his appointment at the last minute. He said his car had broken down. She called his house hoping to speak to him, but instead got his wife, Mabel. She said he was out, but she did not know where. Mabel knew what was going on. Once, she said, she had tried telling George that he must tow the line. Within a month of their conversation, George visited six different specialists and ran up medical bills of $12,000. Mabel said she simply could not afford to risk that again.

That same night, George called the nurse at home. She had no idea how he got her unlisted number. George told a long convoluted story about several different symptoms and how everyone was turning against him. He said that she was the only person to whom he could turn. After a long conversation, George thanked her profusely and apologized for calling her at home.

She never heard from George again until a request arrived three weeks later to transfer his records to a new HMO clinic in town.

This story portrays a man who uses manipulation as a lifestyle. He manipulates his health caregivers, his wife, and probably his friends as well. He uses illness as a substitute for social interaction and as a focus in his life. Subconsciously, he can change his symptoms at will. Who knows which symptoms are real and which are subconsciously motivated? He is dramatically the center of attention. Commiserating volunteers at the hospital are his audience. This is a lifetime game, and as the star player he cannot be beaten. No relationship is likely to give him as much attention as his game. Counseling (to try to get him to realize what he is doing) would likely be yet another game for him. If he found it more challenging, he would switch. But chances are that with his experience and contacts, a medical model gives him more primary and secondary gain. Perhaps a good mental health professional would diagnosis him with a narcissistic personality disorder, but George would first have to seek this help.

What could you, as a health professional in such a situation, do? First, you would have to give the patient the benefit of the doubt. You would have to allow some time to pass for a pattern to establish. Only then could you reliably define the situation. You might accept the situation if the manipulative behavior is mild, or if the behavior is not too detrimental to the patient or to society.

If the behavior exceeds these guidelines, you must be certain to set your boundaries firmly and review them with the patient. You might set some, for example, if the patient calls frequently after hours or frequently fails to appear for an appointment. Discussing such behaviors with a patient may actually be therapeutic for him or her and is likely to be helpful to you as a health professional. Charging for missed appointments is often a good behavior modifier where this is permitted. Charges need not be implemented when the late cancellations are made for credible reasons and are not frequent.

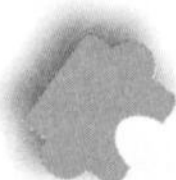

The Patient's World

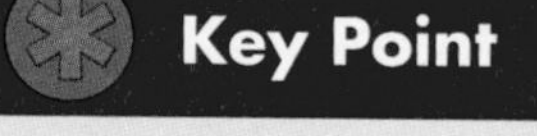

Key Point

Primary relationship closest person with whom you presently choose or are forced to relate.

It is important to think of what life is like for your patient. However, you cannot simply put yourself into a patient's world because you probably would take your own value judgments with you (look back at the section on empathizing in Chapter 2).

An important factor in the patient's world is his or her **primary relationship**. The primary relationship is the closest person with whom a patient presently chooses to relate or is forced to relate on a regular basis in his or her daily life. For most people this is a family member or a friend. But some people have their primary relationships with a dog or cat, with themselves (they may be isolated, depressed, alone, withdrawn, or narcissistic), or maybe with their landlord. As a simple example, an elderly woman whose primary relationship is with her dog is, unfortunately, unlikely to find many health care workers who realize that.

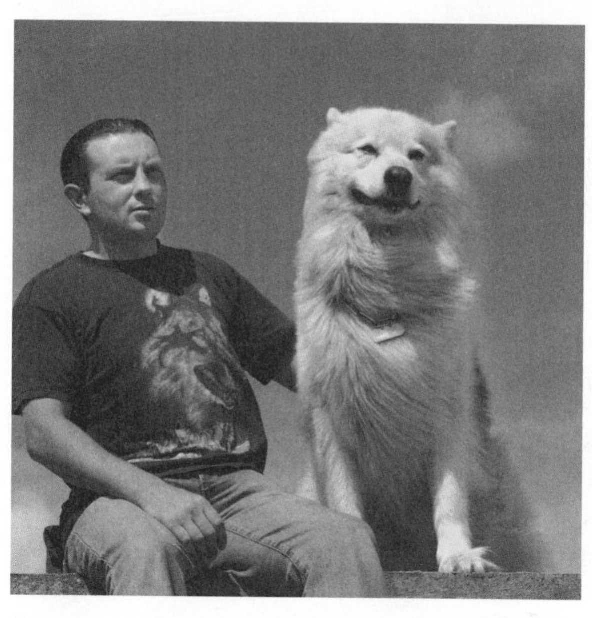

Sometimes a dog is a man's best friend.

One barrier to understanding can be the health practitioner's classic assumption that primary relationships are the most important thing to patients. For some people, the struggle for survival, money, food, sex, or drugs may be most important. Remember the discussion of Maslow's hierarchy of human needs in Chapter 3.

Sensitivity is the key to digesting the information in this chapter. You need to have your ears open to the unique qualities of your patients. You need to build an understanding of the things that all human beings need and value. You need to understand what it is like to be healthy and what it is like to be ill.

Summary

One of the powerful abilities of mental health professionals is to use a few words to describe a patient that are eye opening. Without a knowledge of clinical mental health syndromes, health professionals would be like sailors without a compass. The classification of psychological disease is changing. The most up-to-date expression of this is DSM, currently DSM-IV. This chapter has reviewed the first two axes of the five DSM axes, i.e., clinical syndromes and underlying personality disorders, which were previously labeled as such because they were felt to be immutable but are increasingly seen as changeable.

People are different. They may respond to the same symptoms differently from another person. This is called "illness behavior." It is common knowledge that illnesses become worse with stress, and research has shown that the stressors can be arranged in order of significance.

Family myths and family traditions also affect how people with the same symptoms behave differently. Sick people in contemporary society need to adapt to different roles for optimal recovery. The concepts of primary and secondary gain are discussed. It is important to be careful about who the patient is and what the disease is.

Illness may present in many different ways depending upon the patient's personality, intellect, and how the illness has affected his or her behavior. Some patients use illness as a game (Eric Berne), using appointment negotiating and manipulation. Finally, it is important to keep in mind the patient's primary and secondary relationships.

Chapter Review

Key Term Review

Adaptive regression: Ability to take on the child role when ill as a patient.

Cartesian dualism: A philosophy that states that the body and mind are two separate entities.

Distant relative syndrome: A syndrome in which a distant relative visits, creating a whirlwind of criticism about a previously stable patient's care because she or he does not understand the gestalt.

DSM-IV-TR: A classification of psychological diseases into five axes: Axis I clinical syndrome, Axis II personality disorder, Axis III physical disease, Axis IV severity of stress, Axis V level of functioning.

Illness behavior: Ways different people respond when suffering the same symptoms.

Lonely immigrant syndrome: The substitution of medical care by an immigrant for lack of socialization.

Primary gain: The psychological advantage the illness itself creates.

Primary relationship: The closest person with whom a patient presently chooses or is forced to relate.

Psychosocial stress: Stress most commonly caused by death of a loved one, divorce or separation, jail, and illness.

Secondary gain: A consequence of an illness that has a bonus aspect for the patient.

Sickness role: Adaptive regression of a significantly ill patient to accept treatment.

Type A personality: A personality characterized by a sense of time urgency, striving for perfection, and difficulty in accepting things if they are not the way the person wants them.

Type B personality: A person that is easygoing, accepts people and events as they are without frustration, and feels no compulsion to compete.

Chapter Review Questions

1. Discuss the following idea: "There are no illnesses, only ill people."
2. Discuss the following idea: "Always remember to ask yourself who is really the patient and what is really the disease."
3. Why must you be objective to learn about people?
4. What is the difference between a neurosis and a psychosis?
5. What is an Axis I versus an Axis II disorder?
6. List some examples of psychophysical interaction. Do you have any symptoms that you think could be psychological? Do you have any symptoms that you think are worse when you are under stress?

Case Study Critical Thinking Questions

1. Refer to Case Study 4-1. Do you know any of your friends with a family tradition of illness like this? Tell a story that illustrates this.
2. Refer to Case Study 4-2. How would you have reacted if you were in the identical situation? Can you empathize with the businessperson? What type of personality does he have?
3. What concept does Case Study 4-3 illustrate? Can you think of other examples of a patient accepting treatment when they do not actually have an illness?
4. In Case Study 4-4, what is the primary gain Mrs. Sanger experiences from her illness? What are possible secondary gains she may experience?
5. In Case Study 4-5, who is the patient and what syndrome is this an example of?
6. In Case Study 4-6, what could be some of the explanations for George's personality?

References

1. American Psychiatric Association. www.psych.org
2. American Psychological Association. www.apa.org
3. American Psychiatric Association. *Diagnostic and Statistical Manual of Mental Disorder DSM IV-TR*). Arlington, VA: American Psychiatric Press, 2000.
4. Morrison, J. *Diagnosis made easier*. New York: Guilford Press, 2007.
5. National Institute of Mental Health. www.nimh.gov
6. National Institute of Occupational Safety and Health: Stress. www.cdc.gov/Niosh/stresswk.html

Additional Readings

1. Berne, F. *Games People Play. The Basic Handbook of Transactional Analysis*. New York: Ballantine Books, 1996.
2. First, M. B., Tasman, A. *DSM-IV-TR Mental Disorders Diagnosis, Etiology and Treatment*. Chichester, U.K.: John Wiley and Sons, 2004.
3. *Quick Reference to the DSM-IV-TR Diagnostic Criteria for PDA*, ed. Kindle. Arlington, VA: American Psychiatric Association, 2008.
4. Sperry, L. *Handbook of Diagnosis and Treatment of DSM-IV-TR personality disorders*, 2nd ed. New York: Brunner-Routledge, 2003.

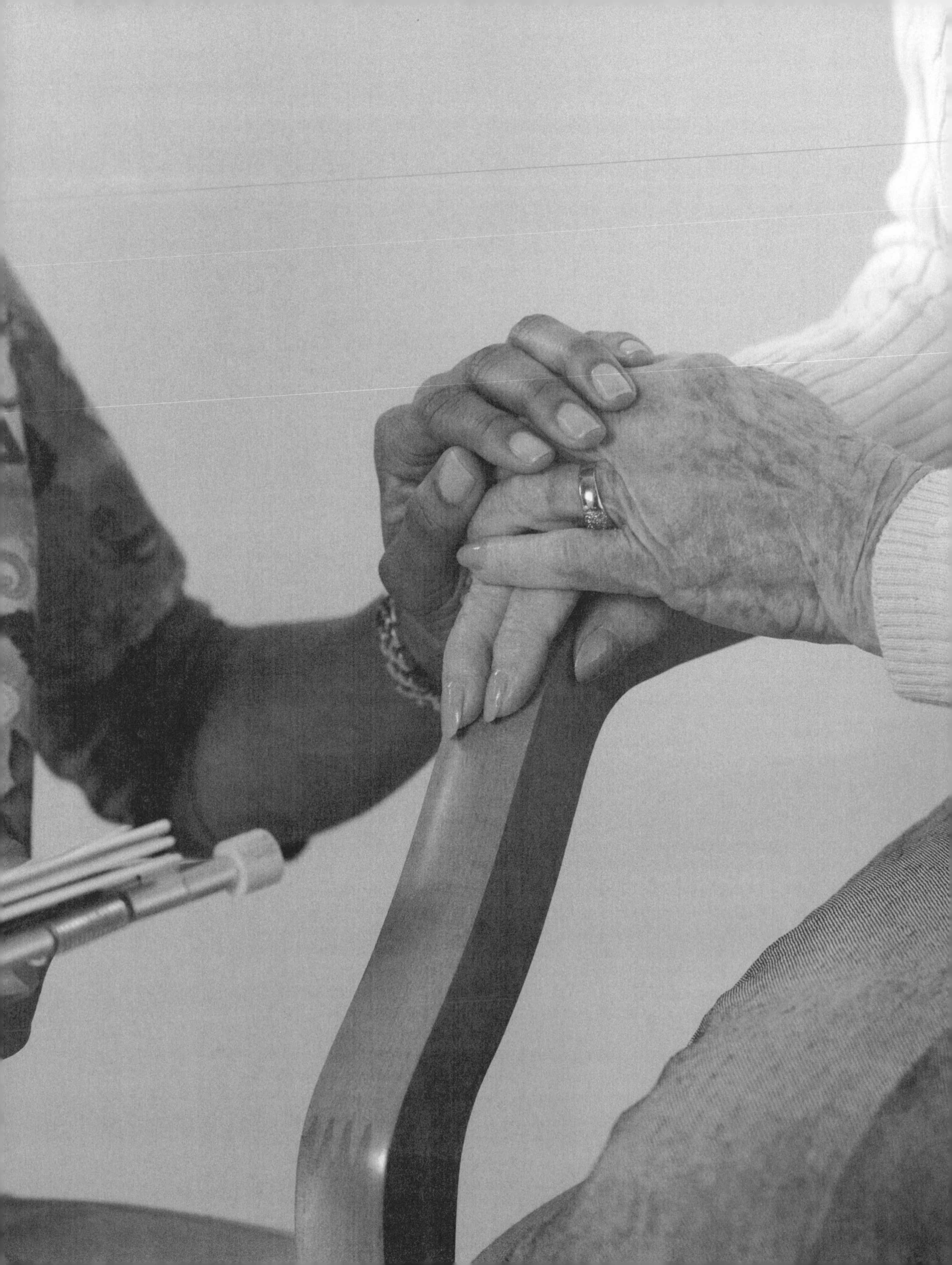

Death and Dying

Learning Outcomes

After reading this chapter, you should be able to:

5.1 Describe the five Kübler-Ross stages of loss.
5.2 Understand denial.
5.3 Recognize anger in a patient and how to deal with it.
5.4 Discuss bargaining and how to work with the patient at this stage, including the use of empathy.
5.5 Identify depression and how to help patients cope with it.
5.6 Recognize when a patient has reached acceptance.
5.7 Discuss reactions and significance to changes in body image.
5.8 Describe the difference between positive and negative euthanasia and philosophies connected with right-to-die issues.
5.9 List five ways to help the dying patient and their family.

Key Terms

Acceptance
Anger
Bargaining
Body image
Defense mechanism
Denial
Depression
Hospice
Negative euthanasia
Positive euthanasia
Stages of loss
Thanatology

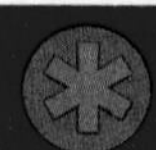

Key Point

Kübler-Ross stages of loss denial, anger, bargaining, depression, and acceptance

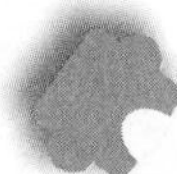

The Kubler-Ross Stages of Loss

Until recently, health care workers generally were not taught to deal with the psychological aspects of loss or death. Curing disease and maintaining life were the primary goals of health care providers. Although people acknowledged death, this harsh reality was seen as a defeat and was thus regarded as unworthy of attention. It seemed more appropriate to focus training on the positive goals than to put valuable time into a negative outcome.

It was not until the 1960s that a physician named Elisabeth Kübler-Ross challenged health care workers to view loss and death as natural. She focused her work on understanding and helping the dying. She pointed out that denying reality doesn't change it. What was being gained by living in a death-denying society? Perhaps the living could avoid looking at reality for awhile, but who then comforted the dying?

Kübler-Ross worked with hundreds of people as they learned of their own terminal illness. She and her staff supported these individuals until the end. What their dying taught them has become a cornerstone for the education of all health professionals. Kübler-Ross's **stages of loss** have far-reaching implications. They enable us to understand and to help not only dying people but all grieving people. They help us to deal with those who are about to die, those who have lost a loved one to death, and those who have lost a body part or the use of their body. Further, they help us gain insight into those who are losing a preferred lifestyle, such as those who face divorce or economic loss. Gaining understanding of these stages will enhance your ability to empathize.

Denial

Key Point

Denial first Kübler-Ross stage of loss: bereaved client uses denial as defense mechanism

Denial is a reaction that commonly follows the first news of impending death or significant loss. It is a **defense mechanism** as studied in Chapter 3. When information is too harsh for an individual to face, denial acts as a psychological buffer. It is an emotional escape hatch, for it tells a person that the thing he or she does not wish to hear is not true. Denial

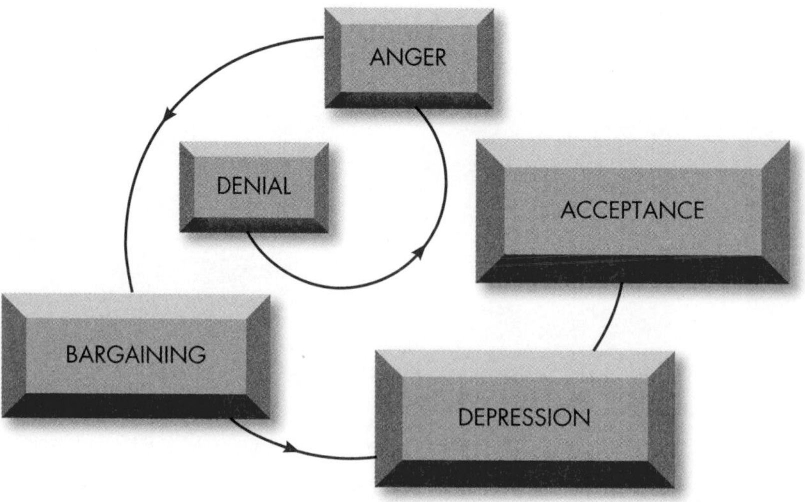

Stages of loss

comes in a variety of degrees, lasts for an unpredictable length of time, and is demonstrated in various forms.

A healthy amount of denial might be described as follows: An individual is told that he has inoperable cancer. His first thought is that this just cannot be true. He seeks a second opinion. While waiting for the retest results, he begins to think about putting his life in order and what he would do if this horrible news were, in fact, true. When the second opinion confirms the first, he begins to let go of his screen of denial and progresses through the other stages.

Sometimes a longer-lasting form of denial is also helpful. An individual who is dying may still need to accomplish many things. For some, only the hope that they will actually live allows them to continue. They may handle situations bravely and be helpful to and encourage family members.

Denial becomes a problem when it goes on too long, makes the patient emotionally fragile ("Please don't say anything that will chip away at my defense"), or gets in the way of positive actions. Some individuals remain in almost a zombie-like state of denial. They cannot make appropriate plans, either for themselves or their family members, and they may engage in a variety of activities designed to convince themselves that they could not possibly be dying. These activities may include making grand vacation plans, buying new cars, having elaborate elective dental work, or procuring new pets. Such individuals focus more on beginning activities than on tying up unfinished business.

Others may be so afraid of facing their illness that they may delay treatment or other help. As mentioned previously, the story is well-known: Aunt Matilda discovers a lump in her breast but says she must have bumped herself and does nothing about it. In some instances, then, denial can cost individuals their lives.

We do not wish to sound judgmental as we discuss denial. Can you sense the panic or fear you would feel if you were to discover a lump that could mean cancer? Can you understand both the power and comfort denial could offer to someone facing something so frightening? See if you can tell which of the following responses (Examples 1 or 2) are empathic. Then practice by creating your own empathic responses to the patient comments. Remember to suspend your judgments.

EXAMPLE 1

Patient: "I know the cancer is in both lungs now, but I won't give up. I'm sure others have been this ill and survived and I'm going to be one of them."

Response A: "You will not stop fighting the cancer."

Response B: "You are desperately determined to live despite the odds."

EXAMPLE 2

Patient: "I don't care how many doctors tell me I will never walk again—I know I will. If I have to leave the country to get treatment, then that's what I'll do."

Response A: "You'll go anywhere in the world to find help in walking again."

Response B: "You're angry with anyone who interferes with your determination to walk again, and you will fight to get the support you need."

* Answers: **A** responses are paraphrasing; **B** responses are empathic.

Anyone associated with a dying person—family members, friends, other patients, and health professionals—may go through denial, as well as through the other stages: anger, bargaining, depression, and acceptance. Sometimes the emotional stages of friends, relatives, and others coincide with the same stage in the patient. Often, however, individuals progress through the stages based on their own personal needs.

CASE STUDY 5-1

For three years a daughter dutifully visited her mother in the nursing home. She came for two to five hours a day. She read to her mother, fed her, and helped to bathe her. Throughout these three years the mother was expected to die any time. Her condition, the result of a stroke, went from grave to critical. The health care providers involved made assumptions about the daughter's preparation for her mother's death. They believed the daughter was devoted to her mother, but they thought she would be tired of caring for her and worrying about her. Further, they reasoned that the daughter had come to accept death as the inevitable release for both. The nursing home staff was not prepared for the daughter's reaction the day her mother did die.

The daughter was called at her home at 7 a.m. She was told that her mother had died quietly during the night. When she heard these words, she began screaming hysterically, "She can't be dead, she can't be dead!" Fifteen minutes later, still wearing a nightgown, she arrived at the nursing home and dashed to her mother's door. There she flung on her mother's bed and sobbed and moaned. It was not until her own daughter was summoned from a nearby town that she was comforted.

Apparently the daughter had been in a state of denial and bargaining. If she took good enough care of her mother, she reasoned, she would never lose her. It was weeks before she attained a level of acceptance. During these weeks she went through the stages of grieving as though her mother's death had been a complete surprise. Perhaps attention to the daughter's needs would have enabled the staff to predict her behavior. Better still would have been intervention before the mother's death. No one realized that this woman was stuck at an early stage of adjustment. What could a health practitioner have said to the daughter in this case? How do you tell a woman that her mother will die soon? (Please see advanced directives and comfort measures in the following chapter.)

Problems like this one can be avoided if family members ask about the future of their loved ones. A gentle but truthful response is then the best one. When family members do not allow themselves to hear the truth, a family conference may be necessary. The conference, which will bring together all close members of the patient's family, not only will clarify health information but also will allow family members to form a support group for themselves as well as for the patient.

In this example, the patient's daughter had a grown daughter of her own. The granddaughter might have become more involved with the patient's care in a way that would have permitted her to comfort her own mother. Or that granddaughter might have helped the staff to identify the depth of her own mother's denial if she had reported the disparity between her mother's comments about her grandmother and her grandmother's actual condition. Even if the patient's daughter had no other family, there might have been ways of detecting her denial. The biggest clue might have been the daughter's intense devotion to her mother's care. Perhaps it was too intense. When anyone seems to do *too well* in a difficult situation, you must be on the alert to discover if this is a form of denial and the extent of the denial.

A nursing home is filled with health care workers of every type. Health care workers who deny feelings for dying patients may, in a sense, atrophy. They can become cold and clinical with the dying. Their technical skills may be excellent, but they hide warmth and humanness from the patients who need it most. The job environment also can affect a health worker's development. Think of a warm, caring, involved provider who works in an environment that is not open to mourning. For how long can a person choke back grief before it causes additional harm? It is not unusual that staff in nonsupportive environments burn out early and leave.

Obviously those who provide continuous care to a patient are most likely to be affected. But even those health practitioners who have less frequent contact with the dying patient may require the right to grieve when a special patient dies.

There is a fine line between professional detachment and coldness. The experienced health practitioner will have developed a skill that permits closeness and understanding without setting up an incapacitating identification with the patient; the practitioner will not cross that boundary. Accepting grief as a necessary part of your work with the dying helps you to deal with it promptly and properly. Unfortunately, you are not untouchable with respect to life's pains. Predicting this helps you to take better care of yourself and of your patients.

Another area of loss with which you may be familiar is that connected with the end of a relationship. When a spouse or family member dies, the remaining family generally receives caring support. There is a formal, prescribed set of social responses connected with death. Friends send flowers, food, and memorial contributions. People come together even from great distances to be there for the survivors. All the people who knew the deceased praise his or her accomplishments.

Proper response to a divorce or the end of a relationship is not as universal, however. Friends often do not know what to say. Yet the dynamics of a breakup are strong and potentially dangerous. A patient who is divorcing may feel both rejected and like a failure. It is very difficult to resume living when self-esteem is so shattered.

Typical responses to a breakup may be well-intended but are not always supportive of the person they're said to. Consider the following responses:

- "Oh, he was no good for you. You're better off without him."
- "You two were never compatible."
- "I knew for years that she was cheating on you."
- "I know you'll be fine; it's just the kids we feel sorry for."
- "I told you you were working too many hours. If you'd been home more, I bet he wouldn't have gotten bored."

This list may sound humorous, but haven't you heard such misguided advice being given? Health care providers need to be more sensitive. Remember that during the first part of a breakup one or both parties may he in a denial state. Typically this means that the persons involved are ignoring any evidence of an impending breakup. A wife may refuse to believe that anything is wrong with the marriage even though her husband fails to come home several nights a week. A husband may not let himself think there is anything wrong at home even though his wife will no longer share a bed with him and is hinting at separate vacations.

When people in denial-like states are hit with reality, they become panicky. Learning that their partner has left brings out feelings of desperation: "This can't be true. I'll never survive without her." The response "I think she'll come back" gives no support.

Understanding the breakup of a relationship is enhanced if examined in the context of the stages of loss. Patient problems and illnesses make more sense when placed with respect to these stages. Remember that there is often overlap between stages. Treatment will improve when focused on how patients are progressing with their grief.

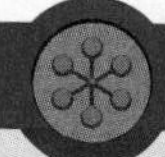

Elisabeth Kübler-Ross, M.D. (July 8, 1926 – August 24, 2004) was a Swiss-born psychiatrist whose book, *On Death and Dying*, introduced what is now known as the Kübler-Ross model. Dr. Kübler-Ross estimated that she had taught 125,000 students in death and dying courses in colleges, medical schools, hospitals, and social-work institutions. She was the recipient of twenty honorary degrees. What distinguished her was not only her soft calm manner of speaking but also her intensity in fighting for sensitive care for the dying and her successful campaign that the health field should reach out to the dying and not deny their existence and needs.

Anger

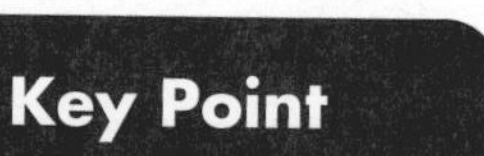

Anger second Kübler-Ross stage of loss: unreasonable anger directed at self or others

Anger generally follows denial. Anger can be detected to some extent in the denial stage. Recall the patient who said "I don't care how many doctors tell me I won't walk again..." This statement shows anger. The way the denials are worded almost screams out that the patient knows the truth.

As the patient breaks out of the denial stage, screaming may, in fact, take place. Facing the harsh reality of a tremendous loss makes most people very angry. This is the "Why me?" stage. There is often bitterness and turmoil as the patient experiences loss and isolation coupled with a sense of unfairness regarding his or her plight.

Patients are angry with their disease and with their poor fortune. Because the objects of their anger are intangible, the anger usually spills over onto other objects. Patients in the anger stage are often difficult to be around. The young, healthy health care worker makes a good target. The worse the patient is feeling and the younger the worker appears to be, the angrier the patient may become. These angry outbursts require caring and gentleness. Responding in anger is most inappropriate; even *not* responding in anger becomes difficult when the patient lashes out as if to blame the health professional for her or his imminent death.

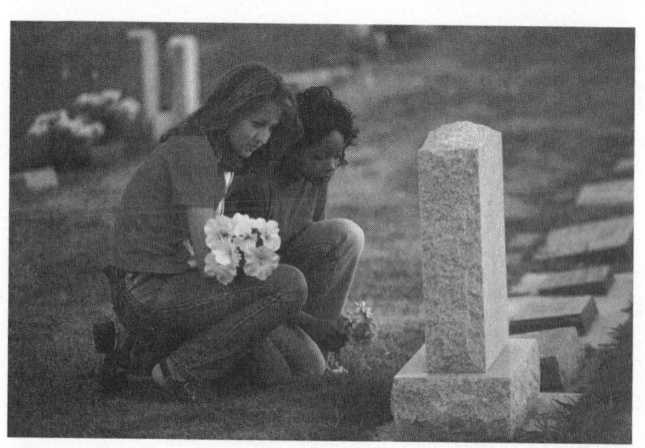

Grief can continue a long time.

When both denial and anger are operating, patients or their families may sue for malpractice because of the terminal diagnosis. "If this or that had been done *or* had not been done *or* had been done sooner, then perhaps Dad would not be dying now." Most such responses are scapegoating. It is so hard to accept loss that anger and blame temporarily ease and divert the involved parties. Unfortunately, this may unduly tax the health care system. After all, Dad may still need help from those who are being blamed.

When health care providers and family members rationally discuss prognosis and possible causes, the patient seems to suffer least. In fact, if health care providers attempt to avoid all dealings with the family's anger, they are more likely to be sued. Stating that you understand the family's grief and pain may help them to fix blame on the disease and not on the bearer of the bad news.

EXAMPLE 3

Patient's Spouse: "Oh, it's easy for you to stand there and say 'we'll do everything possible to make him comfortable. What's it to you? I bet your husband is healthy!"

Health Professional: (Said with warm vocalics and caring facial gestures) "Discussing how to help your husband is critical, but right now all you can probably think of is how terrible the situation is. I just want you to know we really are doing everything possible for him."

By staying with the speaker, you will generally calm them. A defensive remark such as "Where do you get off thinking you're the only one with problems" will only generate more anger. By letting people vent and helping them to feel understood, you decrease their *need* to lash out.

Anger shows up as human beings struggle to understand and accept all types of loss. It may take years to accept a disability. Generally, the more severe the limitations are, the longer it takes to accept them. A 24-year-old who awakes to find that a car accident 10 days earlier has left her a paraplegic probably spends years adjusting to her loss. Think of the number of losses this news involves. Not only can she never walk again, but her **body image**, sexuality and social life, family planning, work ability, general mobility, and long-term health will all be affected. Can she still drive? With what adjustments? How will she control her bowel and bladder? Can her chair fit through the doors of her home? Will she need an attendant? How will her boyfriend and friends react?

Anger and depression can be very strong for those adjusting to loss. Suicide attempts may occur for several years after the loss. The more the individual tries to cope with the disability, the more frustration he or she encounters. When people try and try to make things better, the proportion of effort they must expend is sometimes outweighed by a too-small degree of change. When they feel helpless and frustrated, they sometimes give up. Still others simply become angry at the world. They feel bitter that everyone else appears to "have it all" when they have "lost it all." Until they can deal with their anger, they have little chance of developing independence. Anger will keep tripping them up.

Remember that anger is a natural reaction to loss. When loss is tremendous, anger is likely to be more pronounced. Health professionals need to empathize and respond by acknowledging the patient's anger and the patient's right to feel angry. Who wouldn't be angry facing loss? When a patient holds on to anger for years, more treatment is necessary. Patients will not readjust if they are angry with everyone they meet for not suffering as they do.

Those closest to a breakup often are injured by displaced anger. A mother may not be able to admit how devastated she is at being divorced, but she becomes an overcontrolling, nagging dictator with the kids. She throws her anger and her need to feel in charge on those who are less threatening to her.

Health care providers themselves frequently need a place to be angry. Some facilities, especially those connected with **hospices**, have screaming rooms. These are private, soundproof rooms where individuals can close themselves in and scream. This helps to ease sorrow by releasing the burden of keeping it all in. Remember that anger at a patient's imminent death is common among staff who work closely with the dying. It is difficult to care for a patient while losing her.

The anger stage is painful and difficult for everyone—families, health care workers, and patients. But, like the denial stage, it is normal and necessary to most people. Remember that the dying person is losing everything. While others are grieving over the loss of an individual, the dying person must say farewell to all he has known: people, sunsets, puppies, ice cream, Christmas, music, everything. It is natural and emotionally appropriate to be angry.

Sometimes the specter of malpractice arises. "Why did the therapist say she was safe? We all knew it was only a matter of time before she fell again." Rather than retreating from this or trying to justify this, you now know that you will be less likely to be sued if you paraphrase and empathize and say "I am sorry."

Some elements of the anger stage may remain throughout the dying process. Generally, however, there is an acute angry period followed by considerable calming if the anger is brought out and dealt with properly.

Bargaining

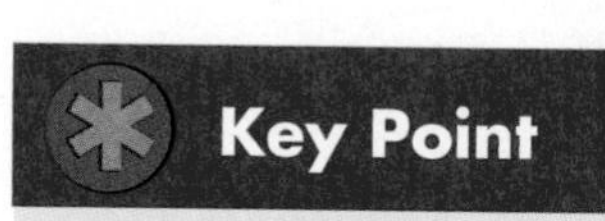

Bargaining third Kübler-Ross stage of loss: delaying tactic to put off need for acceptance

The **bargaining** stage is similar to denial. It is another safety zone or buffer from the full force of unbearable reality. The bargaining stage generally has a religious overtone to it. When faced with death, even the least religious person seems to invoke a higher being. The patient will often offer a sacrifice of sorts if his or her life is saved. If, for example, a patient thinks he has worked too hard and hasn't shown his children enough consideration, he will promise to undo this wrong in exchange for a return to health. "I will spend all my time with my children." Another patient may say, "Please let me live long enough to attend my grandson's wedding." If she should live to the wedding date, she may renegotiate the contract: "Please let me live to see my first great-grandchild born."

Patients may also bargain with the health professional. A dentist gently told a man with terminal cancer that there was no real need to continue his root canal work. She was surprised by the patient's zealous insistence that the tooth must be treated! By convincing the dentist to finish the root canal work, the patient had a sense of gaining proof that he would continue to need his teeth.

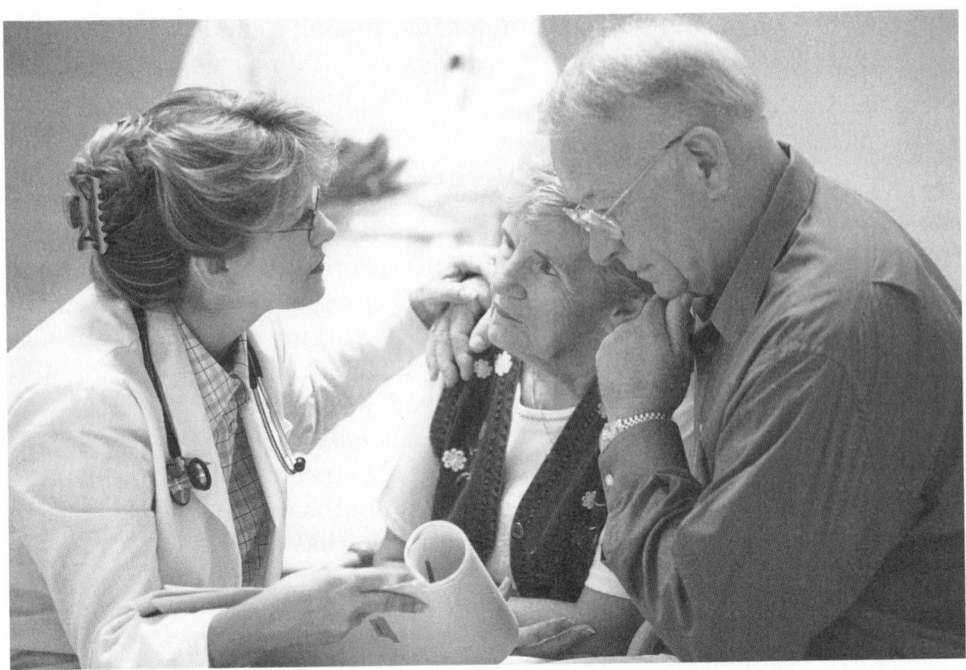

Receiving bad news

Bargaining may provide comfort and hope when all seems lost. Generally, however, the patient sees that the "deal" is not going to be met. This generates feelings of frustration and anger, which usually dissolve into depression.

Depression

Depression occurs when a patient believes that hope is lost. She has cracked through initial denial, raged at the world, and even pleaded with a God in whom she may have had no faith. But everything she has thought and done has been to no avail. She is not getting better and she knows it.

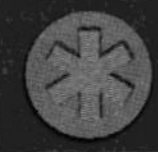

Key Point

Depression fourth Kübler-Ross stage of loss: actual grief from loss

Although you never wish to see a patient suffering through depression, it is a normal and necessary state. During this time the individual examines her life, what she has done, and what she will never do. She becomes introverted and withdrawn and may sit alone in a darkened room. She may refuse most visitors, seeing only a few family and friends who mean the most to her.

Although subdued in tone, the depression stage still contains turmoil. Elements of denial, anger, and bargaining may still creep in. Remember that no previous stage is ever discrete (separate and distinct) or complete. But during depression the patient actually comes to believe in his own mortality and thinks over what he has done and what he has missed.

This stage, like all others, is somewhat mediated by who the patient was before the disease. For example, certain resilient individuals will show similar spunk even when faced with death. Other less emotionally strong people will have more trouble passing through the stages and facing reality.

If depression lingers for a long time, medication and psychotherapy may be indicated. Certainly the patient should receive all the emotional support possible. The threat of suicide is a very real possibility during this stage and mandates referral to a psychologist or psychiatrist.

Behaviors that commonly accompany depression include:

- Reminiscing
- Reviewing life
- Sleeplessness

(These behaviors are reviewed in more detail in the chapter dealing with senescence.)

Life review helps a dying person gain perspective on what she or he has accomplished and will leave behind. Not sleeping well is not only part of depression but also may be the mind's way of working to reconcile the sorrow of grieving and is therefore necessary. For how long is depression normal? Generally speaking, after losing a loved one, a person should be back at work within a month and able to mix socially within six months. Although some sorrow may continue indefinitely, a person who is still having a lot of difficulty handling the loss after six months may need special help and certainly does if grief is acute after one year has passed.

Acceptance

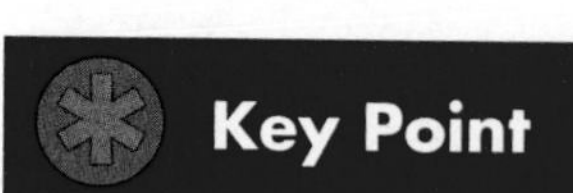

Acceptance fifth Kübler-Ross stage of loss: resignation with fate, return to realistic existence

Acceptance, the final stage in the emotional process, follows depression. Acceptance is not a happy phase, but the patient is generally calm and demonstrates a subdued interest in the world and in attending to unfinished business.

Usually the patient wishes to talk out loud to a trusted friend or two. There seems to be a need to verify many of the thoughts conjured up during depression. And there is a need to touch base with someone who knows about the patient's life and can thus validate his or her worth.

Generally, the more loving the patient's support group is, the easier acceptance comes to the patient. There seems to be a stronger sense of self-worth and of having mattered in the world if many people love you. Such support provides the environment necessary for a patient to face death and to put her or his life together with dignity. Massachusetts Senator Ted Kennedy coped well with his brain cancer diagnosis in 2008, suggesting that he moved quickly to acceptance.

To reiterate, remember that none of these stages is discrete. Although denial will generally come before depression, there are elements of both in each. Some individuals skip stages. Others work through stages very quickly. Passing through stages must be at the patient's own pace. A patient or family member who is suffering because of being stuck at a particular stage may require assistance to progress. If a disease progresses rapidly, the patient may never reach some stages.

Denial, anger, bargaining, depression, and acceptance are the feelings of loss most dying and grieving people must pass through. The more you can learn about these stages, the better able you will be to help your patients, their families, and yourself.

Because denial and anger generally occur at the beginning of the grieving process, they tend to be prominent among the stages. Another reason they are noteworthy is that they can confound and complicate medical treatment. It is essential that you understand both the stages of and responses to denial and anger because they generally entail more of a health challenge than do bargaining, depression, and acceptance. Of course, being familiar with all the stages will enable you to better understand and provide service to your patients.

EXAMPLE 4

See if you can identify the stages in Example 4.

Patient 1: "I've always gone to church and worked hard. This is so unfair. My sister never does a thing for anybody and she is healthy as a horse!"

Patient 2: "I know that if I just eat more carefully this whole thing will reverse itself. No way can I be so sick at my age."

Patient 3: "At this point I want to rewrite my will and fix up the obituary. That will make things easier on my wife."

Patient 4: "If it is God's will that I die, so be it. But I know that he wants me to see my last child through to graduation and I'm going to do it."

**Answers:* Patient 1 = anger; Patient 2 = denial with some bargaining aspects; Patient 3 = acceptance; Patient 4 = bargaining.

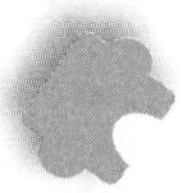

Body Image

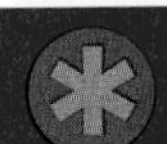

Key Point

Body image mental picture of self including value judgments

The area of **body image** warrants examination. Too often the health professional does not realize the emotional pain involved in a change in appearance. As health care workers, you often reason that if a patient's life is not threatened and there is no pain, that patient is lucky. But burn patients who are fully recovered in terms of physical abilities often remain depressed and suicidal because of the scarring and physical distortion of their appearance. They are acutely aware of the response of others to their scars and frequently compare themselves with how they looked before the burns.

Generally a person with severe scars or other changes in their appearance will see themselves as far worse than do others. It is difficult for the health professional to convince such a patient that they may, in fact, look quite acceptable for the patient holds an image of perfection that they may never obtain. As discussed elsewhere, standards of perfection can only result in disappointment. The patient who is depressed by how they look must be taken seriously and the depression needs to be treated. Failure to treat the depression may have disastrous results.

Some patients refuse a medication because it distorts their facial features, even though taking it would improve the quality of their health. Undoubtedly a breast lump is more difficult for most women to face than other lumps might be. The fear of cancer may remain the same, but the fear of disfigurement is crippling. These examples demonstrate a form of denial that overlaps with other psychological features. As health professionals you need to treat concerns regarding body image as though they are a separate and serious symptom of their own.

For instance, you must be aware that the "typically teenage girl" who is phobic of weight gain will never believe others who tell her she is already too thin. This is part of the pathology of eating disorders. People with anorexia nervosa will literally starve themselves to death as a result, at least in part, of a distortion of body image. This is yet another reminder of the caution health professionals must exhibit when loss of body image is part of the illness or accident that their patients may be facing.

Positive body image is a valuable and fragile commodity. "Loss" is not just about death but loss of a body part (e.g., amputation, mastectomy), loss of ability (e.g., retirement, paraplegia, blindness, or inability to drive) or loss of potential (e.g., infertility).

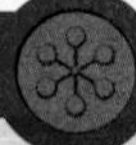

Types of Loss

- Loss of person—Death, Divorce, Empty nester
- Loss of body image—Body part (amputation, mastectomy), Sensory (blindness, deafness), Motor (paraplegia, impotence)
- Loss of social standing—Retirement, Unemployment
- Loss of independence—Inability to drive, Assisted living
- Loss of potential—Infertility

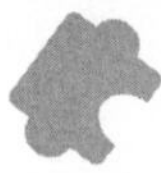

Right-to-Die Issues

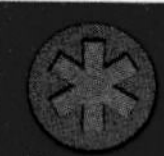

Key Point

Right to die issues quality of human life should be balanced against quantity; leads to concepts of positive and negative euthanasia

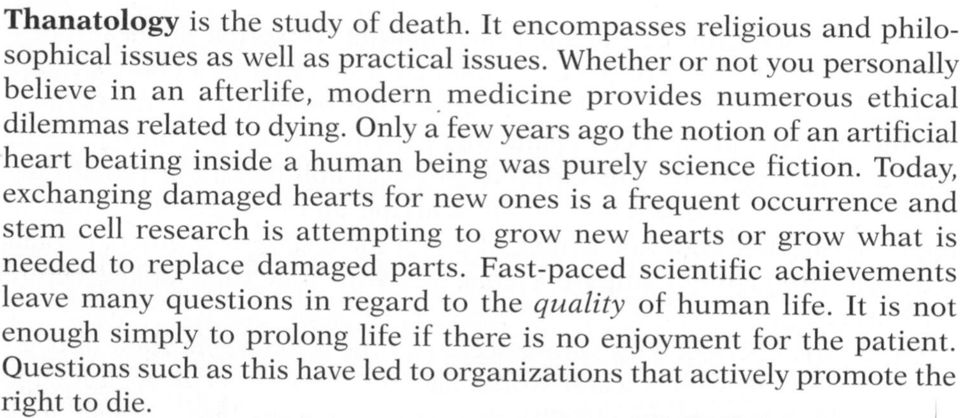

Thanatology is the study of death. It encompasses religious and philosophical issues as well as practical issues. Whether or not you personally believe in an afterlife, modern medicine provides numerous ethical dilemmas related to dying. Only a few years ago the notion of an artificial heart beating inside a human being was purely science fiction. Today, exchanging damaged hearts for new ones is a frequent occurrence and stem cell research is attempting to grow new hearts or grow what is needed to replace damaged parts. Fast-paced scientific achievements leave many questions in regard to the *quality* of human life. It is not enough simply to prolong life if there is no enjoyment for the patient. Questions such as this have led to organizations that actively promote the right to die.

Negative euthanasia is tacit noninterference with the process of death, for instance, leaving pneumonia untreated. Negative euthanasia is an act of omission, for example, treatment may be withdrawn or changed and results sooner in death. (Please see Living Will in the following chapter.)

CASE STUDY 5-2

Terry Schiavo suffered brain damage after she was resuscitated from cardiorespiratory arrest in 1990. This left her in a persistent vegetative state (a beating heart but no higher brain function), and she was institutionalized for 15 years. Her husband petitioned the court to remove her gastric feeding tube after eight years. But Terry's parents felt she was conscious rather than unconscious, so they opposed him. The court said that Terry would not have wanted to be kept alive artificially. Extensive media coverage showed politicians and groups fighting one another about the case until finally in 2005 her feeding tube was removed. This was a case of negative euthanasia.

Positive euthanasia involves *directly* taking a life. The terminally ill are not simply allowed to die but are put to sleep: Positive euthanasia is an act of commission (e.g., giving someone a lethal injection to cause death).

Philosophically, supporters of right-to-die legislation argue that it is inhumane to allow dying human beings to suffer. If there is no hope, why force a patient to die slowly and painfully when one would do more for a beloved pet?

CASE STUDY 5-3

Jack Kevorkian is a pathologist who fought for many years for positive euthanasia, earning himself the nickname "Dr. Death." He felt that a patient whose life had become unbearable should be allowed to end his or her own life. In 1987 he started counseling patients on suicide methods, always careful that the patient was the one who "pushed the button." Over the years he probably assisted in the suicide of more than 100 people. In 1991 he had his medical license revoked, but he continued his work, assisting suicides by using carbon monoxide because he had lost access to intravenous potassium chloride. He went through many court cases. In 1997 the U.S. Supreme Court ruled that Americans have no constitutional right to commit suicide. Kevorkian was jailed from 1999 to 2007. Upon release he announced his intention to run for U.S. Congress and remained on parole until 2009.

In 1993 the Netherlands legislated that physician-assisted suicide was legal, and in 2002 physician-assisted suicide became legal in Belgium. It is not legal in other countries.

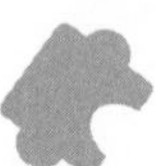

Five Ways to Help the Dying

Obviously, there are more issues surrounding dying than simply providing comfort. Health care workers need to be aware of the legal and ethical ramifications of their treatment of the dying. Some health professionals may even wish to lead the way in finding solutions to death-with-dignity issues. But for most of us, the number one concern is how to help dying patients directly. There are five specific ways in which you, as a health care provider, can help the dying. You can listen, focus through paraphrasing, respond from your own "gut," leave hope intact, and assist the family to be with the patient.

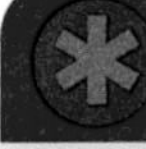

Key Point

Five ways to help dying Listen, focus through paraphrasing, respond from your own gut, leave hope intact, help family to be with patient

Listen

When a dying person wants to talk, *listen*. As part of progressing through the Kübler-Ross stages, the patient needs to gain a perspective on what is happening. Talking can help patients work their way toward acceptance. A big problem for the dying is to find someone who is willing to listen.

Most people freeze up when confronted with a grieving or terminally ill person. They feel ill at ease. They are afraid to say anything lest it be the wrong thing. Health care workers must work very hard to overcome this kind of fear. Students who are just beginning their clinical training often fear dealing with dying people more than they fear any other aspect of patient care. A dying person will often pick a young health care worker to confide in. What should you do if you are the one chosen? First, listen. Take a deep breath. Do not panic. *It is more important to listen than to talk.* Remember that it is okay if a patient needs to talk about dying. You do not have to have years of experience to be of help. You may need to schedule more time to work with such a patient, however. The patient's emotional needs and your ability to respond will be enhanced by extended and frequent visits. Remember, a dying person does not have time to wait.

Focus through Paraphrasing

Listen and then focus through paraphrasing. Stick with what is being said. A typical response to a patient's statement of grief blocks rather than encourages talking.

Patient: "I wonder what it will be like to be dead."

Health Practitioner: "Oh, now don't think about that. Think about getting well."

Such a response is obviously inappropriate. How much easier dying would be if the patient were allowed to talk instead of being closed off.

You do not have to be brilliant, supersensitive, or even vastly experienced to say the right thing. All you have to do is paraphrase.

Patient: "I wonder what it will be like to be dead."

Health Practitioner: "It seems that you are getting curious about death at this point and I'd like to hear your thoughts" Or you can respond as follows if you feel more comfortable: "Yeah" (nodding your head, focusing on nonverbal communication).

Offering either response encourages the patient to keep talking. It says that you understand what the patient is saying and that it's okay to talk with you about it. Once the patient gives more, an empathic response is generally appropriate. But, simply paraphrasing throughout the dialogue is far better than closing off discussion.

An empathic response to this patient's statement is, "It sounds like you're frightened of what lies ahead. Maybe you could tell me what you think death may be like."

Respond from Your Own Gut

Kübler-Ross taught her students to make a gut response. This approach ties in with the use of empathy. Your gut response is an empathic one for you are responding to your patient with an honestly felt emotion. If a patient asks you a question, even a personal or difficult one, you need to answer it. Dying people need to know what you think.

- "Do you believe in a higher being?"
- "Will it hurt to die, nurse?"
- "Will I see my baby brother in heaven?"
- "Are you afraid of death?"
- "Do you think there is an afterlife?"

Problems occur when health care workers have not dealt with these issues for themselves. This is a death-denying society, and health professionals may regard death as failure. How do you as an individual break through denial to share your honest feelings? Your instructor may assign several exercises that will help you feel in touch with your own mortality. Only when you have faced the reality of your own death will you be comfortable in responding from your gut to your patients. Responses that are not honestly felt may seem safe to the giver, but rarely will they fool the receiver.

Leave Hope Intact

There is a subtle difference between denial and hope. Hope can be looked at as a bright spot or an escape hatch. For a dying man to have hope may simply mean that tomorrow won't be taken away from him, even though he has no long-term future. Most human beings, even during stages of depression and acceptance, want hope.

The dying have been asked how they want to be told about their illness and its consequences. They have responded that they want to be told the truth but that they need to believe there is some hope, some reason to fight. If an illness is very serious, then say so. But never convey that it, or a patient's situation, is totally hopeless. Do not lie, but do not give up. In such an atmosphere, the terminally ill can manage to live better until they die. This is increasingly important today as many new target drugs allow patients to live with even stage four cancers for many years.

Most of us will probably not be giving such news directly to a patient. But it is important to understand this frame of reference. Even when you are assisting in the breakdown of denial, you don't want to convey a sense of hopelessness.

You need to be sensitive to the words you select to convey the nature of a patient's illness. Must you always refer to cancer as cancer? Avoiding the word *cancer* may prevent some patients from shutting down their senses and giving in to deep denial. Substituting the word *tumor* may be less emotionally devastating for some patients. Observing patients' body language and concentrating on matching their level of questions may key health professionals in on how best to phrase difficult news. If a patient says, "Is it malignant?" or "Is it cancer?" then the health professional can respond using such words. But if the patient obviously avoids the word *cancer*, then using a less direct term may be in order.

Patient: "Do you think the doctor got it all? They said it was a long operation."

Health Professional: "Well, the surgeon said he got it all, and apparently they are waiting for the examination under the microscope to confirm that."

Help the Family to Be with the Patient

The people who work in hospitals can make a sterile environment less cold and more inviting. Hospitals that are run like hospices are set up to closely simulate the home environment, a difficult task when medical equipment makes up part of the furnishings. The hospice concept promotes home death whenever possible. Dying at home is thought to be more natural. Imagine how much more gentle it might be to die in your own bed, surrounded by familiar things and people who love you, than to die in a hospital.

Unfortunately, dying at home is a luxury that not every family can manage. Some families cannot cope with taking care of a physically infirm loved one. Lifting, feeding, bathing, and bathroom use may present insurmountable hurdles. The physical abilities of the family must be considered along with the condition of the patient.

But the emotional strength of the family is probably the most important consideration. Can the family deal with their loved one and her terminal disease 24 hours a day? How will they react to her pain or nausea? If she becomes severely confused, will they become frightened? How prepared are they for death? Have they enough support systems for their own emotional well-being? If the family wants the patient at home, there is usually a way that home care can be managed. If sufficient community services are available or if money is plentiful, then home care may be possible with even limited family support.

Ideally, medications will be sufficient to keep pain at a minimum. Often medication and other aids to comfort can be adjusted when the health care team makes house calls. The team also can assist family members in making time for themselves away from the patient. If a patient's condition becomes too much for the family, intermittent inpatient care can be arranged.

When hospitalization is constant and prolonged, a patient can suffer a tremendous sense of isolation. He or she may believe that friends and family do not care. When visitors come only infrequently, a long stay in the hospital gives patients a message of rejection or abandonment. Sadly, visitors do tend to avoid the dying. Many people find it painful to acknowledge the possibility of death, especially in a friend. They may fear that the dying person will put them on the spot. Thus your job as a caring health care practitioner must be to encourage supportive visits. You can do this in several different ways.

Encourage the Patient's Family to Let Friends Know What Is Going On

The patient's illness and prognosis need not be a secret if the patient will agree to this. Friends may need to hear that their visits are desired and that the patient is not too ill to want to see them. This may be the time to key in on a family's denial. Not spending time with the sick relative may indicate that the family is blocking the message of how serious the patient's condition really is. The family conference mentioned earlier in this chapter then becomes essential. It is not unusual that the harsh reality has to be spelled out for relatives at such a meeting.

Relative: "When she gets home, will she need a lot of help for awhile?"

Health Professional: "If she gets home, she will require all the help she can get. But she most likely will not be coming home. Have you thought about taking time off?"

Be as Flexible as Possible with Visiting Hours

Don't lock the door on a friend who arrives outside visiting hours unless it is absolutely necessary. It may be difficult for friends to visit during hospital hours. The importance of the visit generally far outweighs the importance of rules.

Be Certain that Friends Receive Positive Feedback

Tell friends how much their visits have meant to the patient. Suggest that they come again. A cheerful reception and a friendly goodbye may keep friends coming for as long as they are needed.

After a loved one is gone, the family continues to need support. They will feel better about themselves if they have been with the patient while he or she was dying. If the family was fortunate enough to have a hospice worker assigned to them, they will be followed for a year after the time of death.

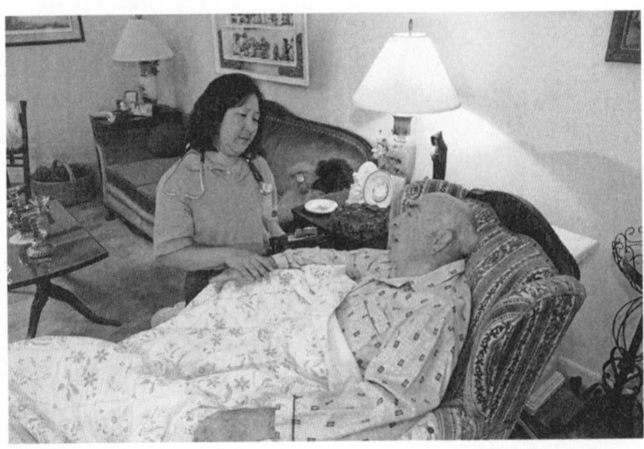
Hospice care at home

A year's follow-up permits the bereaved to have comfort and assistance through all the anniversaries that they connect with their lost loved one. Holidays that were special to the deceased will especially touch those who are left behind. The deceased's birthday and the wedding anniversary when a spouse has died become hurdles to climb. Living through the occasions once permits a natural strengthening.

Having advanced notice of death allows family members to do anticipatory grieving. Writing "This is Dad's last Christmas with us" on all the cards may mean that the next Christmas will be less traumatic. In most cases, having time to prepare for death is easier on the family than is sudden death.

Summary

The Kübler-Ross stages of dying are denial, anger, bargaining, depression, and acceptance. Being familiar with these stages will enable the reader to respond appropriately to patients facing loss. In the first stage, denial, a patient needs a psychological buffer between what his or her mind can accept and harsh reality. The health professional recognizes a problem here if denial lasts too long. Anger generally follows denial. The patient experiences a devastating sense of unfairness in the loss they are facing and is angry with all others who appear *not* to be facing such a loss. Bargaining may have some religious overtones to it as the patient struggles to find a way to change the diagnosis or to at least postpone it. Depression is fairly self-explanatory; the patient now facing the loss more fully feels the pain of all forms of the loss. Acceptance, while not a happy stage, is generally a calmer stage in which the patient is facing what must be accepted and is dealing with the loss, perhaps by saying good-byes, getting his or her will in order, or taking care of important "unfinished business."

Denial and all other stages are true for loss of life but also for death of a loved one, death of a patient, disability, or dissolution of a relationship. This knowledge makes it easier to respond empathically. Losses that alter body image affect human behavior, may be very serious, and also follow these stages.

Concerns about the quality of the life of a dying patient have led to organizations that promote the right to die by supporting euthanasia. *Negative euthanasia* is not providing heroic measures to sustain life in the terminally ill. *Positive euthanasia* is an active measure (a mercy killing)—taking someone's life for the good of that individual. Ethical and legal issues pertaining to these matters are reviewed in the chapter on senescence.

The five ways in which you, as a health care provider, can help the dying are listening, focusing through paraphrasing, responding from your own gut, leaving hope intact, and assisting the family to be with the patient.

Many terminal patients prefer the familiar surroundings of their family and home. For families that can manage it financially, emotionally, and physically, having a loved one at home until death is a more natural process. The home setting is much less intimidating than the hospital, so that other family members and friends are more likely to visit. As a health care provider, you must be aware and supportive of the patient's needs and the family's needs, whether in the hospital or home setting, and be as flexible as possible. End-of-life support is given by hospice in most communities.

Chapter Review

Key Term Review

Acceptance: Fifth Kübler-Ross stage of loss: resignation with fate, return to realistic existence

Anger: Second Kübler-Ross stage of loss: unreasonable anger directed at self or others.

Bargaining: Third Kübler-Ross stage of loss: delaying tactic to put off need for acceptance.

Body image: Mental picture of self including value judgments or psychological distortions.

Defense mechanism: Psychological means of avoiding conscious conflict.

Denial: First Kübler-Ross stage of loss: use of denial as defense mechanism by a bereaved client.

Depression: Fourth Kübler-Ross stage of loss: actual grief from loss.

Hospice: Supportive medical and home care focusing on dying with dignity; an organization that helps the dying and their families.

Negative euthanasia: The tacit noninterference with the process of death.

Positive euthanasia: *Directly* taking a life.

Stages of loss: Kübler-Ross' five stages of bereavement: denial, anger, bargaining, depression, and acceptance.

Thanatology: The study of death.

Chapter Review Questions

1. How is it possible for a patient to experience both anger and denial at the same time?
2. What counseling strategies will help you the most when dealing with dying patients?
3. What must you do to prepare yourself to work with dying patients?
4. What do you think the reason is for the statement "A big problem for the dying is to find someone who will listen to them?"
5. Why might a mastectomy patient suffer more emotional side effects than a patient who has just lost a kidney to cancer surgery (assume the same prognosis for each)?
6. What is it about body image that makes this a serious area of concern?

Case Study Critical Thinking Questions

1. Look at Case Study 5-1. How does bargaining differ from denial and how are they similar? What ideas have you about how to detect when a family member may be in denial?
2. Regarding Case Study 5-2, might you see a time when Dr. Kevorkian's ideas will be accepted as necessary? How do you see society dealing with issues of euthanasia if resources become very scarce? How do you think society will deal with euthanasia if resources are plentiful?
3. Refer to Case Study 5-3. You are living through a period of history in which many American children regularly die of starvation and neglect. How do we, as a society, justify putting financial resources and energy into prolonging the lives of the elderly and terminally ill?

References

1. Kübler-Ross, E. *On Death and Dying*. Englewood Cliffs, NJ: Prentice Hall, 1968.
2. Kübler-Ross, E. *Death, the Final Stage of Growth*. Englewood Cliffs, NJ: Prentice Hall, 1980.
3. LeClaire et al. "Communication of Prognostic Information for Critically Ill Patients." *Chest* 128:1728–1735; 2005.
4. Matsuyama, R., Reddy, S., Smith, T. "Why Do Patients Choose Chemotherapy near the End of Life? A Review of the Perspective of Those Facing Death from Cancer." *J Clin Oncol* 24:3490–6; 2006.
5. Nessim, S., Ellis, J. *Cancervive: The Challenge of Life after Cancer*. Boston: Houghton Mifflin, 1991.
6. Nuland, S. B. *How We Die*. New York: Vintage Books/ Random House, 1995.
7. Redwood, Daniel. "On Death and Dying." Interview with Elizabeth Kubler-Ross. www.doubleclickd.com, 1995.
8. Kübler-Ross, E., Kessler, D. *On Grief and Grieving: Finding the Meaning of Grief through the Five Stages of Loss*. New York: Scribner, 2005.
9. Kagawa-Singer, M., Blackhall, L. "Negotiating Cross-Cultural Issues at the End of Life: 'You Got to Go Where He Lives.'" *JAMA* 286:2993–3001; 2001.

Additional Readings

1. De Kort, S, Willemse, P., Habraken, J., et al. "Quality of Life versus Prolongation of Life in Patients Treated with Chemotherapy in Advanced Colorectal Cancer: a Review of Randomized Controlled Clinical Trials. *Eur J Cancer* 42:835–45; 2006.
2. Holmes et al. "Screening the Soul: Communication Regarding Spiritual Concerns among Primary Care Physicians and Seriously Ill Patients Approaching the End of Life."Am J Hosp Palliat Care 23:25–33; 2006.
3. Welch, F., Winters, R., Ross, K. "Tea with Elizabeth." www.nhpco.org, April 2009.
4. Williams, S., Haskard, K., DiMatteo, M. "The Therapeutic Effects of the Physician–Older Patient Relationship: Effective Communication with Vulnerable Older Patients." *Clin Interv Aging* 2(3):453–67; 2007.

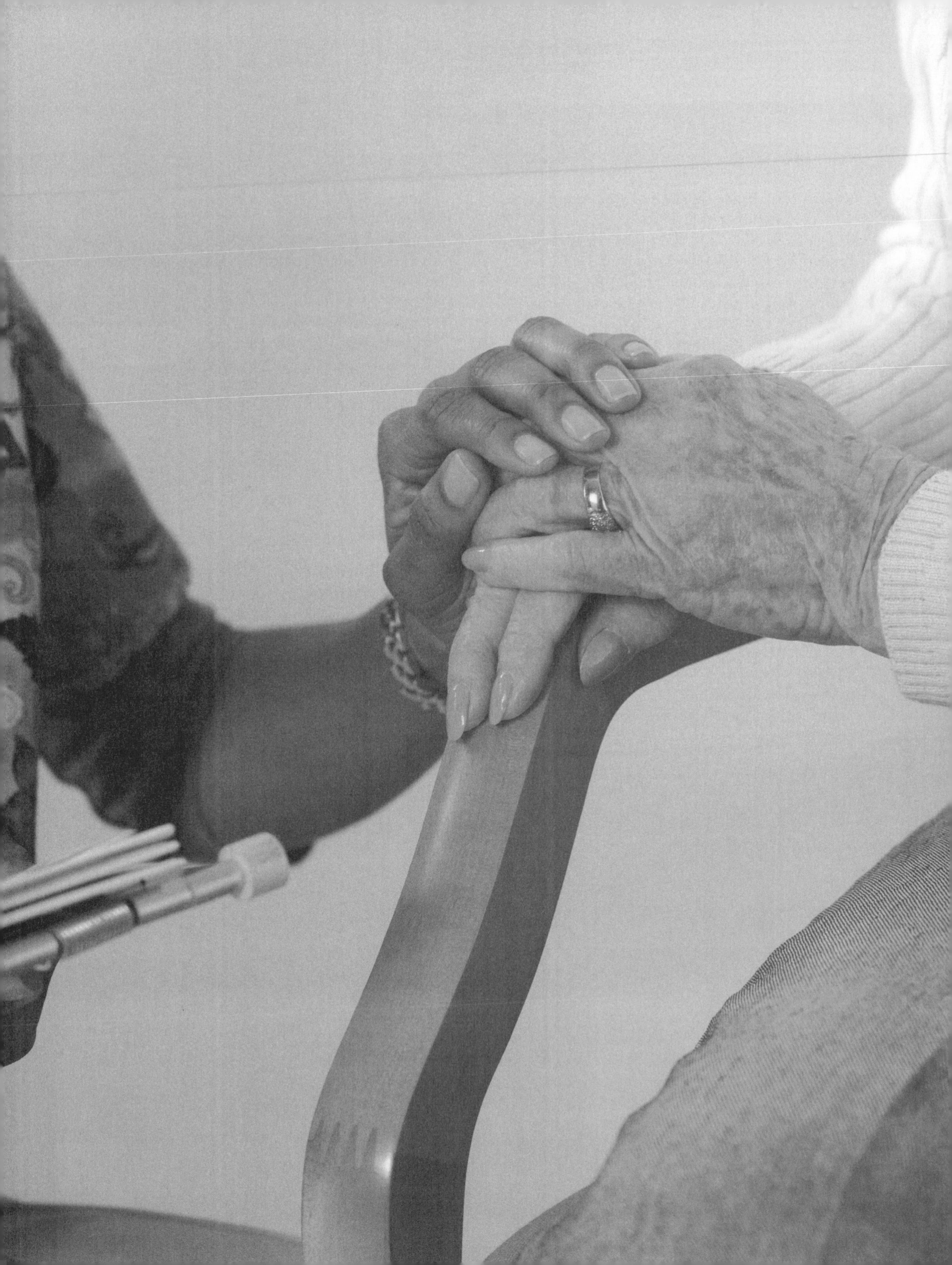

Developmental Issues—Early Childhood and Adolescence

Learning Outcomes

After reading this chapter, you should be able to:

6.1 Explain the concept of parental expectation.

6.2 Recognize bonding relationships and their dependent nature in early childhood.

6.3 Describe separation anxiety and possible ways to involve the parent in its management.

6.4 Understand negativism leading to recognition of self-determinism of young child.

6.5 Summarize how children model themselves after others to achieve competence.

6.6 Recognize why sexual maturation is the most important physiological and social event in the adolescent's life.

6.7 Comprehend that adolescents who feel different have a pronounced sense of rejection.

6.8 Describe issues of teenage pregnancy, early sexual activity, and possible provider limitations when dealing with homosexual adolescents.

6.9 Recognize the need for teens to break away and differentiate themselves from their parents.

6.10 List parental responsibilities when dealing with teens.

6.11 Recognize that teens of a divorced family have a more difficult time adjusting than teens of married parents.

6.12 Describe the balance between the teen having time alone with the health professional and the need for the parent to know.

6.13 List Erikson's developmental stages.

Key Terms

Body schema
Bonding
Developmental assessment
Developmental delay
Developmental milestones
Differentiate
Dyad
Identity
Intervention
Modeling
Negativism
Neonate
Parental expectations
Parental responsibility issues
Positive reinforcement
Primary sex characteristics
Reinforcement
Secondary sex characteristics
Separation anxiety
Stigmatized adolescents
Teens of divorce

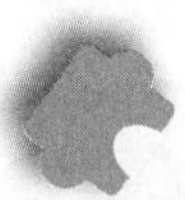

Introduction

In order to provide treatment for a child, the health professional needs to understand different stages of childhood and how to involve the child's parents in the process. It is for this reason that this chapter delves into childhood development. The concepts of bonding, separation anxiety, negativism, and modeling in early childhood will be discussed. The issues of adolescence, including sexual maturation and sexual issues, rejection, and the need to break away, also will be discussed. In early childhood, treatment of children must include their parents, but as children get older they need increasing time alone with the health professional.

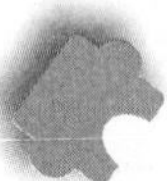

Developmental Issues: Early Childhood

Humans have for generations viewed the birth of a child not only as the astonishing unfolding of new life but also as a challenge to society's caregivers. An array of responsibilities and demands comes with this new life. Dynamic creativity on the part of parents, siblings, educators, and health care workers is necessary. The health care worker's success in meeting the needs of children depends on an understanding and respect for the child's physical, emotional, and cognitive uniqueness.

In early childhood, little can be accomplished unless parents or primary caregivers accept the plan for care and play a role in the child's compliance with the designated plan. For example, the clinical dietitian has little hope of eliminating a particular food from a child's diet unless Mom, Dad, and sometimes Grandma and Grandpa or other significant adults avoid offering the child this food.

Expectancy and Perfection

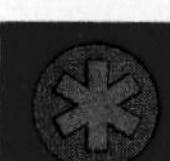

Key Points

Neonate first four weeks after birth

Parental expectations parental vision of the perfection of their offspring which modifies over time

All parents have visions of what their **neonate** will be like: a healthy, happy, physically attractive, well-behaved child who sleeps and eats, sits and crawls, and talks and walks according to pediatric timetables. At some point in the baby's early months, every parent sees his or her expectations of perfection blurred. Expectations can be blurred temporarily by a string of sleepless nights, or they can be all but destroyed by severe illness or disability.

Time and interaction between parent and child modify **parental expectations**, decreasing the discrepancies between expectation and reality. Most of the parents that health care workers encounter are experiencing an ongoing evolution of acceptance. The success of the parent–child relationship depends on the evolution of acceptance, a process that differs little from the stages of loss described in Chapter 5.

Obviously, parents want to be in control of the expectations they have for their child. The greater the gap between reality and their expectations of perfection, the more parents blame themselves and question the observations of others. Discrepant expectations of perfection contribute to parental behaviors ranging from forced feeding to stress-related colic and from verbal abuse to physical abuse. Sometimes little reconciliation occurs between what the parent wants from and for the infant and how the infant acts and reacts to the parent. Conflicts are then set up that affect the health professional's relationship with both the child and the parents.

In high-risk nurseries and in early intervention programs, the health practitioner must help the parents reconcile their discrepant expectations in an empathic, sensitive, and supportive way.

CASE STUDY 6-1

Joey, born three months premature, has been discharged from the neonatal unit of a major research hospital. Despite what the hospital staff has done to prepare the parents, Mary and Dan perceive the discharge from the hospital as a sign that everything is okay. Threats to their expectations of perfection soon arise, however, when family and friends are surprised by Joey's frailty and his lack of head control for a three-month-old. Friends offer comparisons with their children or grandchildren.

Joey's weight and development are not unusual given his premature birth. The reassurance of the hospital staff that Joey was indeed doing "better" than the other infants who continued to stay in the hospital originally decreased Mary and Dan's discrepant expectation of perfection. But the observations of friends and relatives are upsetting. The comparison between Joey and other infants conjure up new fears of imperfection for Dan and Mary. Joey's problems are emphasized by the fact that a home visitor is providing special help for the family. Because parental denial is a reasonable reaction, early intervention providers may find that Dan and Mary don't welcome suggestions. Parents need to feel comfortable about sharing their fears, hopes, and concerns with the providers. Until they can relate openly with the health and educational professionals, efforts to begin a positioning program or feeding schedule will not succeed.

When health professionals focus on the problem and ways to treat the problem, each encounter with the parents is difficult. Why? Because with this approach, health practitioners ask the parents to focus on just those things that are discrepant with their expectations for the child. That is why textbooks recommend a "family-centered" approach. Working hard to build parental trust and listening and incorporating the parents' concerns and priorities into the intervention is essential.

Bonding and Dependency

Even a casual observer sees the special relationship between parent and baby when eye contact and touching bonds a baby to its caregiver. For the baby, the **bonding** stage focuses on basic needs and safety. While being held securely and receiving warmth from the mother's body, both the bottle-fed and breast-fed baby experience a satiation of hunger. The baby is so dependent on this satiation that early in infancy the baby may only be able to fall asleep in the mother's arms.

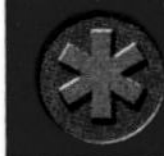

Key Point

Bonding a close mutual attachment between infant/parent dyad, with baby dependent

Although experts agree that this bond develops rapidly under ideal circumstances, bonding is not automatic. Opportunities for fondling and immediate gratification are essential to bonding. Situations that separate the parent from the baby during the first few hours and days of life interfere with bonding for both the infant and the parent. Close proximity, relaxed cuddling, eye contact, and secure handling facilitate bonding.

The necessity for medical intervention such as incubation or use of a respirator makes bonding more difficult. Problems such as cerebral palsy, cleft palate, and respiratory difficulties make feeding a frustrating experience for both parent and infant. Frustration with feeding leads to satiation delay, which has the potential for threatening bonding.

Experts predict that bonding sets the stage for the parent–child relationship. Lack of or delay of bonding can affect the child's eating habits, academic success, and self-esteem. For example, high self-esteem is associated with strong bonding.

Because bonding is so important, early intervention programs focus heavily on this issue. Health care workers and educators become consultants and facilitators, teaching the parent ways to foster physical, emotional, and cognitive growth. While minimizing separation and fostering bonding, this model allows the parent to assume control in the situation without placing unrealistic demands on the parent's skills and resources. Because successful feeding is so important to bonding, clinical dietitians as well as speech, occupational, and physical therapists all encourage programs that help both the infant and the caregiver enjoy feeding.

Separation Anxiety

As a result of bonding, infants perceive themselves as one and the same with their sustainer and nurturer. The infant-parent pair is often referred to as the infant-parent **dyad**. Eventually, either intentionally or because of circumstances, both parent and child find themselves playing a risky game of separation. Light patterns dancing nearby, music in the background, other people in the room, colors flashing past, or hands encountering a textured sweater serve as stimuli luring the infant to give up that tightly swaddled position of comfort. Little by little the intensity of feeding and sleeping is broken by brief periods of concentration on the outside world. Within the trusting relationship of the dyad bond, the child explores new sights and sounds.

> **Key Points**
>
> **Dyad** a couple, a group of two
>
> **Separation anxiety** the anxiety of a young child when separated from person or thing to which he or she has strong emotional attachment, usually parent but sometimes objects (e.g. security object)

The infant soon begins to explore emotional and physical separation from the nurturing adult. He or she begins to develop reaching and grasping ability, allowing contact with more and more environmentally distant objects. The parent's role in presenting the objects diminishes, and the child and the object develop a new and distinct relationship.

While a parent is nearby, the infant tolerates this risky business of exploration well. There comes a time, however, when physical separation is a crisis. When the child sees the nurturing adult leave, inability to understand that the adult will return makes the child ill at ease. Until experience with separation proves that the parent consistently returns, **separation anxiety** occurs. Consider this example:

CASE STUDY 6-2

Jane, a nine-month-old infant, plays happily, exploring toys in the room while keeping watch on her mother. When Mom steps out of the room to answer the phone, Jane searches desperately around the room for her. She is soon screaming shrilly. Others try to comfort her to no avail. Toys that delighted her five minutes ago are now rejected without even a glance. The only thing that calms Jane is Mom's return.

This crisis of separation can interfere with all attempts by health care workers to provide a service. Although separation is difficult for children between the ages of nine months and two years, it can be a problem for children of all ages. With the increased stress often characteristic of encounters with health care workers, even adults find separation from loved ones difficult.

Even very young children respond better when prepared. Preparation can take the form of a simple explanation like "In a few minutes I'll be going out of the room, but I'll be right back." A simple explanation like this can be used for short separations until the child builds confidence that Mom will return. Playing separation games like peek-a-boo and hide and seek when there is no crisis can also help. The child builds trust in the return of the adult through these low-anxiety situations.

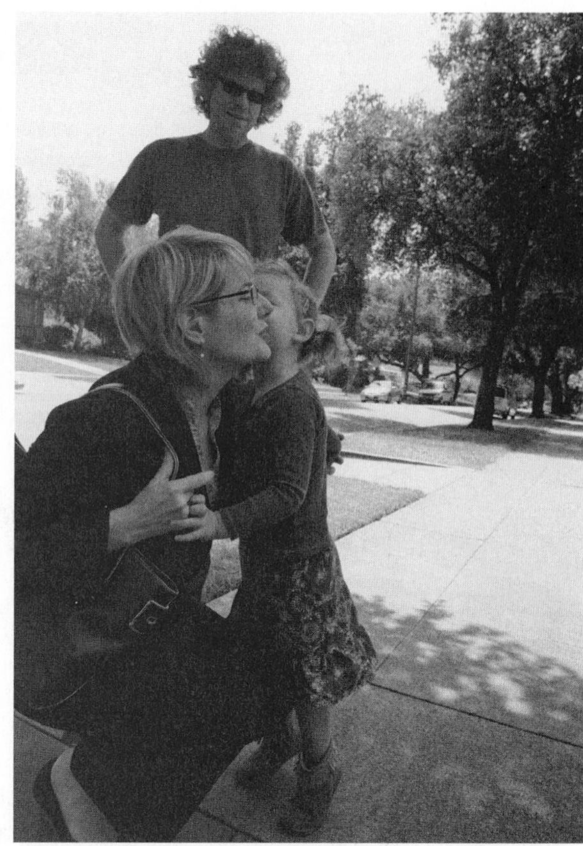

Why is the toddler not anxious yet about separation?

What can health care workers do to prevent separation from interfering with care? For the very young child, health professionals can provide systems of care that minimize separation. Parental overnight stays with hospitalized children are options in many pediatric facilities. When possible, young children can be examined while they are sitting on the parent's lap. Opportunities for preparation, transition, and structured routines allow the child and parent to be more comfortable. Physical spaces can be designed to be more like home environments. A favorite stuffed animal may stay with the child when the family must leave. Sensitivity to separation issues allows the health care worker to integrate an understanding of separation anxiety into a child's plan of care.

Separation anxiety poses a special problem for working mothers. Often care is given outside the home by day care workers, babysitters, or other family members. If the child has a health problem or disability, separation is often more difficult than normal. It is essential, then, that the child's caregivers be competent in positioning and feeding the child and caring for its special needs. Often this means that the health care worker—the physical or occupational therapist, for example—must teach these techniques to day care workers. When substitute caregivers can make the child feel secure and safe, separation will be easier.

Working with the parent and child to make the transition to a day care situation smooth is important not only to the child's emotional security but also to the parent's emotional well-being. Parents often feel guilty when their child cries as they leave. Separation routines help to ease the transition. Preparation followed by some physically structured and consistent routine often helps the child cope with separation.

CASE STUDY 6-3

Bobby, a 20-month-old child, is left at the day care center at 8 a.m. every workday morning. Bobby's mother and his therapist have met with the day care center staff on several occasions to describe the physical care Bobby requires. The therapist has

(Continued)

CASE STUDY 6-3 *(continued)*

taught the staff how to hold Bobby so his lack of head control and muscle weakness does not make him feel insecure. Even with these precautions, Bobby's mom finds that each day she has to force herself to walk out the door while Bobby screams. The day care staff plans a parent conference to discuss ways to work with Bobby and his mother to alleviate this daily crisis. The routine that the staff and Bobby's mother work out goes like this: Bobby and Mom sit together with the center teacher for a few moments while Mom talks quietly with Bobby. She tells him that in a little while she will be going to her office, reminding Bobby that he's been there before! Mom talks about the photograph of Bobby on her desk, creating for Bobby a concrete picture of exactly where Mom will be. This way Bobby can visualize Mom somewhere during the day even though she is not with him. Mom goes on to say that she will be back after his afternoon nap, giving Bobby an easily identified reference for her return. Mom gives Bobby a kiss and hug, gets some in return, and then reinforces her return by saying, "See you after your nap!" as she walks out of the room. Mom walks away; Bobby's teacher picks up on the reinforcements of "permanence and return" that Mom had already introduced. She tells Bobby about Mom going to the office and gets him involved by asking him whose picture is on her desk. She reinforces the fact that Mom loves Bobby and will come back after his nap.

Although this routine may not eliminate the crying on the first day, eventually it will take the place of the crying routine. Separations that occur gradually beginning with a few minutes and then moving up to a few hours are also ideal. They are a weaning process.

Structured routines continue to be important as children get older. If, for example, a 10-year-old child arrives home before her working mom does, she will handle the separation better if a routine can be maintained. A routine might suggest a snack. A phone call from Mom or contact with a neighbor could alleviate concern.

As with most situations that lead to growth, separation is not all bad. Without separation from the nurturing adult, the child cannot develop his or her own identity.

Negativism and Control

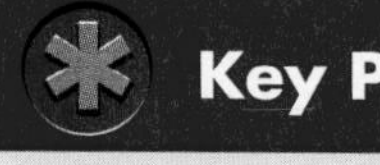

Key Point

Body schema child's ability to use her or himself as a reference for understanding the world; sense of self

Cognitive, language, and motor development all depend on the child's development of **body schema**—the child's ability to use her or himself as a reference for understanding the world. Hands go to the mouth and bring everything from the world to the mouth for exploration. Distance concepts develop from the child's reach for objects close and far. Communication focuses on "me" and "mine," emphasizing the link with the environment. Self-feeding begins, separating nourishment from dependency on adults.

The development of a competent and confident "separate self" ushers in the beginning of self-control. The potential for toilet training and independent choices for food and clothing arises. Parents and health care workers begin to feel this self-directed emphasis in their interactions with the child. They begin to hear that word most feared by all parents of two-year-olds—no!

Somewhere between the ages of 18 months and 4 years, the "terrible twos" descend. A child's relationships with adults and other children are strained. If you call a child who is in this stage, he runs the other way. If you suggest reading a book, he insists on going outside. If you offer his favorite food, he refuses to eat. Parents who have reveled in their child's cautious encounters with independence wonder where their control has gone.

Eating problems are a common manifestation of **negativism**. Fearing that their child isn't being adequately nourished, the parents force the child to eat. The child retaliates. A vicious circle is created. Parents and health care workers need to recognize that young children do not starve through simple negativism. If a child refuses a meal, the quickest way to combat the problem is to accept the child's choice.

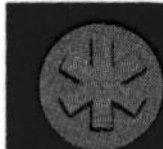

Key Point

Negativism resisting direction from others, which leads to separation and understanding self determinism

This new self-confidence is born out of the battle of separation as the child's understanding of self solidifies. Parents and health professionals must understand and recognize the child's need for control and self-direction. Recognizing the need for choices and presenting acceptable choices or alternatives can save the adult from the wrath of the sometimes defiant two-year-old.

Offering unlimited choices won't work, however. The two- or three-year-old's choice may threaten the child's safety or the parent or caregiver's sanity. Given limited, feasible choices, the child will delight in self-determination, and a new ability to manipulate the world will emerge. "Would you rather have fish and carrots or chicken and corn for supper tonight?" offers acceptable alternatives. "What would you like for supper tonight?" opens the door for disaster. The child could easily choose candy and cookies, leaving the parent no alternative but to try to convince the child to accept a more appropriate alternative. Creating and maintaining the parameters of acceptable behavior is the most important task the parent assumes at this time.

Health care professionals may find working with the negative child particularly challenging. Parent presence may or may not lead to compliant behavior. How should you approach the child? How should you react to negative responses?

Encouraging acceptable behavior for the child at this stage of development includes structuring the setting to decrease opportunities for unacceptable behavior. Remove delicate objects to limit the need to say no. Provide alternative tasks that lead to the behavior you seek. Use "if ... then" statements to mold behaviors. Avoid "don't," which is a command. Remember that the child needs to be in control. "If you ..." sentences give the child the information she needs to make an informed decision. Be sure that the consequence you use is related to the specific behavior you want to avoid. For example, in the statement "If you throw the toy, I will take the toy away," the consequence (removing the toy) is directly related to the behavior. Avoid vague consequences. Consider this example: "If you throw the toy, you will not be allowed to play with these toys the next time you return." The consequence in this example is far too removed in time for the child to see it as an immediate consequence of her behavior. The consequence should be related directly to the interaction between the child and the toy. "If you throw the toy, I will spank you" focuses on a consequence not directly related to the child's interactions with the object. Most authorities think that threats of spanking do not deter future behavior. More importantly, threats of punishment affect the child's self-esteem and interfere with the development of a good relationship with the child. For the health care worker, physical contact must be monitored carefully to avoid any questions of physical abuse.

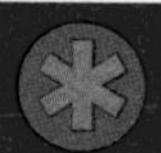

Key Point

Positive reinforcement constant focus on identifying appropriate behavior and praising the child for it while avoiding castigating child for negative behavior

Positive reinforcement is the most effective form of behavior modification for the child at this stage. Remember that a child at this stage is in a mode of rejecting suggestions. Many adults, including health care workers, find that they pay attention to a child's behavior only when it interferes with adult tasks or interactions. Such an approach sets the situation up for failure. Instead, health care workers should focus constantly on identifying appropriate behavior for positive reinforcement. The child who delights in praise and reward will increase the frequency and intensity of those behaviors that led to adult approval. As the frequency of these appropriate behaviors increases, the frequency of inappropriate behavior will decrease.

Positive reinforcement is especially effective when you deal with more than one child at a time. Consider this situation:

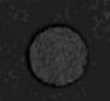

CASE STUDY 6-4

Maria and Hector are siblings brought to the outpatient laboratory by their mother for blood tests. As the medical technologist begins to tell them what she will be doing to perform the finger prick blood test, Maria listens intently while Hector begins to talk loudly and interrupt. If the medical technologist stops the instruction and tells Hector to stop talking and listen, Hector is likely to reject this adult control and continue to talk and interrupt. But, instead the medical technologist says quietly to Maria, "What good listening, Maria, I really like the way you are paying attention," Hector may stop his ranting for a moment. At that moment, the medical technologist could say to Hector, "What good listening, Hector. Now let's see if you remember what we were talking about."

In this example, the health care professional used positive reinforcement of Maria's behavior to indirectly point out the importance of good listening. As soon as she saw an approximation of appropriate behavior in Hector, she rewarded him. For some children, a verbal reward is enough to mold behavior; for others a more concrete reward may be necessary.

Any rewards you use must he considered appropriate by the parents and the agency in which you work. For example, the small objects like the tiny figures often found in the treasure chest at the dentist office are hazardous for the children under three.

It is sometimes impossible to control behaviors through positive reinforcement. When the child's safety or property in the room is threatened, it may be necessary to gently restrain the child. In all situations, however, both the child and the parent must still feel your acceptance and respect. Even when you must express disapproval for some action, your disapproval should be specific to the behavior so that it cannot be perceived as general dislike for them as persons. Communication skills are especially important here. Paraphrasing the child's or parent's response, so they can further define their wants and needs, can clarify the situation and may prevent conflict.

The rebellious stage can create ambiguous feelings for the parent of an ill or handicapped child. There is a tendency for the parent to rejoice in the

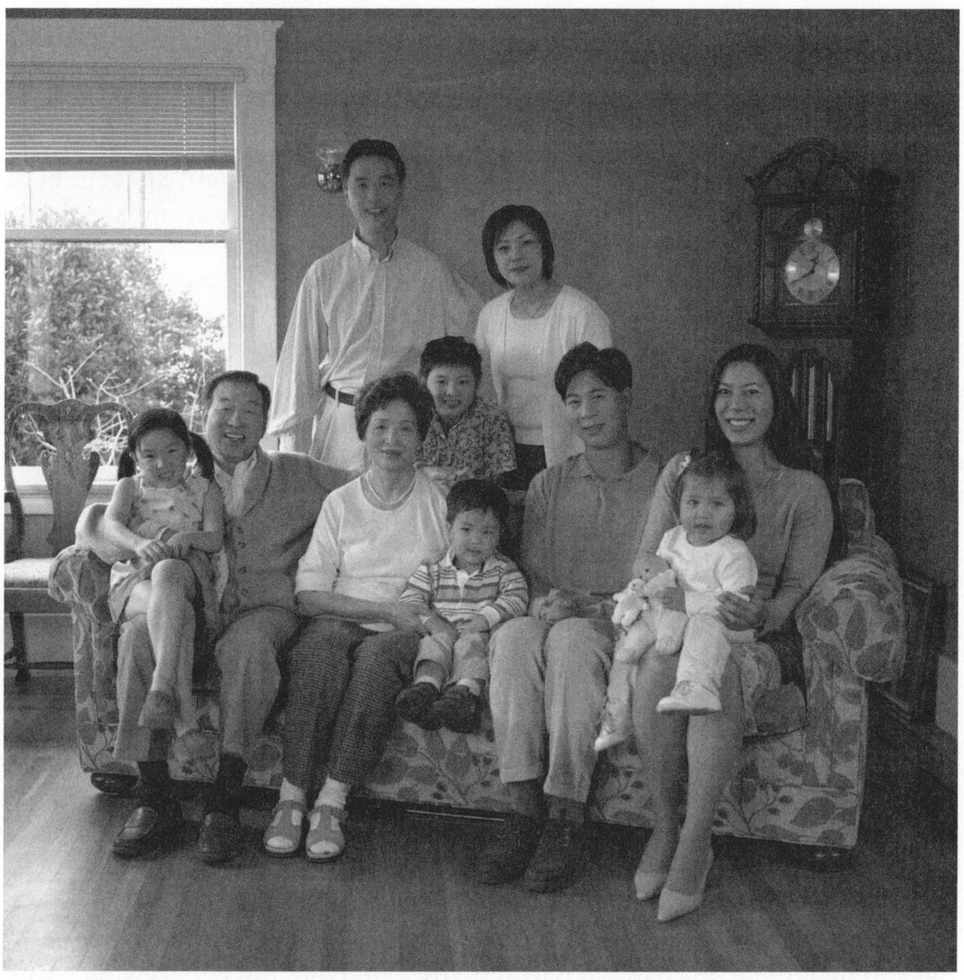

Multi-generational families have many people to help with negativism and positive reinforcement.

child's attempts at interacting with the world even if the child's behavior is manipulative and inappropriate. Spoiling the child by giving in during conflict deprives the child of the consistency and structure that can assist him or her in organizing the cues from the world. Adults should guide the alternatives offered to the child in a way that allows for choice but that structures or limits the child's alternatives. Given some practice with structured decision making, the child will grow in ability to make appropriate decisions that support safe and productive actions. Without such experience, a child's interactions with the world are likely to be compromised.

The health care professional needs to recognize when the parent may need help in determining appropriate behavior and applying limits consistently. Inability on the part of the parents or the health care professional to deal with a child's negativism may affect the overall success of any necessary evaluation or treatment. Making referrals for help in handling behavior problems that interfere with health care may not only be appropriate but essential. All children of any age normally have times during their development when behavior is a problem. The health care professional who recognizes and understands the parents' struggle can provide helpful modifications in the health care program to make the interaction more successful for the child, the parents, and the health professional.

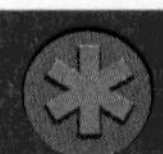

Key Point

Modeling children basing behavior on activities of others to achieve competence by imitation, practice, and peer or adult feedback.

Modeling and Competence

When the young child learns that within acceptable behavior many options for control exist, adults and other children become strong models. The young child watches the activities of others and then imitates the activity and practices the skills necessary for success in movement, speech, play, and feeding. This is called **modeling**, and successful imitation is exciting for the child.

As the child imitates the action of others, the relationship between the action and the outcome (cause and effect) intrigues the child. Persistent repetition of tasks is often a focus of the young child's activities. Even the nine-month-old shows signs of persistent repetition during throwing activities. You have all seen the child in a highchair or playpen who throws all the toys or objects onto the floor for the sheer delight of hearing them hit. The action (throwing) is reinforced by the outcome (the toy hitting the floor), and the child repeats the action over and over again. Adult and peer feedback reinforces attempts at dressing, eating, and construction type tasks. Through this reinforcement and repetition the child gains competence.

Being competent means meeting a goal. Nine-month-old John works diligently to remove his shoe and shrieks with delight when he succeeds. His mother puts the shoe back on, and John takes it off again. Sometimes parents misinterpret this repeated goal-directed activity. A fine line exists between negativism and the stubborn persistency to be independent and competent.

An adult must make allowances for competence development. A successfully completed task for the child need not be at adult standards. Sharon, age three, diligently works at spreading peanut butter on bread for her sandwich that she can eat without any help from the supervising adult. Acceptable behavior for the adult may include a clean counter, no peanut butter on Sharon's shirt, and evenly spread peanut butter without any holes in the bread.

School-age children are particularly influenced by other children as well as adults and may imitate their behavior. This may include social mannerisms, experimenting with drugs, smoking, hobbies, social cliques, and behavioral issues like truancy. Social rejection at this time can be particularly devastating, and children may model their behavior on anyone to gain acceptance into a group.

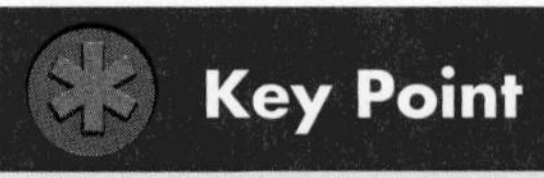

Key Point

Developmental milestones usual age ranges for the child to sit, walk, talk, copy shapes, etc.

Developmental Milestones

As health professionals we are likely to be asked to give our opinions on the appropriateness of a child's abilities at a particular point. Usual age ranges for the child to sit, walk, talk, copy shapes, etc., are called developmental milestones. Lists and charts showing age ranges and skill criteria for **developmental milestones** are used as a reference by health professionals, parents, and educators in evaluating the development of a child. If as health professionals you need to communicate with parents of children, you need to be aware of normal developmental milestones.

These lists and charts can guide us in setting realistic expectations. Developmental testing also meets the parents' need to know that their child is making good progress toward competencies expected at each age level.

Additionally, the sequence of one task followed by another gives us cues for structuring the child's environment to maximize the potential for growth.

The Denver Developmental Screening Test (II) is one such guideline used by a variety of health professionals to assess a child's progress in successfully completing age-appropriate tasks. The Denver II includes test forms in pads, each sheet of which can be marked with the child's results. The exact administration of the test is very important.

The purpose of the chart is to give the health care provider specific tasks to observe and criteria for indicating whether a child is competent in the task. The Denver II allows the professional to draw a vertical line through the adjusted age of the child (chronological age minus any weeks of prematurity). The adjusted age line will intersect on the chart with those skills typical of a child at that age. After short periods of observing the child, the health care practitioner can determine whether the child is performing below or above average for her or his age.

Using such a chart is especially appropriate when an inexperienced health care worker is asked by a parent whether his or her child is slow in some areas. When used to measure strictly against a standard or to compare one child's performance with another's, the chart can strip a child of the unique competence he or she has been developing. Developmental testing is, after all, only an approximate estimate of a child's level of skills in various areas. It can be helpful, however, in discussing and planning opportunities for a child to grow in areas where competence is still evolving. Other instruments also exist to measure whether the child is developing normally.

Developmental assessment may be necessary to validate a need for special services that offer the child additional opportunities for developing skills. Unfortunately, labeling a child as **developmentally delayed** may be necessary to receive special services. And labeling can have a permanent effect on the child's access to services and the child's social acceptance. A health care provider makes this determination only after careful, repeated assessments and full consideration of medical problems that might be affecting skill development.

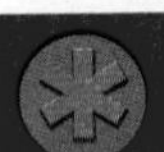

Key Points

Developmental assessment evaluation by professional to determine child's personal-social, fine motor, gross motor, and language abilities

Developmental delay delay in any one of key milestones, sometimes necessitating labelling child as delayed to get services

Determining language delay in a young child is a good example of the need for careful and comprehensive assessment. "Failing" items on the chart related to speech sounds may indicate mental retardation, or it may indicate that the child has a hearing impairment resulting from repeated ear infections. The courses of action in each of these cases, of course, differs dramatically. In one case, repeated and expanded testing might indeed show a tendency for the child to have difficulty in many related skills, resulting in a diagnosis of mental retardation. In the other case, treatment of the ear problem might resolve the speech problems, making formal speech therapy services unnecessary.

The health practitioner must be careful to discuss his or her assessment of any developmental milestones supportively and positively. Emphasis on isolated deviations from the norm can stifle both the child's and the parent's confidence in other skill areas and can decrease the child's feelings of self-worth. Questioning competence is especially crucial when the child already perceives himself or herself as different. Children with visual, hearing, physical, or learning disabilities tend to receive special services to assist them in gaining the competence to become productive adults. In providing those services, educators, parents, and health care workers find themselves in the role of evaluator, teacher, and enabler. As helpers they must support the child's intact competence.

Helping a child to become more competent often involves the painfully difficult task of pointing out inadequacies in the child's approach to a task. In other words, what the child is doing "wrong" must be pointed out. Making concrete suggestions for substitute strategies is more successful than directing the child to avoid doing something. Consider the following case study:

CASE STUDY 6-5

Sharon holds the spreading knife in a cutting fashion. Her mother says, "Sharon, you are making holes in the bread. Don't hold the knife that way!" Sharon continues just the same.

Liz, a friend of Sharon's mom, says nothing until Sharon starts on the next slice. Then Liz says, "Sharon, when you hold the knife flat like this, the peanut butter spreads better." As Sharon starts doing this, Liz says, "Hey! Great going, Sharon! It tastes better that way, doesn't it?"

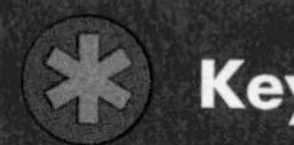

Key Points

Reinforcement praising child for success, which builds child's self-esteem

Intervention stepping into health problem issues in order to facilitate change

Reinforcement for what is successful builds a child's self-esteem. Criticism for unsuccessful attempts destroys a child's energy and enthusiasm for seeking competence.

Communication with parents about developmental milestones requires tact, sensitivity, and an understanding of parental expectations of perfection. The parent bond with the child makes it inevitable that comments about a child's performance will be interpreted as criticism of the parent. It may help to remember that the child who focuses on cognitive tasks in school and motor skills in sports uses the same competence-seeking behaviors as does the infant who is learning to walk or talk. In fact, adults who choose to continue growing in skills and developing in areas of competence use these same behaviors as well. Linking act with outcome, persisting with repetitions and practice, and being sensitive to criticism of success at the task are competence-seeking behaviors characteristic of all age groups.

Health care students who anticipate primary involvement with children or who fear interactions with young children should work on gaining a basic understanding of the forces responsible for the typical behaviors seen in children. The first 12 years of life entail a fascinating array of complex interactions with people and objects. The health care provider who understands the stages of child development will be better able to understand the actions and reactions of children and their parents and will develop skills that motivate children to participate in health care activities, allowing successful **intervention**. Such a professional can transcend the accomplishment of tasks associated with the role of professional and focus on unique and rewarding relationships with the children and their parents.

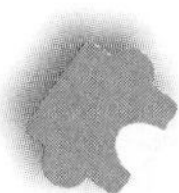

Adolescence

The transition from childhood to adult life is often difficult. Adolescents are still dependent on their parents but must struggle to prove otherwise. Much of what one needs at age 15 must still come from parents: permission and approval is required every step of the way. Parents subsidize outings with friends, the adolescent's wardrobe, the ability to train for the future, and eventually even auto insurance.

Ideally, parents recognize and reward teenagers with increased privileges as they demonstrate increased ability to take responsibility. This approach allows for some stability and emotional support. Adolescents are in conflict, wanting to be independent yet needing emotional support. No single aspect of adolescence illustrates these difficulties better than puberty.

Puberty and Sexuality

Following the advent of walking, the transition to sexual maturity is undoubtedly the most important physiological and social event in a child's life. The hormones work in ways that produce both longed-for developments like pubic hair and breasts and embarrassing developments like increased sweating and acne.

Changes in **primary sex characteristics** refer to changes in the reproductive organs. These changes soon lead to the possibility of reproduction if sex were to take place. In males, wet dreams (the nocturnal emission of semen) generally characterize reproductive readiness. In females, the onset of menses (the menstrual period) generally indicates reproductive readiness. If reproductive readiness coincided with social and emotional readiness, life would be a lot simpler. Sadly, the adolescent usually experiences a strong attraction to the opposite sex at the same time she or he feels awkward and insecure.

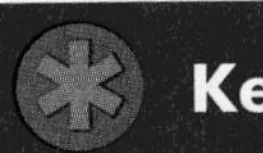

Key Points

Primary sex characteristics features of the reproductive organs

Secondary sex characteristics other physical features associated with reproductive readiness

Peer groups of the same sex serve a valuable function as adolescents learn from each other. Experienced peers may be admired for their knowledge of what sex is really like. Less experienced peers serve as a baseline of support. Peers encourage one another through the heroic tasks of meeting possible mates. They brag and joke about the aspects of sexuality that make them nervous. They comfort each other in the face of romantic rejection.

Discussion and valuation of **secondary sex characteristics** are among the most important roles of the peer group. Secondary sex characteristics are other physical features associated with reproductive readiness. Both males and females develop pubic hair by puberty. Males now also develop facial hair and a deepened voice. Females take on the characteristic hourglass shape with an increase in hip size and breast development.

Although secondary sex development is normal, it is a time fraught with insecurities for the adolescent. The recently developed female may feel self-conscious in settings that call attention to her body. Going to the beach, for example, may create a pronounced discomfort. Further, the female who develops later than her peers is generally perplexed and unhappy over her fate.

Males are anxious for the outward signs of manhood to appear. But when an adolescent boy's voice first cracks in public or his kid sister teases him about peach fuzz, these signs may feel humiliating. The boy who is slow in developing is doubly humiliated; he fears that nature has played a cruel trick on him.

Peer pressure is toward conformity at this age. Everyone wants to be recognized as normal. Early adolescents often dress alike, talk alike, buy the same music, worship the same heroes, and generally imitate all possible characteristics of their group. As adolescents become more mature, they begin to make decisions on their own. Conformity during the early stage has given them enough stability to become more individualized in the later stages. Still, the peer group is very influential.

Adolescents Who Are Different

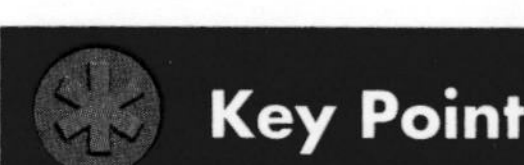

Stigmatized adolescents adolescents often rejected by peers

What about those who are different? **Stigmatized adolescents** are often rejected by their peers. Children who are too fat, too short, or too tall or children who are truly disabled in some way suffer acute anguish, especially during early adolescence. Imagine already being insecure and not thinking of yourself as normal. Then add the difficulties of puberty. These children are often rejected by peer groups. Rejection is so strong that they may fail to date. They tend to withdraw from events like school dances, events that are designed for their developmental benefit. They may spend years feeling ostracized and depressed. Kids who feel the "outsider" role most strongly are likely to end up in serious trouble.

What does this mean as a health care worker? Well, adolescents must be assessed for any emotional or developmental damage that is being inflicted. Diseases in general threaten a potentially frail self-concept. Any health problem visible to others (the loss of a limb, facial disfigurement, hair falling out, skin problems) threatens the adolescent's self-concept further. When the body image of an adolescent is threatened, the psychological stress is devastating. When a patient is a child who has grown up with a disability, puberty may signal the temporary loss of stability. The onset of sexual issues, which demand normalcy and acceptance, may make kids who are already different feel terrible and could trigger clinical depression. For a discussion of suicide the reader is referred to the next chapter on senescence.

CASE STUDY 6-6

Gloria felt especially proud to be developing breasts at the age of twelve and realized that she was attractive to boys at school, who would often stop and talk with her. But within a year she developed a severe case of acne. The boys no longer talked to her. She knew the reason. What made it even worse was that her older sister had beautiful skin and a beautiful figure and was constantly the center of attention for all the boys.

Gloria thought about seeing the school nurse but it was even more humiliating for her to have to see someone about it so she decided just to wait, hoping that it might go away by itself. One day she summoned up the courage and saw the school nurse, who just said, "Don't worry about it; lots of teenagers get acne." Gloria was devastated but said nothing. She just silently left the room. That night in bed she cried.

Sexual Activities in Adolescents

Teenagers who are aggressive or hostile usually feel rejected, inadequate, or too dependent. They may get into trouble in numerous ways as they struggle to prove themselves. Drinking, using stronger drugs, and having sex are favorite activities of adolescents who feel inadequate. What better way to prove maturity than to drink a lot and make a baby!

Moral values around sexual activities differ from culture to culture. Even within our own society, various groups view sexual behavior in differing ways. If the peer group believes that only a fool is still a virgin at 15, then there is extraordinary pressure on young adolescents to become sexually active. If sex is considered appropriate only between those who intend to marry, then permissive behavior is looked down on. "Well-adjusted" behavior, then, has to be seen in the context of its subculture. Teenage pregnancies fortunately have declined over the last 15 years but are still too high. This creates a cycle of poverty in which an impoverished single mother struggles to raise a child only to have that child, filled with insecurities of his or her own, also reproduce before reaching full maturity. Pregnancy rates in 15–19-year-olds fell from 117 per thousand in 1990 to 75 per thousand in 2002. For women 14 or younger, pregnancy rates fell from 17.5 to 8.6 from 1990 to 2002. But these figures are still too high. National Vital Statistics Reports (CDC) showed teenage childbearing increased, interrupting the decline from 1991 to 2005. The birth rate for teenagers 15–19 increased by 3 percent.

While the median age for first having sex is 17, we know many teenagers begin having sex much younger. A review of sex education programs by *Mathematica Policy Research* showed that "abstinence only sex education" had no effects on the rates of sexual abstinence in young people or on the average age of first sexual intercourse.

Homosexuality is thought to be practiced by approximately 10 percent of the population. Although having sexual relations with someone of the same sex is considered a sexual preference rather than a mental illness, homosexuality still carries stigma in many communities. This causes some individuals who have homosexual feelings to hide them or to hide their true selves. Suicide attempts are common among adolescent gays who find no acceptance in their homes, schools, or communities.

Health care workers need to cope with their own beliefs because what one believes may have an impact on others. Counseling or guiding an individual whose sexual practices differ from the professional's can be a challenge. If the clinician is straight and must help a person who is exploring his or her own gay feelings, the professional may need to know his or her own limitations. At times, referring a patient to someone more like themselves may be a tremendous help.

In any event, being homosexual in our society is not easy. Professionals must be careful that patients do not perceive referral as rejection. Adolescents are, of course, extremely fearful of homosexuality. Since all adolescents struggle to "fit in," the fear of being rejected by society is enormous. Males whose voices fail to change on schedule or who have the misfortune of a feminine appearance live in dread of being pointed out as a "faggot." Females who don't feel feminine because of their size or shape may shrink with terror at being called "butch." Yet adolescents who know they are gay yearn for acceptance.

These issues are especially pronounced as each adolescent goes through the normal phase of feeling homosexual. Feelings of sexual attraction for a close friend are both pleasant and frightening to the adolescent. Not infrequently, sexual experimentation occurs. In the straight adolescent, such experiments usually occur before age 18 and are short-lived. When they occur frequently and well beyond age 18, the individual is usually homosexual or bisexual. Because bisexuality is also different from the norm, it raises additional obstacles. Acceptance by family and friends is badly needed by all who are different.

Identity and Breaking Away

A 16-year-old boy slams the bedroom door, shouting, "I wear the same crummy clothes everyday! The other kids must think we're on welfare!" A 15-year-old girl exclaims, "Don't you know anything about nutrition, mother! You serve so much cholesterol and salt we'll all be dead in 10 years!" Another adolescent shouts, "Sure, you'll let me get my license if I make the honor roll. By then cars will be out of style and you'll have kept me nice and trapped!"

Identity sense of self; differentiation and separation from parents

These youths are all complaining about the same thing. They are struggling for their own **identity**. They want to **differentiate** or separate themselves from their parents; they are struggling to break away. Rejecting the clothes and food the family provides is symbolic of demonstrating independence. Anger at, or rejection of, family values is another expansion of independence.

Most adults view this as destructive, rebellious behavior. It is difficult for a family to accept the rejection of family values, and the adolescent knows it. The more parental resentment and hostility the youth has built up, the more she or he will try to destroy the values she or he has been raised with. This is the time that a child raised in a religious home is most likely to reject God, whereas the child of agnostics might embrace a cult. Staunch Republican parents may find their child on a Democrat's campaign committee. Avid hunters and fishers may have children joining Greenpeace. And whatever hair style looks best to the folks, John and Jane are certain to wear the opposite.

"The acorn never falls far from the tree," but don't tell a 16-year-old. Although most children eventually end up not too dissimilar to their parents, they will put on a good act of being opposite as they struggle to break away. This is normal and healthy. Without this struggle between parents and child, differentiation would not take place. The child's message is, "I am not you. I have to find my own way of doing things, even if you don't approve of my way." Obviously, this is a difficult time for parents as well as the adolescent. The more the parent understands the dynamics of the adolescent's behavior, the better the family unit survives.

Without parental understanding, rejection of parental values may be carried to extremes and cause real trouble. In homes where the young person's sense of self or identity is weak, pathology may emerge. Such teenagers seek to define themselves by doing what they think will get peer approval. The more impact these approval-seeking behaviors have on parental control, the better they look to such youngsters. The overuse of alcohol gets peer approval. Show the group what a daredevil you can be while intoxicated. If Mom and Dad are devastated, so much the better.

Adolescence is also the prime time for eating disorders to emerge. The young women (primarily) who fall victim to eating disorders define beauty and perfection by the impossible quest for thinness. The only way they know who they are is if they push themselves to be perfect. Naturally no one can define, let alone achieve, perfection. Such young women may make themselves vomit to lose weight. The control issues at the core of most eating disorders also provide fuel for the adolescent. Perhaps Mom and Dad have always been in charge. The young woman with an eating disorder may not have found ways to strike out on her own or to be in charge of herself. With food and purging, she finds a way to gain control.

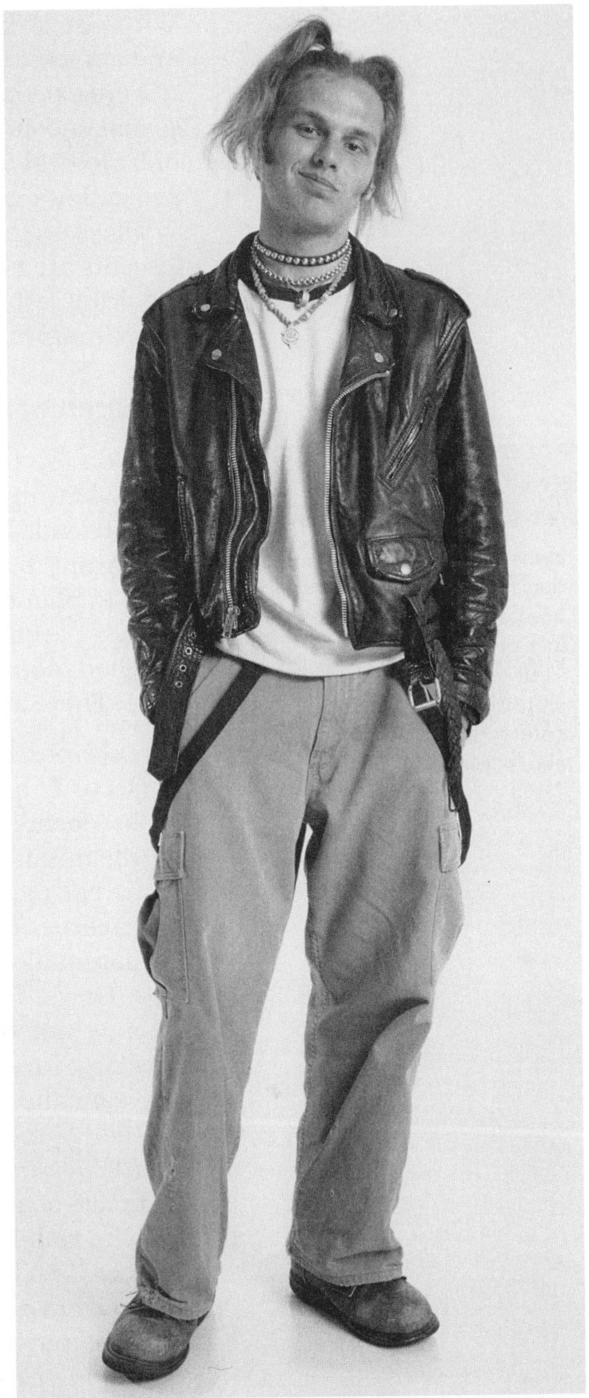

Breaking away

Parental Responsibilities and Dilemmas

The experiments of the adolescent who is struggling to find maturity can spell disaster and create parental nightmares. Does a parent allow a teenager to drive? At what age? How does the parent gauge when the child is mature enough to avoid speeding or drinking and driving? For that matter, what does a parent say to a child about drinking? Can the child be trusted to attend parties where alcohol will be used? Does the parent have to check up on the adolescent's stories? Can the parent believe it when a child says, "Of course Johnny's parents will be home"? How does a parent deal with sex and birth control issues or information about sexually transmitted diseases (STDs) and human immunodeficiency virus (HIV)?

For decades, parents stuck their heads in the sand when it came to the sexual activities of their children. Parents simply could not deal honestly with this topic. If their son got a girl pregnant or if their daughter became pregnant, they would then find some way to cope. Otherwise, **parental responsibility issues** involved the ostrich approach, or "no news is good news."

More recently, enlightened parents have told their adolescents about birth control. Some parents have helped their children obtain birth control and thus avoid unwanted pregnancies. But the issue of adolescents practicing birth control has been fraught with controversy. Much of society believes it is wrong to condone teenage sexual activity. Many people believe teenagers should be told that sex is wrong before adulthood or marriage.

With the advent of HIV, a disease transmitted through bodily fluids, the only absolutely safe advice that can be offered to any age group is to abstain from sexual relationships. More reasonable advice is to have only one sexual partner in a mutually monogamous relationship. Many adult couples now both get HIV testing before sex. The use of condoms is the best protection against STDs, but there is still some risk even with condoms.

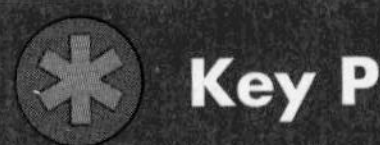

Key Point

Parental responsibility issues trust, driving, drinking, drugs, sex, birth control, venereal disease

With one risk now being a debilitating, as yet incurable disease, parents and adolescents have new nightmares with which to grapple.

Some people think that the chance a condom will be used in initial sexual encounters in teenagers is so small that the contraceptive pill is the most logical choice for preventing pregnancy. The pill, however, offers no protection from STDs.

There are no easy solutions to such parental dilemmas. Remember, adolescents are healthiest when their responsibilities are increased as rewards for prior responsible behavior. Generally, until teenagers reach the age of 18, parents may have to serve as gatekeepers for their children.

Children of Divorce

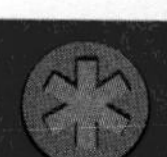
Key Point

Teens of divorce adolescents dealing with parents' divorce; have difficult time because of lack of security, mistrust of family ethic, uncovered repressed anger, playing parents off against each other, and loneliness.

How do the **teens of divorce** cope with separating themselves? Consider first what it is that adolescents need to do. At 15, children want to have their friends accept them. They want to build their own social network. They want to attract and be attracted by a potential sexual partner(s). They want to plan their own future, look forward to a driver's license, and prove to their parents that they are capable and trustworthy.

When mom and dad have separate addresses, additional difficulties may arise. There are several reasons.

1. *Lack of security.* Security is the springboard for independence. If early security has been shaken by divorce, children may have had to become independent at an early age. Often the oldest child is left filling in for the missing parent. Sometimes a grandparent becomes a substitute for a real parent. Conversely, a lack of security may decrease a child's eagerness to break away. Such a child may express fear of leaving a parent alone but in fact may be afraid of aloneness.
2. *Mistrust of the family ethic.* The idea of forming their own families may not hold much appeal to children of divorce. Their attitudes about love and marriage may show a cynicism inappropriate for their years and stage of development. They do not wish to be like the adults they've seen.
3. *Uncovering repressed anger.* Children of divorce may choose adolescence as a time to act out the rage from bygone days. Perhaps Mary, who was 10 when her parents divorced, was overwhelmed by anger at that time but never let her anger show. At 17 she may still be angry and now has a strong urge to demonstrate her rejection of her parents. This urge may elicit far more than the average aggression.
4. *Playing parents off against each other.* Children of divorce may use animosity between their parents as a powerful weapon. Parents who communicate well together have a chance of surviving their children's teenage years. Parents in separate households who do not often speak with each other may become victims of their separateness. The adolescent may use misinformation from one parent to the next to get what she or he wants. When all else fails, such a child may threaten to leave one parent for the other as emotional blackmail for power and control.
5. *Loneliness.* Whether the family is intact or not, teenage isolation is a serious problem. Isolation may mean rejection by the peer group and the family. The family may be too busy to notice. Teenagers generally do not do well when consistently left alone and ignored. Even in homes that give every appearance of normalcy, a family member may feel very

much alone. Isolation and depression contribute heavily to the high suicide rates of adolescents. Although adolescent suicide is rare, it is strongly correlated with depression and substance abuse. Health professionals should be particularly sensitive to an adolescent who talks about suicide and this needs immediate referral.

Treating the Adolescent

Parental Involvement

When health professionals treat adolescents, they need to think to what degree parents should be involved. Some parents will not trust a minor child to represent his or her symptoms accurately. The parent thinks that she or he must be present to explain the child's problems or the health care worker will never understand what is going on. Most treatment plans require parental consent and understanding. However, when, how, and even if parents must be involved can be controversial. Such decisions often depend on the situation. Generally, young patients are more comfortable and open if they are treated alone. Health professionals should be assertive in making some alone time for the adolescent unless the child appears to be afraid or unless the disease or situation make time alone unnecessary.

A health professional who has good communication skills can usually well understand a teenager. Having a parent present may actually lead to confusing or conflicting information. If hostility exists between parent and child, the child may deny the accuracy of what the parent says simply to get even with the parent. Or the child may be hiding information from the parent and will not give the health practitioner accurate information while the parent is present.

Topics that are especially likely to be distorted when the parent is present involve sexual behavior and the use of alcohol and other drugs. A teenage girl was brought to the doctor's office because she had been menstruating for six weeks. It wasn't until her mother left the room that the girl told the nurse she'd had an abortion six weeks before. This example is only one of many that could be used to demonstrate how important it is to question adolescents privately. Also, if parents are present, children may simply be afraid to ask the questions they need to ask.

Gauging Maturity

Health care workers must be careful not to put too much responsibility on the adolescent patient. Don't be fooled into thinking that a physically mature

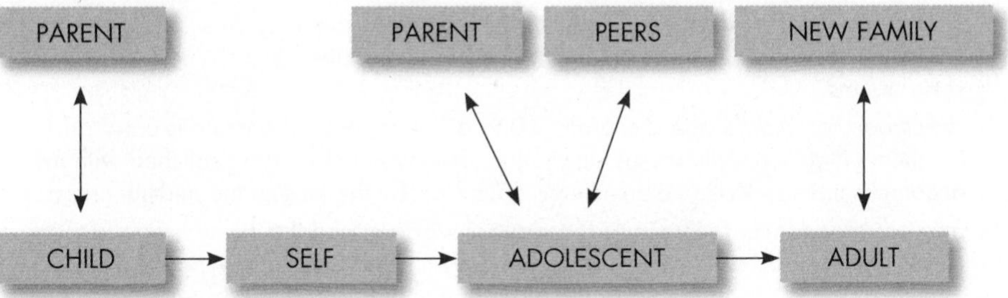

Significant individuals at different developmental stages

person is an emotionally mature one. Take extra care to ascertain to what extent the adolescent is really aware of her responsibilities and the consequences of her behavior. Consider how to appropriately involve parents as a safeguard or backup. Remember that it is easier to work with parents if the treatment does not involve possibly controversial social issues.

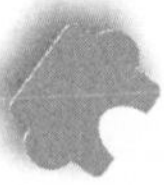

Erik Erikson's Developmental Stages

A popular developmental sequence is Erik Erikson's developmental stages (see Table 6.1). These stages pull together and summarize the stages that have been discussed. The stages extend from infancy into old age, which is dealt with in the next chapter on senescence.

Erikson (1902–1994) was a German-born psychoanalyst with a particular interest in children and developmental stages in life. He emigrated to the U.S., where he studied Native American children and developed an eight-stage model of life stages. Erikson focused more on adolescence, whereas Freud had focused more on early childhood. The eight stages included a "virtue" for each stage, and the "yin and yang" of each stage.

It should be stressed that each stage does not necessarily have a specific age associated with it but more a role in life. For example, adolescence may start at any time from say 11 to 16, especially with the variability of onset of secondary sexual characteristics. The late adulthood stage may start at early retirement at 50 or be delayed by a mid-life crisis at 70 when the adult decides to take on a new career.

Table 6.1 **Erickson's Developmental Stages**

1. *Infancy* (prewalking and speech): The virtue is hope, and the theme is trust versus mistrust. The infant thinks, "Can I trust my parent?"
2. *Early childhood or toddler* (walking): The virtue is will, and the theme is autonomy versus shame and doubt. The child explores its world.
3. *Kindergarten or preschooler* (four to six years old): The virtue is purpose, and the theme is initiative versus guilt. The child plans and does things on its own.
4. *School age* (six to puberty): The virtue is competence, and the theme is industry versus inferiority. The child recognizes disparate abilities of other children.
5. *Adolescence or teens* (puberty, often legally construed as 12 in girls and 14 in boys, to adulthood): The virtue is fidelity, and the theme is identity versus isolation. Erikson was the inventor of the phrase *identity crisis* to explain how adolescents found their place in the world as adults.
6. *Young adulthood:* The virtue is love, and the theme is intimacy versus isolation. The young adult asks, "Who will my friends or lovers be?" and "When will I settle down?"
7. *Adulthood, or middle age* (generally 40 to 60 years old): The virtue is care, and the theme is generativity versus stagnation. The adult asks, "Am I satisfied with my accomplishments? Will I help society?" This may be the time of the mid-life crisis.
8. *Late adulthood* (after retirement): The virtue is wisdom, and the theme is ego identity versus despair. The retiree reflects on the past with satisfaction or with despair.

Summary

This chapter discussed various developmental milestones. While these milestones provide valuable cues, they are best interpreted individually and with caution.

Parents often expect a perfect child. Often they have to be helped to accept a child who does not meet their expectations of perfection. Bonding is a close mutual attachment between infant and parent. Bonding and dependency lead to appropriate body schema and the development of a separate self.

The young infant going through the "terrible twos" becomes negative; this is an expression of the child's sense of autonomy and ability to control its environment. Here, the health practitioner is encouraged to use positive reinforcement and to encourage parents to do the same. Modeling and competence are further ways that young children will develop. Adults are cautioned to remember that the child's expectations may not match the adult's expectations.

The life of adolescents can be difficult as they feel a sense of rejection and struggle to deal with their changing bodies and new found sexuality. Puberty causes rapid physiological and emotional changes. Coping with these changes involves family and social support. The more different the teenager feels, the more support is required.

Differentiating from parents nearly always means a struggle on the home front. No matter how well things are going at home, adolescents fight for independence by rejecting what their parents offer. Rejection is especially difficult for parents when they see their values being trampled. The more problems a child has had in the past, the more he or she is likely to act out aggressively during this breakaway phase. Families survive best when they have provided long-term stability and offer the adolescent emotional support. Adolescents should be rewarded on the basis of responsible behavior.

Parents frequently have a difficult time dealing with teens who are "acting out." The health professional needs to be vigilant about guiding teens as well as the parents on issues of divorce's influence on the teenager, teenage sex, depression, and substance abuse. It is also important to spend time alone with the teen that may now have found his or her place in the world.

Erikson developed an eight-stage model of life stages for infancy through old age. The infant balances trust versus mistrust in bonding with the parent. The toddler cultivates autonomy counterbalanced by shame and doubt. The preschooler develops initiative in the face of guilt. The school child explores industry versus inferiority, and modeling plays a big part in ego development. Adolescents strive to find their own identity. Young adults explore intimacy versus isolation. Middle-aged adults ask whether they are productive versus stagnant, and retirees reflect on life with either satisfaction or despair.

Chapter Review

Key Term Review

Body schema: Child's ability to use her or himself as a reference for understanding the world; sense of self.

Bonding: Close mutual attachment between two people (e.g., maternal or paternal bond, male or female bond).

Developmental assessment: Evaluation by professional to determine child's personal-social, fine motor, gross motor and language abilities.

Developmental delay: Delay in any one of key

milestones, making it necessary in some cases to label child as delayed to get services.

Developmental milestones: Usual age ranges for child to sit, walk, talk, copy shapes, etc.

Differentiate: Making distinct, making separate.

Dyad: A couple, a group of two.

Identity Differentiation and separation from parents.

Intervention: Stepping into health problem issues in order to facilitate change.

Modeling: Child looks up to and imitates actions of another person.

Negativism: Resisting direction from others, leading to separation and understanding self determinism.

Neonate: First four weeks after birth.

Parental expectations: Parental vision of the perfection of their offspring which modifies over time.

Parental responsibility issues: Topics such as trust, driving, sex, birth contol, and venereal disease.

Positive reinforcement: Focusing constantly on identifying appropriate behavior and praising the child for it while avoiding castigating child for negative behavior.

Primary sex characteristics: Changes in reproductive organs.

Reinforcement: Praising child for success, which builds child's self-esteem.

Secondary sex characteristics: Changes in shape, body hair, and voice that accompany primary sex development and that occur at puberty.

Separation anxiety: Anxiety of a young child when separated from person or thing to which it has strong emotional attachment, usually parent but sometimes objects (e.g., security object).

Stigmatized adolescents: Adolescents who are often rejected by peers.

Teens of divorce: Adolescents who have a more difficult time than other teens because of lack of security, mistrust of family ethic, uncovered repressed anger, playing parents off against each other, and loneliness.

Chapter Review Questions

1. Describe the effect of parental expectations on the developing infant, toddler, and young child.
2. How is differentiation related to body schema?
3. What is the difference between developmental assessment, developmental delay, and developmental milestones?
4. Every third time that four-year-old Andrew writes his name, he draws an "M" where the "W" should be. What advice would you give his mother to help her handle this?
5. What are the conflicts for both parents and adolescents that typically arise over differentiation?
6. What is the most important event in a normal teenager's life?
7. Give examples of adolescent stigma.
8. Why do adolescents who are children of divorce have such a difficult time?

Case Study Critical Thinking Questions

1. Read Case Study 6-1. How would you feel if you were Mary or Dan? What would you say to your spouse? How would you feel about the health care system? Whom would you blame?
2. What theory does Case Study 6-2 illustrate?
3. What phenomena do Case Studies 6-3, 6-4, and 6-5 demonstrate?
4. How would you have handled Gloria in Case Study 6-6 if you were her health professional? What would you have said to her? If she just left saying nothing, what would you have said?

References

1. American Academy of Pediatrics. www.aap.org/
2. Developmental Stages. www.aap.org/healthtopics/stages.cfm
3. Developmental Assessment. http://apt.rcpsych.org/cgi/reprint/7/1/32.pdf
4. Developmental Milestones. www.cdc.gov/ncbddd/actearly/milestones/index.html
5. Teenage Pregnancy. www.nlm.nih.gov/medlineplus/teenagepregnancy.html
6. Teenage Pregnancy. www.cdc.gov/nchs/fastats/teenbrth.htm
7. *Statistical Abstract of the United States.* Washington, DC: U.S. Bureau of the Census, 2004.
8. Vital and Health Statistics Series 13, Number 152, June 2002.

Additional Readings

1. Bierman, K. *Peer Rejection*. New York: Guilford Press, 2004.
2. Braselton, T. B., Greenspan, S. I. *The Irreducible Needs of Children: What Every Child Must Have to Grow, Learn, and Flourish*. New York: Perseus Books, HarperCollins, 2000.
3. Craig, G. *Human Development* Upper Saddle River, NJ: Prentice Hall, 1999.
4. Edgette, J. *Stop Negotiating with Your Teen. Strategies for Parenting Your Angry, Manipulative, Moody, or Depressed Adolescent*. New York: Berkley Publishing Group, 2002.
5. Eisen, A. R., Schaefer, C. E. *Separation Anxiety in Children and Adolescents: An Individualized Approach to Assessment and Treatment*. New York: Guilford Press, 2005.
6. *US Teenage Pregnancy Statistics*. New York: Guttmacher Institute, 2006.
7. Horvat, M., Block, M. E., Kelly, L. E. *Developmental and Adapted Physical Activity Assessment*. Champaign, IL: Human Kinetics Publishers, 2006.
8. Jackson R., et al. "Qualitative Analysis of Parents' Information Needs and Psychosocial Experiences when Supporting Children with Health Care Needs." *Health Info Library J* 25:31–37; 2008.
9. Masters, W. H., Johnson, V. E. *On Sex and Human Loving*. New York: Little, Brown and Co., 1988.
10. Pipher, Mary. *Reviving Ophelia*. New York: Ballantine Books, 2005.
11. Schab, L. M. *The Divorce Workbook for Teens: Activities to Help You Move Beyond the Break Up*. Oakland, CA: New Harbinger Publications, 2008.
12. Van Servellen, G. M. *Communication Skills for the Health Care Professional*. Boston: Jones and Bartlett Publishers, 2008.

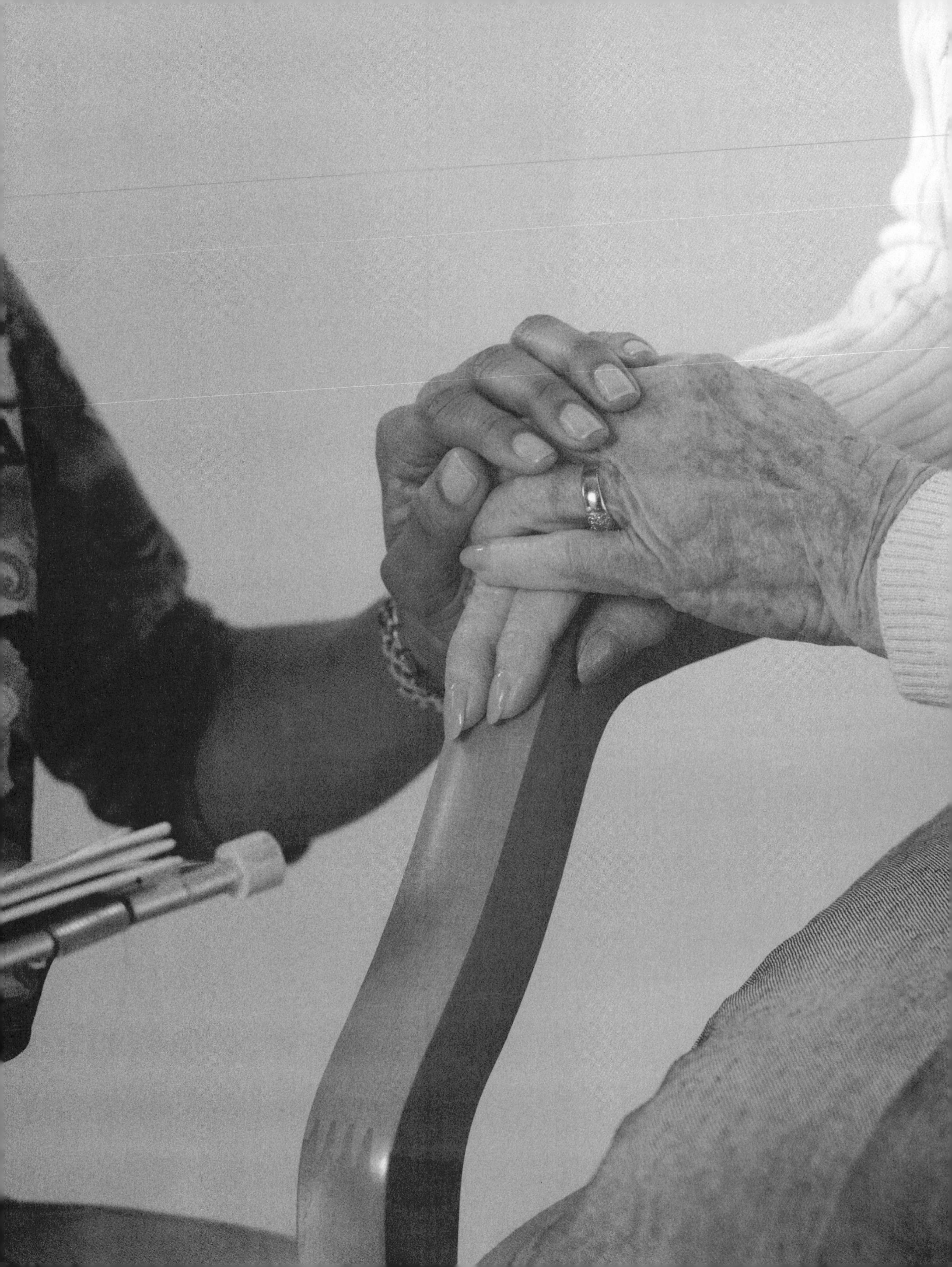

Developmental Issues: Senescence

Learning Outcomes

After reading this chapter, you should be able to:

7.1 Discuss the decrease in biological adaptability in older patients.
7.2 Describe retirement as a time of disengagement from society with opportunities and risks.
7.3 List the top three causes of death.
7.4 Explain dementia and its symptoms.
7.5 List activities of daily living.
7.6 Understand the ways that the elderly are often stigmatized.
7.7 Explain the most feared loss for most elderly patients.
7.8 List six important risk factors for suicide in the elderly.
7.9 Describe advance directives.
7.10 Define the philosophy of Comfort Measures Only.

Key Terms

Activities of daily living (ADL)
Advance directives
Baby boomers
Chronic suicide
Comfort Measures Only (CMO)
Competent
Compliance
Confabulation
Dementia
Dialysis
Disengagement theory
Disorientation
Gastric feeding tube
Health care agent
Incidence of illness
Incontinent
Institutionalization
Intravenous (IV)
Intubate
Lack of biological adaptability
Living will
Parasuicide
Resuscitate
Senescence

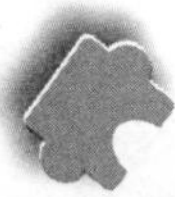

Senescence

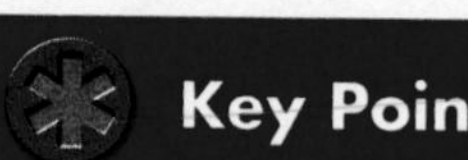

Key Point

Senescence aging, growing old; study of aging.

Senescence is defined as growing old, or aging. In a society that worships youth, it is easy to forget that the older person has a lot to offer. Although the elderly are held in high esteem in many societies, in American society there is a wide range of value for the aged. The first lesson for those working with the aged is to be open to learning from and respecting the older person. Health professionals must remember that, despite the changes and difficulties that can arise, this time of life still offers enjoyment for many of the elderly. Clinicians must remember that older people still have the adaptability to deal with problems because they can draw on their experiences in life.

Health professionals must refrain from thinking of the elderly as collections of "worn out parts" and instead look at issues that are important to older people. People who are over 65 are not necessarily "over the hill." On the contrary, most senior citizens continue to live happy, healthy, and socially useful lives. Remember that 95 percent of people over 65 live at home, many continue to work, and many continue to live active lives. In fact, some people say life begins at 65.

Remember, too, that many people over the age of 65 are high achievers. Consider these examples:

- Grandma Moses started painting at the age of 78. She painted every day for 23 years, until she was 101.
- Harland Sanders retired at the age of 65. He then started a franchise we all know as Kentucky Fried Chicken.

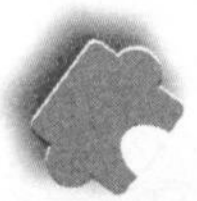

Adaptability

There are two reasons that the body eventually wears out: because of wear and tear and because of built-in obsolescence. It is now known that certain cells are genetically programmed to age in order to ensure reproduction and adaptability. If a species lives too long, it becomes too unadaptable in evolutionary terms.

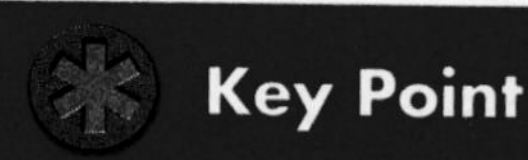

Key Point

Lack of biological adaptability decreased physical, social and psychological ability to change with aging.

In general, elderly people show a **lack of biological adaptability** across the board: physically, socially, and psychologically. A young person quickly adapts to an artificial limb; a 90-year-old may never adapt. Young people make friends easily, something the older person may find difficult. Young people may adapt well to life in close quarters, to a serious infection, to the loss of a loved one, or to surgery. But an older person cannot adapt so easily.

Mentally, this lack of adaptability often manifests as rigidity. Older people are said to be "set in their ways." There may be reasons for this; the elderly person may be afraid of failure, or their rigidity may give them a feeling of security.

Older patients are often physically and *sometimes* mentally slow. By working within their system and showing some patience for their slowness, we can better help them. A physically slow patient usually responds to "take your time" better than to "come on, hurry up."

On the other hand, many older persons have superior adaptive skills when compared with younger persons. The following phrase reflects this:

"He's mellowed since he's gotten older." A lifetime of experience teaches many things, such as better ways of handling people, how to get around shyness, and confidence in one's own decision making.

Much has been made of a fall off of cognitive skills with age. However, the drop in intelligence quotient with age starts several decades before the age of 65. The decline is very small and is more than compensated for by experience. Some areas of cognition apparently improve in older age, for instance, the ability to learn foreign languages.

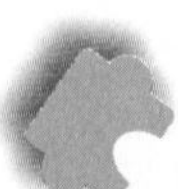

Retirement

Although transition to old age generally begins at 65, there is no biological reason for setting 65 as retirement age. It started in Germany before World War I, when the government decided the old could retire. An investigation into the financial cost of such a program led to picking the arbitrary age of 65, and it has been with us ever since.

Seventy-six million **baby boomers** (born between 1946 and 1964) are now forming a huge retirement cohort and a huge economic and societal force. Retirement changes lifestyle. A place of work—like a family— gives a person a role, a purpose, time-structuring activities, and a circle of friends and acquaintances. Retirement removes all this in one fell swoop. Is it any wonder, then, that retirement often causes stress? If the patient still has a good relationship with her or his spouse or has another work interest after retirement, then retirement may be less of a blow. If retirement has been planned in advance, the shock may be less.

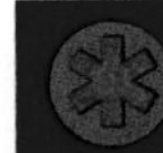

Key Point

Baby boomers people born between 1946 and 1964 in the post–World War II marriage boom.

Who you are before retirement is a good predictor of who you will be after. Sociable, adaptable people with multiple interests are likely to remain so. For many, however, the hobbies and activities they have put off until retirement never materialize. Instead, a sort of boredom or a feeling of having been put out to pasture sets in. Such feelings may turn into a chronic grief reaction. The elderly person may feel that his or her self-image has been stolen and cannot adapt to a new life. Instead of exploring and savoring a new environment, such a person withdraws.

Further fuel is added to the fire when societal attitudes become manifest if retirees see themselves as a burden on society because they are economically unproductive.

If one thinks of the retiree's experience and the lifetime of work she or he did for society, then the retiree becomes a person to be honored. Looking at the retiree in terms of his or her own life situation can help direct the patient. For the patient who is well-motivated to keep him or herself occupied, and who has strong primary relationships and a strong social support system, retirement may be a joy. But the patient who has a poor primary relationship, has lost his or her social support system through retirement, and isn't motivated to occupy his or her time needs help. Volunteer work is often a good choice because it can strengthen self-image. For some, becoming a parking lot attendant, a clerk, or a janitor may fill the bill; others may find such a job damaging to their self-image. Activities that may help are clubs for the elderly, exercise groups, bridge groups, sports, senior centers, religious work, travel, and education.

For the children of the elderly, who often need help with their own children, grandparents can offer considerable stability. Children who have significant relationships with their grandparents often benefit considerably. And grandparents thrive with the young. Grandparents who have contact with their grandchildren remain happier and healthier than do those elderly people who are isolated from the young.

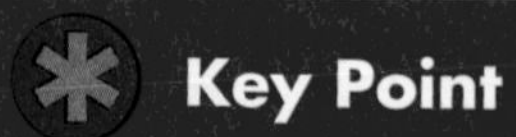

Disengagement theory theory that elderly sever friendships by as part of a more general disengagement from society.

The **disengagement theory** postulated by E. Cumming and W.E. Henry states that the elderly sever friendships as part of a more general disengagement from society.

They may disengage because of stigma. They may feel, for instance, that drawing Social Security and no longer being productive is how they are viewed by the people around them. Thus they may feel that they no longer "belong" in their former circle of friends.

They may disengage because they feel they will soon die. Why bother learning new skills or games or making new friends if they may be dead in a few years anyway? Or their hearing has faded and communication is too much of a struggle.

They may disengage because fewer roles are allowed in friendships. Roles formerly may have included workmate, boss, helper at work, mother, father, or confidante. When the children are grown and live in other cities and the elder is retired, many of these roles are lost.

Discrimination and withdrawal of the elderly may intensify this role reduction. The roles left may be grandmother, grandfather, money giver, or money needer. This smaller number of roles may reinforce the elder's disengagement.

Society has deprived older people of their right to be "village elders." In part, this is because of a socially and geographically mobile society. For some elderly people, however, mobility becomes their salvation. They travel around the country in their mobile homes (when gas prices permit), or they join retirement communities. They may disengage from the rest of society but not from one another.

Primary relationships remain important as people age. Once the children are gone, the husband and wife may draw closer together. But sometimes they withdraw from each other, or they may have problems relating to their now adult children. Couple or family counseling may be essential for seniors in maintaining their primary relationships.

An unmarried person often maintains close ties with a brother or a sister or perhaps a cousin. If such a tie is a person's primary relationship, health care providers need to know about it. If a patient's spouse dies, a grief reaction of some severity is expected. But health professionals may discount grief behavior after the death of a cousin unless they realize that the patient has lost his or her primary relationship.

Separation from others is a part of life. For the child who leaves home, for the parent whose child grows up, or for the person who loses a dear friend, separation drives home a new reality. As the names of more and more old friends appear in the obituaries, the elderly person becomes increasingly aware of separation. The finality of death hits home. Sometimes an elderly person feels regret about what feels unfinished in a relationship with a deceased friend. As time goes by, some older people withdraw from making new friends.

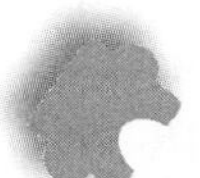

Illness

The **incidence of illness** in the elderly is much higher than for the young. Although people over 65 accounted for only 12.4 percent of the population in 2000, over half of the hospital costs for that year were for people over 65. By 2030, 19.6 percent of the U.S. population will be over 65. People may, however, have an unnecessarily pessimistic view of life expectancy for the elderly. Consider the survival figures in Table 7.1. A 75-year-old woman who thinks she is too old to have an operation might be amazed to learn that, statistically speaking, she may live another 13 years.

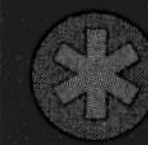

Key Point

Incidence of illness the frequency with which disease occurs; heart disease cancer and strokes top three causes of death. Majority not institutionalized.

Another view many people have of the elderly is that they are all **institutionalized** in nursing homes. Not so. Even in their 90s the great majority of elderly persons are independent. Only about 4.5 percent of people over 65 and 18.2 percent of people over 85 live in nursing homes. The vast majority of elderly who live in nursing homes are there because of dementia, which is discussed later.

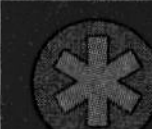

Key Point

Institutionalization the placement of a person in an institution, where he or she eats, sleeps, and spends working time (or what should be working time).

What do the elderly die from? In order of frequency for both men and women over 65, leading causes of death are:

- Heart disease—sudden death, heart attack, and heart failure.
- Cancer—in men, lung, prostate, and intestinal cancer are most common; in women, lung, breast, and intestinal cancer are most common.
- Strokes.

Table 7.1 Life Expectancy by Age.*

Exact Age	Male	Female
0	74.83	79.96
10	75.55	80.58
20	75.88	80.76
30	76.58	81.05
40	77.08	81.46
50	78.46	82.25
60	80.36	83.53
70	83.27	85.72
80	87.62	89.22
90	93.8	94.6
100	102.02	102.36
110	111.11	111.2

*SOURCE: Social Security Administration, 2004.

Table 7-2 presents the 10 most common causes of death in the population.

Although disease is common among the elderly, most elderly people are still independent and healthy even in their 80s and 90s. Disease is a fact of life to some, however, and it is often chronic disease. People who have chronic diseases often have multiple problems. One patient may, for instance, have diabetes, heart failure, high blood pressure, and osteoarthritis. The CDC Health Data for All Ages (HDAA) in 2006 reported a limitation in activity in 7 percent of people under 17, 13 percent of people over 18, 25 percent of people 65–74, 38 percent of people 75–84, and 60 percent of people over 85 years old. Limitation of activity was defined as a long-term reduction in a person's capacity to perform the usual kind or amount of activities associated with his or her age group because of at least one chronic condition.

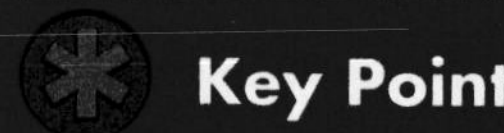

Compliance following directions, especially as given by health care provider for patient health.

Compliance is the ability and willingness to follow directions, especially from the health professional. The medication regime for a person who has multiple problems is often highly complex and may change frequently. It is not uncommon for such patients to be on 5 or even 10 medications on a regular basis. The fact that elderly people can adhere to such regimes is evidence that they have been able to adapt to their illnesses. Younger people would be less likely to comply with or consent to such regimes.

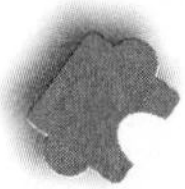

Dementia

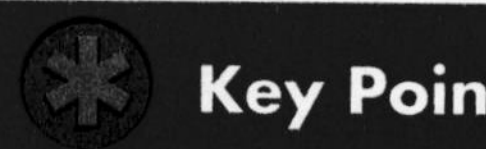

Dementia chronic diffuse mental deterioration in a conscious patient, manifested primarily by memory loss and secondarily by behavioral and emotional changes.

Dementia is a common syndrome in the elderly most often caused by Alzheimer's disease. Many patients describe it as "going senile." The initial problem in **dementia** is a loss of recent memory, which gradually leads to a loss of orientation. The patient cannot remember what year, month, date, and day it is because he forgets what he was told this morning. If he is at home and has lived there many years, he will know it is home. But if he is brought to the hospital, he may say it is the pharmacy or home. He has no memory of being told where he was going.

Table 7.2 Top Ten Causes of Death*

1. Heart disease	27.2%
2. Cancer	23.15%
3. Stroke	6.3%
4. Chronic lung disease	5.1%
5. Accidents	4.7%
6. Diabetes	3.1%
7. Alzheimer's	2.8%
8. Pneumonia and flu	2.5%
9. Kidney disease	1.8%
10. Septicemia	1.4%
11. Others	22.2%

*SOURCE: Center for Disease Control, 2004.

If a health care worker asks a victim of dementia whether she recognizes the worker, she may say yes. If she is asked what the health professional's name is, she may ask, or she may pause and say that the name escapes her at the moment. If asked what the health professional does for a living, she may say something like "sell ice cream." If asked what she had for breakfast, she may say cornflakes, waffles, and coffee. Her attendant may well disclose that she had scrambled eggs, doughnuts, and orange juice.

This example describes disorientation and confabulation, two characteristics of dementia.

Disorientation is a loss of memory for time, person, and place. **Confabulation** is a cover-up in which the patient fabricates, or makes up, events. It is similar to the lying a small boy does in telling his mother where he has been. But the patient with dementia is not lying, nor is the patient using some subconscious defense mechanism. Confabulation is a natural process that is part of dementia and other organic conditions such as stroke or toxic states.

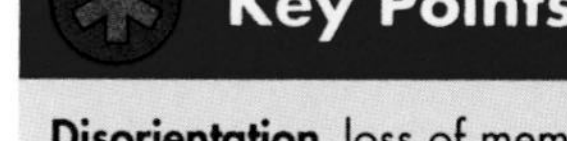

Key Points

Disorientation loss of memory for time, person, and place.

Confabulation cover-up in which the patient fabricates or makes up events.

It is typical for the patient with dementia to cover his or her disorientation. If instead of covering up, however, a patient you work with constantly answers questions that evaluate memory with "I don't care," you must suspect depression. Sometimes, demented patients—often with a tinge of paranoia—will answer questions with such replies as "You think I'm crazy, don't you?" or "You're just trying to trick me, aren't you?" or "I'm not going to answer these questions." Often correct answers will come only from the spouse, who may try to cover up their loved one's intellectual deterioration. (See Table 7.3)

Table 7.3 Memory Evaluation

Question	Testing Recall
Where are we now?	Place
Where is this place located?	Place
What day is it?	Time
What is today's date?	Time
What month is it?	Time
What year is it?	Time
How old are you?	Recent or remote memory
What is your birthday?	Recent or remote memory
What year were you born?	Recent or remote memory
What is your spouse's name?	Recent or remote memory
How long have you been married?	Recent or remote memory
What are your children's names?	Recent or remote memory
Who is president of the U.S.?	General information–memory
Who was president before him?	General information–memory

CASE STUDY 7-1

A health care worker visited a woman with dementia at home. Earlier in her life, this woman had an obsessive-compulsive personality. As the worker walked through the hallway, he noticed that the entire living room was covered with tiny scraps of paper. In places they were several layers deep. They covered the top of the television set, the mantel, the sofa, the chairs, and the tables. On each scrap the woman had written a brief instruction to herself: "Put garbage out this morning." "Put the cat out tonight." "Bundle up the newspaper." On her coat she had pinned another message that said, "Glasses appointment this morning." This woman was mostly disoriented, but as her intellect had started disorganizing, her compulsive personality had obviously started organizing.

Dementia is often accompanied by paranoia, agitation, or depression.

Preservation of distant memory in a dementia victim may trick you into thinking that there is nothing amiss. A person with dementia may be able to recount with amazing detail and accuracy the history of his hometown before World War II, but he does not know where he is or who you are. Recent memory is lost: Patients with dementia cannot remember current affairs or what you or their spouse told them five minutes ago.

As the process of dementia advances, more of the brain is involved and long-term memory begins to be affected. Victims lose the ability to speak, become spastic, and lose control of both bowels and bladder. They cannot coordinate swallowing so that food goes down the wrong way. In terms of the nervous system, the dementia patient gradually becomes similar to a newborn.

The complete scientific story behind dementia remains unknown at present. It is most commonly a result of Alzheimer's disease, a degenerative process that affects the cerebral cortex, the part of the brain that coordinates thinking, memory, and other higher activities of the nervous system. Less common causes of dementia are multiple strokes and Lewy body disease. Sometimes depression can masquerade as dementia (pseudodementia). Occasionally dementia is mimicked by unusual conditions like an underactive thyroid gland, a brain tumor or blood clot pressing on the brain (subdural hematoma), water on the brain (hydrocephalus), or a lack of vitamin B_{12}.

In the early stages of dementia, a victim usually lacks insight but may know that he or she is becoming demented and will compensate with defense mechanisms until no longer aware of what is happening to him or her. Some patients become depressed or withdrawn. They may become cranky so that people will not ask them questions and expose their dementia. Many patients become paranoid. One reason is that when a dementia patient puts an item down, he or she cannot remember where it was placed and so presumes that someone stole it.

The caregiver, usually the spouse or a daughter, has to continue caring long after the patient has forgotten even who the caregiver is. It is extraordinary that so many caregivers are able to continue so long. But, as a senior nurse once said, "Our parents never abandoned us when we were helpless children, so why should we abandon them when they become helpless?"

The example that follows illustrates how difficult dementia is for both the victim and the family (in this case, the spouse).

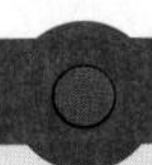

CASE STUDY 7-2

One day Ben noticed that his wife, Sally, 10 years his senior, was becoming less concerned about her appearance. The forgetfulness that he ascribed to inattention, disinterest, or simple absentmindedness was gradually becoming a real problem. The previous evening, when he'd told her to get ready to go out for dinner with friends, she had gone upstairs, but, when he checked on her a few minutes later, he found her sitting on the edge of the bed looking at old photos. When he told her they were going out, she acted as though he had never said that before.

Ben soon discovered that unless he gave Sally a shower, she would never shower herself. Every time she wanted a cookie, Ben had to fetch the cookies, no matter how many times he told her where they were. He found this behavior particularly irritating despite the explanations the visiting nurse patiently offered him. Unable to accept that she forgot within seconds of being told, he would argue with Sally, saying "I already told you where the cookies are!"

Eventually Sally began to get up in the middle of the night and start dressing herself (thinking it was morning). Often she would get upset because she could not pull her stockings on over her head like a pullover (dressing apraxia). Sometimes she got up to go to the toilet and urinated in the clothes hamper (either she could not find the toilet, or mistook the clothes hamper for a toilet).

Ben now had to start cutting back on his own activities. He could no longer count on sleeping through the night. He had to install a high lock on the bedroom door so Sally wouldn't fall down the stairs in the middle of the night. When she did fall or bump herself and a bruise appeared, she would ask repeatedly how she got it.

Sally would turn on the gas stove and leave the oven door open or turn on the iron and leave it on. She began to wet herself more often and to wander outside after dark. Twice she was picked up by neighbors and once by the police when she wandered into the road and couldn't find her way back.

All of this Ben could put up with. But when Sally started accusing him of stealing from her, he could take no more. It was painful enough that the person he once loved was slowly becoming like a toddler who needed constant watching. The suggestion of distrust was too much. When all the rewards for coping seemed to be gone, Ben gave up and put Sally in a nursing home.

Fortunately, dementia affects less than 5 percent of people over 65. More than 95 percent continue to live their lives with their mental faculties fully intact.

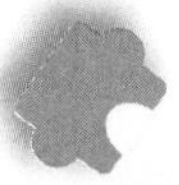

Disability among the Elderly

Because they are susceptible to disease, the aged are more likely to suffer serious disability. An important factor with the elderly is that they suffer from multiple pathologies, so their disabilities compound. Arthritis in the knees and hip caused by aging may prevent walking; cataracts (clouding of the lens of the eye) may cause blindness; weak heart may cause chronic tiredness and shortness of breath. One person may have all these afflictions together. The patient may also live alone, be below the poverty level in terms of income, and suffer from severe obesity.

For the person with such a complex list of disabilities, the important questions are not what sort of arthritis she has or how bad is it or which joints are affected. Rather, they are: Can she walk through the supermarket?

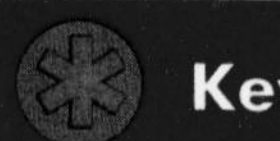

Key Point

ADL acronym for activities of daily living: getting out of bed, walking, dressing, washing, toileting, and eating.

Can she read the labels on cans? Can she get on and off the toilet? These **activities of daily living (ADL)** become the new standard. Whether the patient can do them determines whether she can make it alone. Independence is as important to the elderly as working or parenting is to the young adult.

The elderly also suffer from what has been called the "bits" syndrome. Maybe Uncle Jack can make it with his cane, despite his arthritis, but if his cataracts get worse, he can't see his way so well. If he also gets dizzy because of his high blood pressure pills whenever he walks, he may not make it. Now the nerves to his legs are wearing out and he feels as if he's walking on cotton wool. He has arrived at the point at which he cannot make it on his own. A single disease or symptom may not be too much, but all the "bits" together create a problem. Sometimes one little bit cured can make a remarkable difference, however. Examples include:

- Cutting painfully ingrown toenails and removing corns.
- Getting a new prescription for glasses or simply fixing broken glasses or cleaning them.
- Fixing a hearing aid or getting new batteries for it or removing wax from the ear
- Arranging for a high toilet seat so the patient can use the toilet alone.
- Lining a patient's dentures so they fit better.
- Getting a pair of shoes that fit properly or getting shoes with Velcro, not laces.

Health practitioners need to question the elderly or those who care for them about falls, abuse, continence, ADL, and memory, for such information is seldom offered spontaneously. Falls may cause a loss of independence. The patient may fall and then be afraid to walk because of a fear of further falls. Falls can have medical causes (low blood pressure from too many medications) or be accidental (tripping over a scatter rug or a small dog or slipping on a polished floor or in a wet bathtub).

If an elderly patient's injuries appear to be unnatural or cannot be accounted for, or if the patient seems generally fearful, abuse should be suspected. Approach the patient gently and in private with your questions. (Abuse is discussed in Chapter 12.) Continence and ADL are integral to a patient's independence. Review the ADL activities in Table 7.4 and the short memory evaluation material in Table 7.3 previously presented.

Table 7.4 Activities of Daily Living

Activities of Daily Living	Instrumental ADLs
• Getting out of bed alone • Walking • Toileting • Bathing • Dressing • Eating	• Doing housework • Making meals • Taking medications and arranging appointments • Shopping • Using telephone • Managing money

One important point to keep in mind when working with the elderly is that they require patience. Do not rush older patients. Allow them to prepare themselves with their wigs, dentures, hearing aids, jewelry, and canes. Remember that they may not feel right without these normal aids to their everyday existence. Hospitalized patients in particular should not be expected to respond without these accoutrements of existence. The equivalent to a young person would be to converse with them while they were still in the nude without having had a chance to get dressed.

It is sometimes difficult to strike a balance between treatment of every symptom and dismissal of every symptom with "you're just getting older."

CASE STUDY 7-3

Mrs. Olshaw, aged 84, lived alone in the country. She was a little confused and quite nervous about her nine different medicines for high blood pressure, breast cancer, heart failure, and arthritis. But despite this, she still smoked about 15 cigarettes per day because she said: "I would be nervous if I stopped." She shopped once a week. For eight years she had used Meals on Wheels on which she relied for a daily meal. (She depended heavily on Meals on Wheels and ate virtually nothing else.) One night she was awakened by severe shortness of breath, was admitted to the hospital, and was told that she had had a heart attack. Sandra, a dietitian, was called in to see her for a low-cholesterol diet. Mrs. Olshaw's cholesterol was mildly high at 238 mg percent. What should the dietitian do?

She could treat this new finding or she could view the patient in a different perspective and realize the difficulties a dietary change would involve, then discuss the situation with the physician. The dietitian could tell the physician that since Mrs. Olshaw's Meals on Wheels does not have a low-cholesterol diet, the patient should be advised to avoid butter- and egg-containing products if they are served. Sandra had found out from the patient that she would try to stop smoking if she could keep her Meals on Wheels. In the greater scheme of things a low-cholesterol diet was a low priority for Mrs. Olshaw.

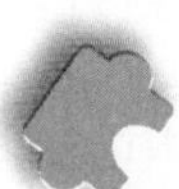

Stigma

Stigma is another important problem in the elderly. Stigma is an integral part of disability and further compounds disability in the aged. Stigma against the elderly is called "ageism," analogous to "sexism" or "racism." East Asian societies and some other groups often honor their elders, but in American society the elderly are not so revered.

Stigma is associated with:

- **Retirement**—As discussed earlier, retirement brings with it a loss of image as a useful and productive member of society.
- **Economic loss**—9.4 percent of the elderly live below the poverty level. This percentage is similar to the percentage of 18–64-year-olds who live below the poverty level.
- **Social isolation**—About 5 percent of people in their 20s live alone, 10 percent of people in their 50s live alone, and 30 percent of people over 65 live alone. Part of this reflects a loss of social mobility with the loss of adaptability in the elderly.

- **Touching**—The elderly, some with wrinkled, spotted skin, are often seen as unattractive, not to be touched. As a health care provider, you will quickly find that a handshake often turns into handholding. Sometimes the therapeutic effect of touching will be the major content of a patient's visit to you. It is also made easier because touching the elderly does not have the social connotation of a sexual advance, which it may with young people. Touching is of particular importance in the elderly, and even more so in terminal illness, HIV, skin disease, and cancer patients. A recent study contrasted formal massage with therapeutic touch in hospitalized patients and found no significant difference.
- **Sex**—Sex among the elderly is rarely seen on television or in the movies. Instead, the elderly are seen in comfortable nightclothes and a safe distance apart. Many jokes are made about the elderly having sex. The expression "dirty old man" attests to a feeling of disgust that the elderly should even be interested in sexual matters. But, although the frequency of intercourse often declines as people age, many elderly people still have sex regularly.

Discrimination and prejudice against the elderly are subtle and pervasive. If health professionals can shake off their prejudice, older patients will respect them, and they can be more effective in helping the patients.

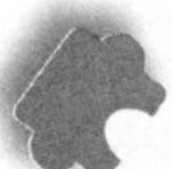

Loss

To the elderly, the loss of friends, acquaintances, and loved ones is a part of life. They also anticipate their own death as the time draws nearer. How an elderly person accepts the prospect of dying depends on many factors. If the person has a disease or disability that makes the quality of life low, death may not be unwelcome. To some, the approach of death is neutral, expected, even longed for. Many old people say they've lived long enough or ask why God doesn't take them. Others say, "I'm no good to anyone" (indicating a loss of positive self-image) or "I've been through enough." Because pneumonia is so often the cause of death, it has been called the old person's friend.

To many old people, loss of independence is actually a greater threat than death. Some individuals fiercely maintain independence even in seemingly dangerous circumstances. An elderly person who has had recurrent dangerous falls may stubbornly insist on continuing to live alone. Even accepting help may signify a loss of independence to such a person.

Loss of health and vigor is also part of aging. Aches and pains last longer and come more frequently. As one elderly physician put it, "It's not the heart that wears out first, it's the knees!" Joint replacement surgeries give new life to many.

As already discussed, the elderly also face loss of occupation, which can be attended by boredom or a state of suspended animation. Another kind of loss can arise from the realization that all those jobs and hobbies the person was going to get done one day are never going to be completed. The elderly may go through the same stages of grief discussed in Chapter 5, but they may also use other coping mechanisms.

Common coping mechanisms for the multiple losses of growing old include:

- **Excessively defensive behavior**—"I don't need a visiting nurse because I don't have high blood pressure."
- **Withdrawal**—An elderly person may shun contact with others because she or he is afraid of exposing loss or suffering further loss or being reported as incompetent and losing independence.
- **False humor**—Such a defense keeps the interaction from getting too close to the real issues.
- **Dependence**—An elderly person usually depends on a spouse or a relative. Occasionally the dependence is on a friend. "I can't be left alone at night," the dependent person may say; "I may have a heart attack." Many older people are not as afraid of dying as they are afraid of dying alone.
- **Depression**—Depression is a state of chronic grief, often with physical as well as mental symptoms. Symptoms can include sleep disturbances, weight loss, mood changes, slowing of thoughts and actions (psychomotor retardation), loss of drive, loss of sexual drive, and somatization (converting concerns to bodily symptoms).
- **Reminiscing—**This behavior can be explained in many ways. The elderly person may be undergoing a review of his or her life in preparation for dying. Reminiscing may allow an older person to reorganize her or his attitudes, which may be beneficial, given the older person's rigid and more obsessive thought system. Or rather than think about her current miserable status, an elderly patient may want to identify with proud moments in her past that she can relive. Reminiscing may also simply be an equivalent of daydreaming—a device to counteract boredom. A rigid person may feel more comfortable thinking about what is familiar. In contrast, the young are more likely to explore with their daydreaming.

  Using reminiscence therapy is something positive health workers can do to help the elderly. Ask about their photos, their life when younger, or their knickknacks. Ten minutes looking at their photo album with them may have immensely more therapeutic benefit than hours of our professional skills.

All humans must face loss. Recall the Kübler-Ross stages from Chapter 5 as you review the common coping mechanisms. The vast majority of elderly people can accept losses as part of life. Most lead fulfilling and satisfying lives. Just take a look at AARP magazine to see how engaged older people are and what fun many of them are having!

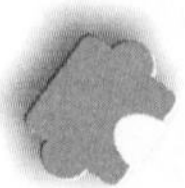

Suicide

The young are sure they are immortal, but the elderly often have a realistic view of death. The older person may say, "I've lived my life. It's time to go now." According to legend, when Eskimos reached this point they walked off into the snow and lay down to die.

Dying from a broken heart is another phenomenon in the elderly. Studies show a high mortality rate in the first year after the death of a lifetime mate.

Some patients seem to decide that they have had enough and simply go downhill. The psyche can cause death, albeit slowly. This is not really suicide but more a subconscious speeding up of the end of life.

An aspect of living and dying that health professionals must keep in perspective is that quality of life is just as important, if not more important, than quantity (length) of life. This same distinction may arise when there is concern about an elderly person's safety. The issue may be loss of independence versus risk of death. Health professionals might help guide a patient by pointing out, for instance, that a fall and a fractured hip would most likely bring a loss of independence, whereas using a walker might enable the patient to hold on to his or her independence.

Religious questions inevitably enter into the older person's attitudes toward dying, often easing the passage from this world to the next. Some cannot wait to join their previously deceased spouse, believing that death will reunite them.

Suicide is common among the elderly. It is the eighth most common cause of death in all age groups. An elderly person may commit suicide for:

- Altruistic reasons: "I've lived my life; I'm just a burden now."
- Loneliness: The person may be tired of living which has increasingly become lonely and a struggle.
- Chronic disease: Diseases take their toll more because they are chronic than because they are severe. The cancer patient may wait for the end to come naturally. The isolated blind man with severe arthritis may be unwilling to wait.

Depression, alcoholism, and accidents also are common among the elderly; all are associated with suicide. Who is to say whether the elderly alcoholic who falls down a flight of stairs does so intentionally? Any attempted suicide must be taken very seriously. The likelihood of repetition and success are very high in those over 40. People over 65 rarely fail to succeed the first time.

The annual incidence of suicide is 11.1 per 100,000 persons (in 2004 that translated to 32,439 successful suicides with approximately 10 times that many unsuccessful attempts). Men are three times more likely to be successful than women, but women attempt suicide three times as often as men do. This means that women may outnumber men by nine to one in unsuccessful suicide attempts. These figures refer mainly to adolescents and young adults, however. Older persons who attempt suicide are all *much more likely* to be successful.

The risk of suicide increases with independent risk factors as listed in Table 7.5.

The elderly widowed retired man living alone is at high risk for suicide.

Not all suicide is death-seeking. The patient may be crying out for help, trying to communicate psychic pain, seeking revenge ("see what you made me do"), or trying to relieve boredom or physical pain.

Suicidal patients often talk about it. Actually, 80 percent of those who commit suicide tell someone about it beforehand. Fifty percent see a health professional within a month of suicide; seven percent see a health professional the same day of suicide.

Health practitioners must ask about suicide. There is no evidence that asking about it puts any ideas in a patient's mind. Ask the patient whether he feels that life is worth living or whether he ever feels like ending it all. If he asks what is meant, respond "Have you ever thought of doing away with yourself?" To establish whether suicide is a real risk for a patient, you must

Table 7.5 Risks of Suicide

- Sex and race: White males over 65 (31.1 per 100,000 in 2004) versus African American females over 65 (0.7 per 100,000 in 2004)
- Separation, widowhood, or divorce
- Living alone or dependent on others
- Unemployment or retirement
- Depression or personal or family history of suicide
- Substance abuse
- Chronic pain, physical or emotional
- Terminal illness
- Loss of body part or function
- Alternative sexual lifestyle
- Career: Physicians (especially psychiatrists), psychologists, police, and attorneys

ask a question such as "Do you think you would ever actually kill yourself?" Once suicidal risk has been established, appropriate referral or hospitalization is mandatory.

The cause of suicide is not "being crazy"; it is not "just in your genes"; it is not just an effect of the weather or the phase of the moon. Rational people commit suicide; psychotic people usually do not. Depression, which may have a genetic influence, may dispose a person to suicide, but most suicides are not the result of depression. Male suicide often is associated with financial concerns for those that will survive him.

Once the crisis that may have precipitated the suicide has passed, the patient is still at risk and needs continued support.

For some, suicide is simply one component of self-destructive behavior. **Chronic suicide** is a term used to describe chronic self-destructive behavior. Examples of such behavior include alcoholism, drug abuse, refusal to comply with an important medical regime, and morbid obesity caused by overeating. **Parasuicide** includes chronic suicide, dying from a broken heart, giving up, and living life dangerously; in some situations, it may include accident proneness. Some of these behaviors are common in the elderly and can be regarded as the equivalent of suicide.

As health professionals, you cannot condone suicide, but you might permit a patient to take risks if it allows continued independence. When a patient develops a terminal illness, she or he may want to be allowed to die should God decide it—a sort of Russian roulette.

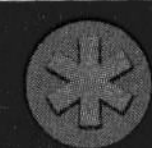

Key Points

Chronic suicide chronic self-destructive behavior.

Parasuicide mentally allowing death when death need not occur, including chronic suicide, giving up, and dying of a broken heart.

Advance Directives

Advance directives include a living will and appointment of a health care agent. The Uniform Rights of the Terminally Ill Act of 1985 allowed people to make a **living will,** which lists patients' wishes should they be unable to express their desires at a later date, and to name a **health care agent**, who can legally decide what efforts should be made on the patient's behalf to

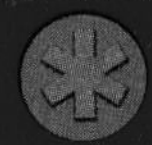

Key Points

Advance directives Living will and appointment of health care agent made while patient is competent in case patient is unable to express his or her wishes in future.

Living will document expressing patient's wishes on resuscitation, intubation, and artificial means of sustaining life like artificial hydration or nutrition.

Health care agent person named in advance to have power of attorney for health care decisions if patient is incompetent.

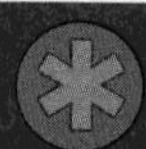

Key Points

Competent person mentally capable of making legal decisions.

Resuscitate Restore to life by squeezing heart, inflating and ventilating lungs, and giving chemicals intravenously after patient has stopped breathing (cardiopulmonary resuscitation [CPR]).

Intubate put tube down windpipe in order to ventilate lungs.

Intravenous (IV) within a vein.

Gastric feeding tube plastic tube usually placed through the abdominal wall into the stomach for artificial feeding

Dialysis circulation of blood through a machine to take over functions of the kidney.

prolong or continue life. This allowed negative euthanasia for the first time in the U.S. However each state has slightly different legislation, and right-to-die issues have been fought out in the legislature in nearly every state.

The Patient Self-Determination Act (PSDA) of 1991 *requires* hospitals at the time of admission to ask patients whether they have an advance directive.

Patients now often draw up living wills while they are **competent**. Competency is the ability to understand relevant risks and alternatives and to make a decision that reflects the patient's own choice. Typically they will list DNR (do not **resuscitate**), DNI (do not **intubate**), and no artificial hydration or nutrition, either through an **intravenous (IV)** or a **gastric feeding tube**. If they wish they may add other desires (e.g., no **dialysis**).

More important than the living will is the appointment of a health care agent (also called health care proxy or health care power of attorney). This health care agent (HCA) form designates one person to be the legal agent to direct what medical decisions should be made. However, if the patient can still express themselves, the agent has no say. The living will, by contrast, is simply an expression of the patient's wishes to guide the health care agent. Health care agents may make whatever decision they think fit. Indeed, not uncommonly, they go against the wishes expressed in the living will.

CASE STUDY 7-4

Hugh draws up a living will that says DNR/DNI. Five years later he is admitted with a huge cerebral hemorrhage and is comatose. The physician says that death is inevitable. His son Albert, also his health care agent, is so shocked that he cannot bring himself to agree to DNR/DNI. Hugh's heart stops beating. Hugh is resuscitated and spends two weeks on the intensive care unit on a ventilator. The problems of a persistent vegetative state are discussed with Albert. Finally Albert agrees to DNR but not to withdrawing the ventilator. A DNR order is entered into Hugh's hospital chart. Two evenings later Hugh's heart again stops beating. This time he is allowed to pass on.

This example shows how the living will applies only when patients' disease processes are unlikely to improve (e.g., permanent paralysis confining the patient to a nursing home), *and* the patient cannot express his or her wishes (e.g., because they are unconscious, unable to speak, aphasic, or too confused). It also demonstrates how the living will may assist the family in their time of denial.

However, if Hugh had had an acute appendicitis, he might reasonably want to suspend the DNR/DNI instructions during his acute illness as he could express his wishes and did not have an irreversible or inevitably progressive illness. His hospital chart would then be labeled "Full Code Status" during the perioperative period.

Resuscitation means that, if the heart and/or breathing stop (called "a code" in hospitals), external cardiac massage, electric shocks to restart the heart, and mouth-to-mouth breathing are performed. Studies vary, but in situations where the patient is severely ill, meaningful survival from resuscitation is less than 10 percent and often less than 5 percent. If the attempt is even briefly successful, a large tube will usually be placed through the patient's mouth into his or her trachea (intubation) and the patient will be

Living Will

DECLARATION

This declaration is made this ______ day of ______________________ (month, year).

I, ______________________, being of sound mind, willfully and voluntarily make known my desires that my moment of death shall not be artificially postponed.

If at any time I should have an incurable and irreversible injury, disease, or illness judged to be a terminal condition by my attending physician who has personally examined me and has determined that my death is imminent except for death delaying procedures, I direct that such procedures which would only prolong the dying process be withheld or withdrawn, and that I be permitted to die naturally with only the administration of medication, sustenance, or the performance of any medical procedure deemed necessary by my attending physician to provide me with comfort care.

In the absence of my ability to give directions regarding the use of such death delaying procedures, it is my intention that this declaration shall be honored by my family and physician as the final expression of my legal right to refuse medical or surgical treatment and accept the consequences from such refusal.

Signed ______________________

City, Country and State of Residence ______________________

The declarant is personally known to me and I believe him or her to be of sound mind, I saw that declarant sign the declaration in my presence (or the declarant acknowledged in my presence that he or she had signed the declaration) and I signed the declaration as a witness in the presence of the declarant. I did not sign the declarant's signature above for or at the direction of the declarant. At the date of this instrument, I am not entitled to any portion of the estate of the declarant according to the laws of intestate succession or, to the best of my knowledge and belief, under any will of declarant or other instrument taking effect at declarant's death, or directly financially responsible for declarant's medical care,

Witness ______________________

Witness ______________________

History
(Source: P.A. 85-1209,)
Annotations
Note, This section was III Rev Stat, Ch. 110 1/2, Para. 703.

APPOINTMENT OF HEALTH CARE REPRESENTATIVE

I understand that, as a competent adult, I have the right to make decisions about my health care. There may come a time when I am unable, due to incapacity, to make my own health care decisions. In these circumstances, those caring for me will need direction and will turn to someone who knows my values and health care wishes. By signing this appointment of health care representative, I appoint a health care representative with legal authority to make health care decisions on my behalf in such case or at such time.

I appoint ______________________ to be my health care representative. If my attending physician determines that I am unable to understand and appreciate the nature and consequences of health care decisions and to reach and communicate an informed decision regarding treatment **my health care representative is authorized make any and all health care decisions for me, including the decision to accept or refuse any treatment, service or procedure used to diagnose or treat my physical or mental condition and the decision to provide, withhold or withdraw life support systems,** except as otherwise provided by law which excludes for example psychosurgery or shock therapy.

I direct my health care representative to make decisions on my behalf in accordance with my wishes as stated in a living will, or as otherwise known to my health care representative. In the event my wishes are not clear or a situation arises that I did not anticipate, my health care representative may make a decision in my best interests, based upon what is known of my wishes.

If ______________________ is unwilling or unable to serve as my health care representative, I appoint ______________________ to be my alternative health care representative.

This request is made, after careful reflection, while I am of sound mind.
_____ /_____ /_____ (Date) X ______________________

WITNESSES' STATEMENTS

This document was signed in our presence by ______________________ the author of this document, who appeared to be eighteen years of age or older, of sound mind and able to understand the nature and consequences of health care decisions at the time this document was signed. The author appeared to be under no improper influence. We have subscribed this document in the author's presence and at the author's request and in the presence of each other.

x ______________________
(Witness)
x ______________________
(Number and Street)
x ______________________
(City, State and Zip Code)

x ______________________
(Witness)
x ______________________
(Number and Street)
x ______________________
(City, State and Zip Code)

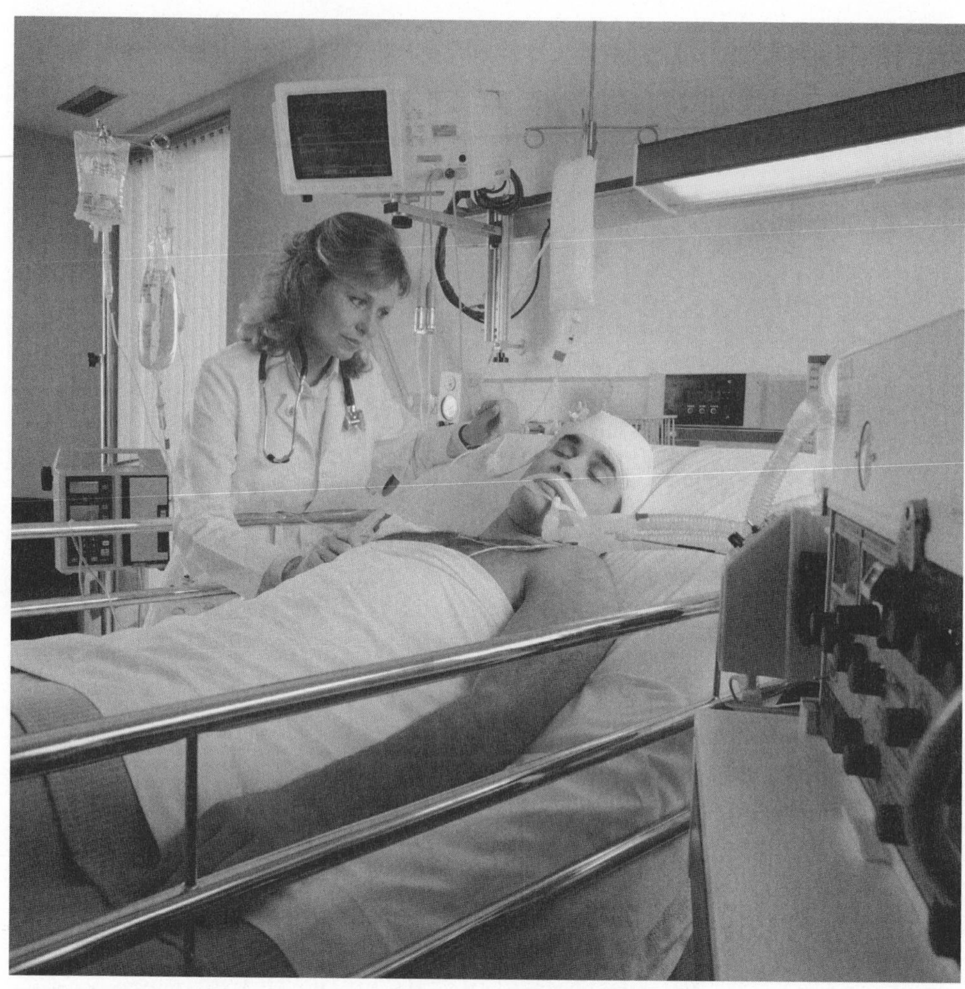

Patient on a ventilator

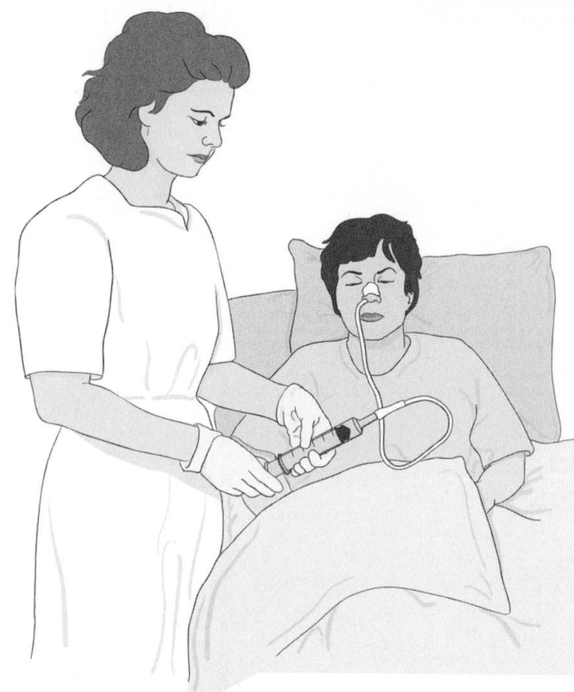

Nasogastric feeding tube

placed on a ventilator to keep his or her breathing going. Sometimes the patient will stay on the ventilator for weeks until someone has to make the agonizing decision of whether to remove the patient from the ventilator rather than continue artificial life support on a patient in a persistent vegetative state (often irreversible brain damage was caused when the heart stopped beating in the first place).

No artificial hydration or nutrition means that, if the patient is unable to express his or her wish *and* is unable to swallow (for example from a stroke or Lou Gehrig's disease), he or she does not want intravenous or gastric tube feeding. Again, this is an expression of the patient's desire, and health care agents may override that wish if, for example, they feel the patient may recover.

Unfortunately, the actual care that takes place depends on the ability of the health care agent to face reality at a time of his or her own anticipatory grief (a difficult situation) rather than the patient's previously expressed wishes. The area of advanced directives is complex and often not well understood even by health care professionals.

Nevertheless, advanced directives are still best discussed with health professionals involved in that field. Forms are available on the Internet or in hospitals or doctors' offices, and patients do not need to see a lawyer for this.

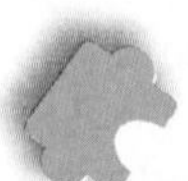

Comfort Measures Only

When illness is advanced and prolonged, there often is a point when the family, health care agent, and caregivers feel the quality of life is gone. Those nearest to the patient believe that extending life further is both cruel and futile.

CASE STUDY 7-5

Matilda, an 88-year-old with Alzheimer's disease, has had recurrent pneumonia caused by aspiration of food into the lungs (Alzheimer's also affects the coordination of swallowing). She is a resident in a skilled nursing facility. Over the last three months she has lost 18 pounds. Matilda can no longer talk or walk and no longer engages in eye contact. She is transferred daily from bed to chair and back again by a Hoyer lift. She is **incontinent** of urine and feces. She needs an aide to feed her specially prepared food to reduce the chances of aspiration. She takes only about 25 percent of her meals, and liquid intake has dwindled to 600 of 800 mL of fluid a day. She has frequent episodes of fever, coughing, and vomiting. The nursing director, Matilda's nurse, speech pathologist, physical therapist, nursing aide, and social worker meet with the family and suggest **Comfort Measures Only (CMO)**.

They explain this means that Matilda will be treated primarily to keep her comfortable rather than to prolong life. Care will be focused on quality of life rather than length of life. For example, when she is short of breath, oxygen will be administered. When she has a fever, Tylenol will still be administered. All distress or symptoms will be treated even if they result in earlier death.

However she will no longer be treated with antibiotics each time she has pneumonia as that would prolong death. All medicines that are preventative only (multivitamins, blood pressure pills, calcium pills, osteoporosis pills, cholesterol pills, B12 shots, etc.) will be stopped. She can now have her favorite foods (once prohibited because of her diabetes), and her finger stick sugar tests four times a day will be stopped, as these also do not provide comfort.

The family listens carefully. Some members are in absolute agreement, saying that this is a great relief for what they feel must be torture for Matilda. They feel her quality of life is zero and that the time has come to say goodbye. However, Matilda's daughter Sarah, who is also her health care agent, is against the idea, saying that she wants to keep Mom going as long as possible. After an hour of discussion, they agree to meet again next week.

The next week Matilda has pneumonia again. She has a fever of 103 and is coughing and vomiting. At the meeting Sarah's brother says to Sarah, "Do you really think Mom would have wanted to live like this?" Sarah breaks down crying and shortly agrees that CMO should be instituted.

CMO keeps the patient from undue discomfort but do not strive to extend life. The decision to offer CMO is a team decision usually involving the family when the patient is no longer able to participate in decision making.

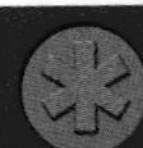

Key Points

Incontinent unable to control flow of urine or feces, resulting in urination or defecation at any time.

Comfort measures only (CMO) treating for comfort only, with no attempts to prolong life (i.e., quality, not quantity, of life).

Summary

Older people have a wealth of experience that historically others looked up to or revered. This is true even though age brings increasing loss of biological adaptability. Such loss is demonstrated physically, socially, and psychologically. Mentally, this lack of adaptability is seen as rigidity. However, despite many seemingly depressing changes, the great majority of the elderly still cope well with life's problems, leading fulfilling lives.

Seventy-six million baby boomers will soon retire. Disengagement theory says that the elderly sever friendships as part of a more general disengagement from society. Without work the retired begin to narrow their contacts. This may be due to stigma, discrimination, or shrinking roles.

Illness is common among the elderly, especially heart disease, cancer, and strokes. Yet, Americans are living longer than ever before and must plan for an old age. Compliance to medications is important to living well.

Dementia is the most common reason for institutionalization to a nursing home. With loss of memory comes disorientation to time, people, and places. A demented person uses confabulation to mask his or her problems for as long as possible. Dementia may also be accompanied by paranoia, agitation, or depression. Dementia is caused by a degenerative process in the cerebral cortex, a series of strokes, or other diseases. Some causes remain unclear.

With disabilities among the elderly, ADLs become the new standard for independence, so jealously guarded by the elderly. Falls are a major concern for loss of independence. Health professionals must also be alert for signs of abuse of the elderly.

Stigma is associated with retirement, economic loss, social isolation, touching, and sex in the elderly. The elderly must frequently deal with loss—particularly the death of family and lifelong friends. Common coping mechanisms are defensiveness, withdrawal, false humor, dependence, depression, and reminiscing.

Suicide is common among the elderly: they may think they are a burden, be tired of living, or be worn out by multiple diseases. Depression, alcoholism, and accidents are also common among the elderly. Attempts at suicide are most common among the young, but the elderly are far more likely to be successful. Suicidal patients will often talk about their suicidal ideation.

Documents called advance directives include a living will, which expresses wishes about "do not resuscitate" status, and appointment of a health care agent to make decisions in the patient's best interest. Both of these can be created while the patient is competent. If the patient does these in advance of needing them, it helps the family and health care workers to understand the patient's wishes.

End-of-life decisions are frequently disregarded by health care agents when the situation demands CMO. These measures keep the patient from discomfort but do nothing to prolong life. The decision for CMO is arrived at when it is clear that the quality of life has completely deteriorated.

Chapter Review

Key Term Review

ADL: Activities of daily living.

Advance directives: Living will and appointment of health care agent made while person is competent in case person is unable to express his or her wishes in the future.

Baby boomers: People born between 1946 and 1964 as a result of post–World War II marriage boom.

Chronic suicide: Chronic self-destructive behavior.

Comfort Measures Only (CMO): Treating for comfort only, with no attempts to prolong life (i.e., quality, not quantity, of life).

Competent: Mentally capable of understanding relevant risks, benefits, and alternatives.

Compliance: Following directions, especially as given by health care provider for patient health.

Confabulation: Cover-up in which the patient fabricates or makes up events.

Dementia: Chronic diffuse mental deterioration in a conscious patient, manifested primarily by memory loss and secondarily by behavioral and emotional changes.

Dialysis: Circulation of blood through a machine to get rid of waste chemicals and circulate the blood back to body—typically taking several hours three times a week for maintenance, or needed only during serious illness

Disengagement theory: Theory that the elderly sever friendships as part of a more general disengagement from society

Disorientation: Loss of memory for time, person, and place.

Gastric feeding tube: Plastic tube usually placed through the abdominal wall into the stomach for artificial feeding

Health care agent: Person named in advance to have power of attorney for health care decisions if patient incompetent.

Incidence of illness: The frequency with which disease occurs; heart disease, cancer, and strokes are top three causes of death. Majority of those diagnosed not institutionalized.

Incontinent: Unable to control flow of urine or feces, resulting in urination or defecation at any time

Institutionalization: The placement of a person in an institution, where he or she eats, sleeps, and spends working time (or what should be working time).

Intravenous (IV): Within a vein.

Intubate: Put tube down windpipe; tube is hooked up to machine called a ventilator to keep breathing going.

Lack of biological adaptability: Decreased physical, social, and psychological ability to change with aging.

Living will: Document written before death expressing patient's wishes on resuscitation, intubation, and artificial hydration or nutrition.

Parasuicide: Mentally allowing death when death need not occur; includes chronic suicide, giving up, and dying of a broken heart.

Resuscitate: Restore to life by squeezing heart, inflating and ventilating lungs, and giving chemicals intravenously after patient has stopped breathing (cardiopulmonary resuscitation [CPR]).

Senescence: Aging, growing old.

Chapter Review Questions

1. Make a distinction between the terms *differentiation* and *disengagement*.
2. List predictors of successful retirement.
3. List adverse events associated with retirement.
4. What is the disengagement theory?
5. Independence is as important to the elderly as working or parenting is to the young adult. Discuss.
6. Why do you think many elderly are more afraid of dying alone than of death itself?
7. Why is reminiscing important for the elderly?
8. What is the difference between advance directives, a living will, and health care agency?
9. What are Comfort Measures Only?

Case Study Critical Thinking Questions

1. From the observation made by the health care worker in Case Study 7-1, we can see how "who we were before the illness" influences who we are during an illness. Please elaborate on this point from the case. What do you think of the client's coping strategy?
2. Read Case Study 7-2. At what point is it advisable to institutionalize a loved one? What stages of loss was Ben, the husband, going through?
3. Read Case Study 7-3. If you were instructed to give Mrs. Olshaw a low-salt, low-cholesterol diet, what

would you have told the patient? What would you have told the daughter? Would you do anything else?

4. Refer to Case Study 7-4. Albert engages you as one of his father's health professionals and asks what you think. What would you say?
5. Refer to Case Study 7-5. When Sarah finally breaks down crying and agrees to comfort measures only, one of your associates objects for religious reasons. How would you handle the situation? What would you say to Sarah? What would you say to the rest of the family? What would you say to your associate who objects?

References

1. Caring for an aging loved one. www.pueblo.gsa.gov/cic_text/family/aging/lovedones.htm
2. Caring for aging parents. www.buzzle.com/articles/caring-for-aging-parents.html
3. Cummings, E., Henry, W. F. *Growing Old: The Process of Disengagement*. New York: Basic Books, 1961.
4. Jones, A. *The National Nursing Home Survey 1999 Summary*. Vital Health Stat 13(152). Washington, DC: Department of Health and Human Services, 2003.
5. Eldercare Locator: www.eldercare.gov/Eldercare.NET/Public/Home.aspx
6. Moody, H. R. *Aging: Concepts and Controversies*. Thousand Oaks, CA: Pine Forge Press, 2010.
7. *Statistical Abstract of the United States*. Washington, DC: U.S. Bureau of the Census, 2004.

Additional Readings

1. Craig, G. *Human Development*. NJ: Prentice Hall, 1999.
2. Glenner, J. A., et al. *When Your Loved One Has Dementia: A Simple Guide for Caregivers*. Baltimore, MD: Johns Hopkins University Press, 2005.
3. Kendrick, K. *Their Rights: Advanced Directives and Living Wills Explored*. London: Age Concern Books, 2002.
4. Masters, W. H., Johnson, V. E. *On Sex and Human Loving*. New York: Little, Brown and Co., 1988.
5. *Deciding to Forego Life-Sustaining Treatment*. Washington, DC: President's Commission for the Study of Ethical Problems in Medicine, 1983.
6. Roy, A. *Suicide*. Baltimore, MD: Williams and Wilkins, 1986.

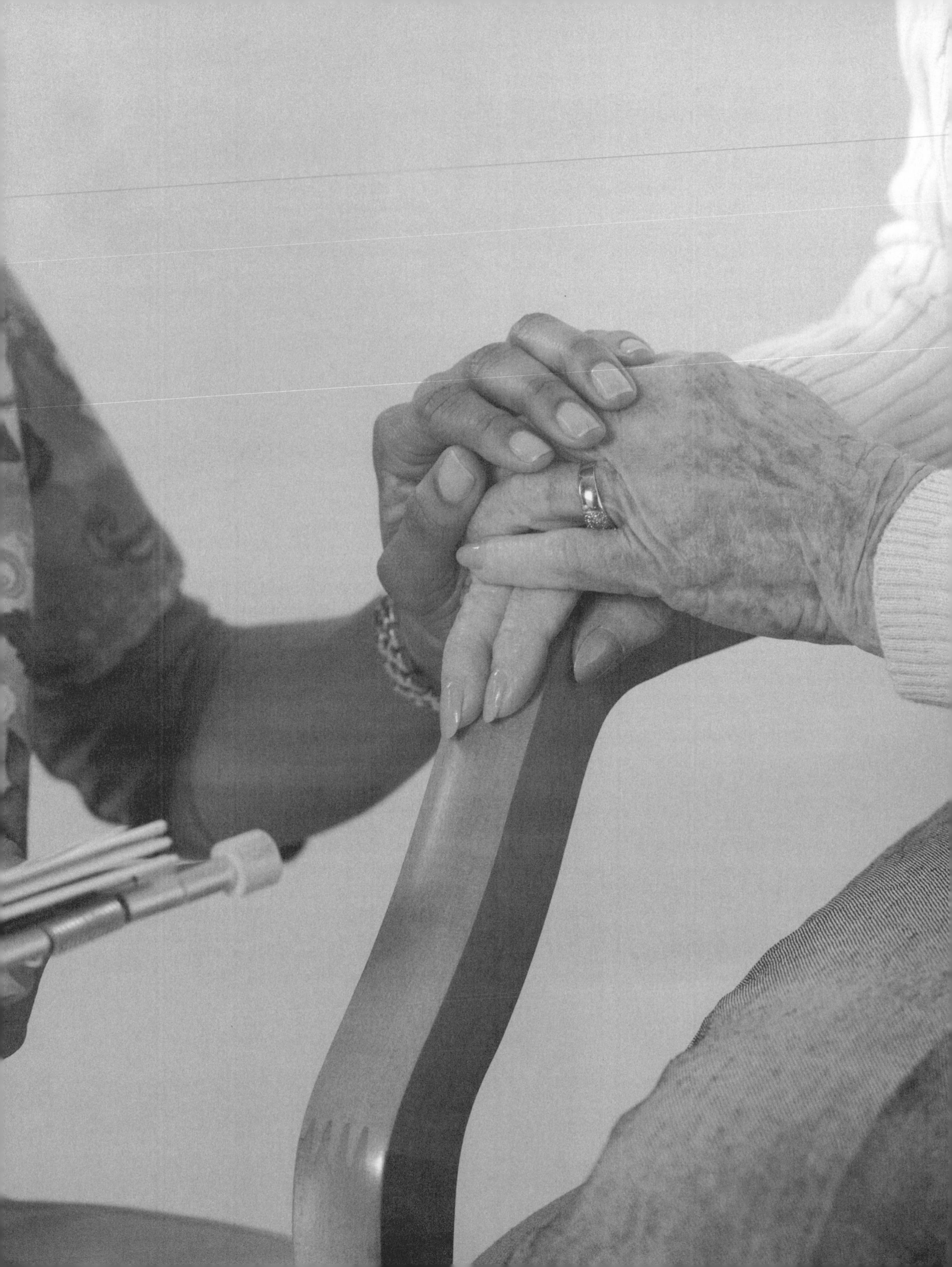

Addiction

Learning Outcomes

After reading this chapter, you should be able to:

8.1 Define addiction and alcoholism and differentiate between addiction, dependence, habituation, tolerance, and cross tolerance.

8.2 Assess genetic, psychologic, and cultural theories of alcoholism.

8.3 Interpret signs of alcoholism in patient examples.

8.4 Discuss the psychologic consequences of alcoholism.

8.5 Recognize the physical consequences of alcoholism.

8.6 Summarize treatments of alcoholism.

8.7 List the major classes of addictive drugs and comprehend the impact of the epidemic of prescription drug abuse.

8.8 Discuss the consequences of substance abuse.

8.9 Describe strategies for the prevention and treatment of substance abuse.

8.10 Recognize the largest preventable cause of death in the United States and describe the addictive factors of smoking.

8.11 Describe the physical consequences of smoking and evaluate the national cost of smoking.

8.12 List the steps necessary to help people to give up smoking.

Key Terms

Addiction
Additive effect
Alcoholics Anonymous (AA)
Alcoholism
CAGE
Cognitive behavioral therapy (CBT)
DARE
Downregulation
Emotional augmentation
Fetal alcohol syndrome
Moderation Management (MM)
Neurotransmitter
ONDCP
Physical dependence
Polysubstance abuse
Problem drinkers
Psychologic dependence
Psychologic treatment
Substance abuse
Substance dependence
Substance use disorder
Tobacco dependence
Treating addiction
Treatments of alcoholism

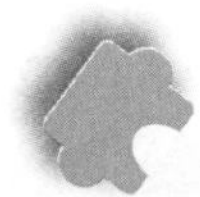

Introduction

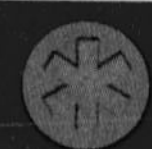

Key Points

Alcoholism chronic consumption of alcohol that continues despite significant interference with a person's physical, economic, or social health.

Addiction physical and/or psychologic dependence on a substance (often leading to drug-seeking behavior).

Alcoholism and all addictions are common problems in health care. **Addiction** refers to physical and/or psychological dependence on a substance (often leading to drug-seeking behavior).

Physical dependence means there is a physical withdrawal syndrome (for example, convulsions, fever, and hallucinations) when the substance is not being used. With physical dependence, there is an actual physiologic "need" for the drug.

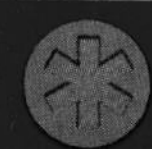

Key Point

Physical dependence physiologic need for a substance, resulting in a withdrawal syndrome when substance is ended.

Tolerance is when a patient needs higher doses of a drug to have the same physical effect. That is, the more a person uses a drug, the more of it he or she needs to experience the same high because the liver has learned to accommodate the toxic substance, decreasing its effect.

Psychologic dependence results in a psychologic withdrawal syndrome, for example, anxiety, insomnia, or an irresistible craving to take more of a drug. *Habituation* is psychologic dependence on a substance. A habit-forming drug causes psychologic dependence but involves no tolerance. Marijuana was once felt to cause only psychologic dependence but is now known to cause physical dependence as well, and many experts believe it is a pathway to more serious drugs and thus it is referred to as a "gateway" drug.

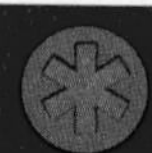

Key Point

Psychologic dependence (habituation) addiction to a substance leading to a psychologic withdrawal (e.g. anxiety, insomnia, irresistible urges to take more of a drug).

An addictive drug is associated with physical and psychological dependence and tolerance. Examples include narcotics, alcohol, and sedatives. Stimulant drugs (and activities like sex, sports, and gambling) flood the **neurotransmitters**, especially dopamine receptors in the limbic system or reward circuits in the brain, and this is felt as pleasure. Intense stimulation causes intense pleasure, with 2 to 10 times the levels of dopamine that normal psychologic rewards do. Suddenly stopping the drug causes withdrawal. But the addicted brain **downregulates** the dopamine receptors in response to such high levels of dopamine so that the abuser's brain now gets even scantier stimulation from normal psychosocial rewards. Additionally, the receptors overworked by drugs can no longer uptake or receive the dopamine or serotonin even when the body has replenished its own supply. The receptors are blocked because of drug damage and may never fully recover, depending upon the amount of damage that has been done. Thus addicts feel flat and lifeless and can't enjoy things they previously could. The mental illness of mania simulates the arousal felt with stimulants.

Other neurotransmitters are also involved in addiction, including glutamate, gamma amino butyric acid (GABA), serotonin, and endorphins.

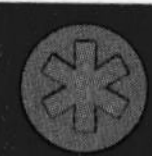

Key Points

Neurotransmitter chemical substance released from nerve endings to stimulate other nerves.

Downregulation decrease in number of receptors (e.g. for dopamine) on surface of cell making it less sensitive to further stimulation (e.g. by dopamine)

Sex, infatuation, and mystical experiences cause dopamine and serotonin stimulation of the neocortex of the brain. Abuse of hallucinogens and schizophrenia also simulate this.

Food, relationships, shopping and TV cause GABA and endorphin stimulation of the limbic cortex of the brain. Alcohol, sedatives, opioids and depression also simulate this.

One drug of particular seriousness is methamphetamine, especially in the West coast, rural West and Midwest. Ten million Americans have admitted to using it, and half a million are currently addicted to it. It totally takes over its users, breaking down or aging their bodies rapidly. Unfortunately, it is easy to manufacture and instantly addictive—a most dangerous chemical.

Addiction occurs in people with psychologic problems, but it is also a biological problem. Animals can be induced to become addicts, so there has to be a nonpsychologic component. Addiction, then, is seen as learned behavior in those with a physiologic predisposition; addicts become physiologically dependent on the substance.

Alcoholism is an addiction that can be defined as a chronic consumption of alcohol that continues despite significant interference with a person's physical, economic, or social health. Important elements of the definition of alcoholism are the following:

- The person's drinking is having significant ill effects on his or her life socially, psychologically, and/or physically.
- The person cannot stop despite the ill effects.

The amount of alcohol the person consumes relates not primarily to any absolute quantity but rather to significant ill effects.

CASE STUDY 8-1

Jack is a 24-year-old white male who lives next door to his parents in rural Colorado not far from a small city. He is self-employed as a carpenter, and his girlfriend and her three children have recently moved out of his house, citing his temper and roughness as their reason for departing. He is seeking counseling following his second arrest for a DWI (driving while intoxicated). (Some states refer to this as DUI, or driving under the influence.) He also has a police record for domestic violence against the girlfriend. His parents attend Jack's second session of substance abuse treatment as they want to be supportive and Jack agrees to involve them. When the counselor uses the word *abstinence* (refraining from alcohol and all nonprescribed substances.) Jack's father becomes very defensive and angry. He makes it clear that he wants his son to be able to "enjoy a few beers" with him after work. Think about Jack as you read this chapter.

According to the National Survey on Drug Use and Health (2007) slightly more than half of all Americans aged 12 or older, or approximately 127 million people, currently consume alcohol. About 23 percent of these people admit to binge drinking at least once in the past 30 days from the time of the survey and just under 7 percent report heavy drinking. There is a "fine line" between problem drinking and alcoholism. Alcoholics typically consume over 50 drinks a week, and **problem drinkers** typically consume 15–30 drinks a week. Approximately 60 percent of drinkers are social drinkers consuming typically fewer than 14 drinks a week. One drink is defined as 0.6 ounces of pure alcohol (e.g., 5 ounces of wine with 12 percent alcohol or 12 ounces of beer with 5 percent alcohol). A preventive model urges moderation.

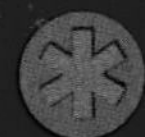

Key Point

Problem drinkers drinkers who have high alcohol consumption but may stop of their own volition without treatment or peer group support. May progress to alcoholism.

Suddenly stopping a drug causes withdrawal. The alcoholic may develop serious withdrawal signs or symptoms from alcohol cessation (e.g., seizures, hallucinations, nervousness, insomnia, or fever). That is why alcohol withdrawal is ideally medically managed in a process known as *detoxification,* which provides medication and nutrition in a safe environment. Alcoholism is viewed as a disease and most sufferers "hit bottom" (have nothing left) before they are able to respond to treatment. At least in "detox" patients are protected physiologically while they go through withdrawal and then may better begin treatment.

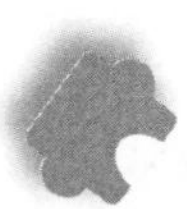

Causes of Alcoholism

Alcoholism has multiple causes, and at the top of the list is an inherited predisposition to alcoholism. Whether personality traits or genetic traits cause alcoholism and whether personality is a cause or effect in alcoholism remains the subject of continuing debate. Societal pressure also has an important impact on alcoholism. *As you read below, how do you see Jack from the above case study matching up against these markers?*

Key Point

Theories of alcoholism genetic, psychological, and cultural.

Genetic Theories of Alcoholism

In 1960, E. M. Jellinek, based on a questionnaire of 98 alcoholics, initiated the disease model of alcoholism. Subsequently the disease/habit debate took over. It is currently felt that genetic factors weigh more heavily in alcoholics and behavioral factors weigh more heavily in problem drinkers.

One study looked at 55 men from alcoholic biological fathers who had been adopted in infancy. By their late 20s, 18 percent were alcoholic (interestingly, their brothers who stayed with their biological fathers had a similar rate). By contrast, 5 percent of 78 adopted men from nonalcoholic parents were alcoholic. Although it involved a rather small sample, this study suggests that alcoholism is partly inherited.

In another study of nearly 1800 Swedish adoptees, two types of alcoholism seemed to emerge. Type 1 was the young person who began drinking seriously in the teen years. They are called *male-limited types*. They were almost all male and became severe alcoholics before the age of 25. About 25 percent of all alcoholics are Type 1. The Type 1 alcoholics had bad work habits and police records; many had been in jail one or more times. This finding suggests that teenagers and children may become addicted very fast. Having an alcoholic parent was an important factor.

The Type 2 alcoholics were called *milieu limited*. Of all alcoholics, 75 percent are Type 2. These individuals drank heavily after age 25, but they had good work and legal records. They often stopped drinking successfully.

According to the genetic theory of alcoholism, the patient starts drinking for the same reason that nonalcoholics do. But the person who becomes an alcoholic may experience more pleasurable effects, loss of control, alcoholic blackouts (loss of memory while drunk), and greater tolerance right

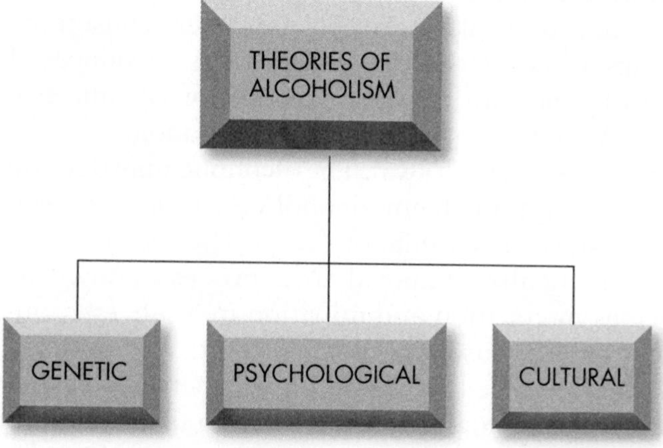

Factors related to alcoholism

from the beginning. These are early constitutional manifestations of alcoholism that lead ultimately to addiction. If there is a strong family history of alcoholism and a young patient has not yet started drinking, it may be helpful to point out that it would be a good idea to remain abstinent.

The following facts support the genetic theory of alcoholism and also account for differing ethnic influences of alcoholism. Those from Jewish backgrounds seem to have a high resistance to alcoholism, with rates of about 1 percent, and their alcoholism starts late in life. Jews have consumed alcohol since antiquity. Northern Europeans started drinking alcohol over the last 1,500 years, have medium resistance, and their alcoholism begins in middle age. North American Indians and Eskimos have been exposed to alcohol for only 200 to 300 years, have alcoholism rates up to 80 percent, and have an early age of onset of alcoholism. These differences suggest that groups most recently exposed to alcohol are constitutionally more prone to alcoholism.

Psychologic Theories of Alcoholism

Psychologic testing of alcoholics frequently reveals a number of common psychologic traits: denial, aggression, depression, regression, low self-esteem, and paranoid thinking. Although a group of traits alone may not cause alcoholism, in a genetically predisposed person it may. Add to this the possibility of peer pressure or a familial culture of drinking, both of which place stress upon an individual to fit in. *Think about the case study of Jack in this context.*

Other psychologic factors can play a part in alcoholism. If a person has difficulty socializing and alcohol has a disinhibiting effect, that person will tend to drink whenever socializing. "Social phobia" is a common diagnosis among alcoholics as the life of Bill Wilson, co-founder of **Alcoholics Anonymous** (AA) brings to light (Cheever 2004). Similarly, if a patient becomes depressed but finds that his mood is elevated by alcohol, he probably will continue to consume because he has discovered a drug that works. He feels better and continues to medicate himself with alcohol. Many alcoholics self-medicate their depressive feelings, not knowing they have a treatable condition such as bipolar disorder or posttraumatic stress disorder. Use of alcohol works only in moderation when the alcohol acts to suppress inhibitions; greater amounts of alcohol result in more depression.

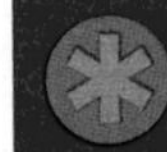

Key Point

Alcoholics Anonymous (AA) informal meetings for recovering alcoholics wanting to achieve and maintain sobriety.

Cultural Theories of Alcoholism

It is easy to dismiss cultural explanations for alcoholism as racism when applied to a culture and as bias when applied to an individual. Nevertheless, differing cultural incidences of alcoholism are real and, as mentioned earlier, American Indians and Eskimos have a high alcoholism rate, the Irish somewhat less, the English lower, the Jews and Chinese lowest.

Culture plays an important part in attitudes toward alcohol consumption. In Portugal, for example, 15 percent of the population lives by making or selling wine. It would be difficult to imagine antagonism toward drinking in such a country.

Some demographic groups—persons in the armed forces, bartenders, salesmen, and entertainers, for instance—have higher rates of alcoholism. Availability of alcohol definitely seems to have an effect. Underage drinking in the United States is very common. In one survey of teenagers, grades

9–12, 50 percent had a drink within the last week; among 12–17-year-olds, nearly 10 percent reported use of illicit drugs (SAMHSA 2007).

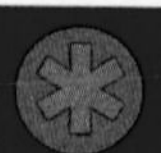

Key Point

Diagnosing alcoholism open-ended questions to test for denial and a review of social history.

Diagnosis of Alcoholism

How does a nurse, psychologist, counselor, social worker, or other concerned health care worker know whether a client is alcoholic?

Because denial is so common and so pervasive as part of the disease of alcoholism, it has diagnostic value. How a person answers the questions "Do you drink?" or "How much do you drink?" is highly important. If the person's answer is straightforward, she or he probably is not an alcoholic. Straightforward answers are answers like these:

"I take two highballs after dinner."

"I drink two glasses of wine about four nights a week"

"I am a teetotaler."

"Oh, I probably have four beers with my friends on Friday nights and maybe an occasional glass of wine otherwise."

"I haven't had a drink for twelve years—it was becoming a problem."

These appear to be upfront answers. The patient may have nothing to hide, or he or she could be an accomplished bluffer, having learned this behavior to protect his or her addiction.

Alcoholics typically underestimate the amount they consume. As a health practitioner, you need to watch for answers that contain an element of denial. Such answers will sound vague, unfinished, defensive, or paranoid. Examples include the following:

"I only drink beer."

"I only drink on weekends."

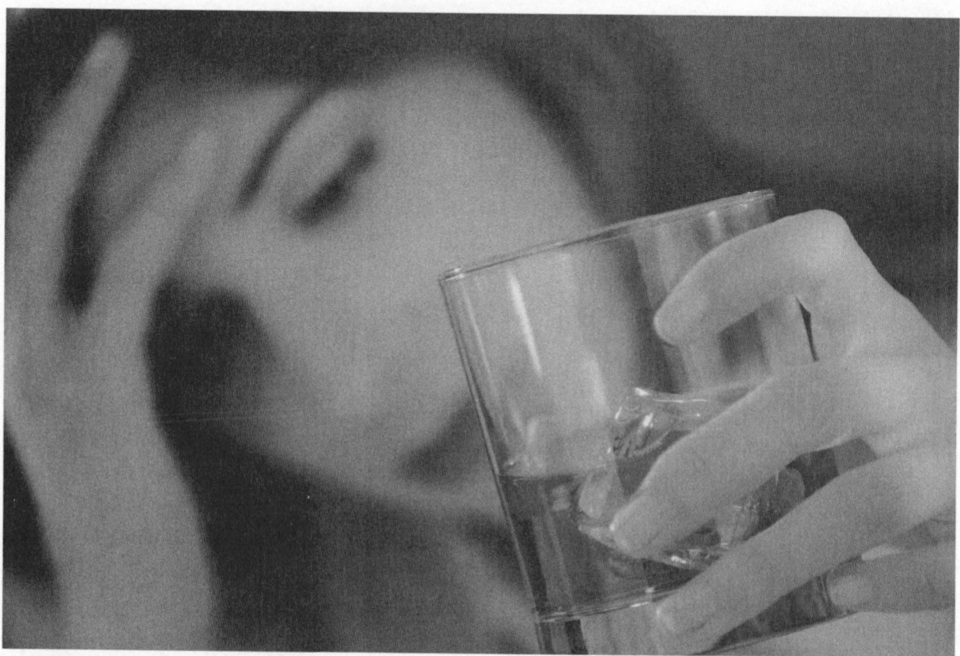

The alcoholic continues to drink, despite enormous physical, psychological, and social consequences.

"Oh, I can hold my liquor all right."

"I don't drink so much now."

"I gave it up."

Answers like these suggest that the patient has something to hide. Note that alcoholics may say, "I gave it up" to cover the fact that they have stopped drinking only a few hours ago.

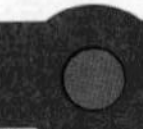

CASE STUDY 8-2

A 40-forty-year old emergency room intake nurse, Amanda, sees a young man with chest pain that sounds like a fractured rib. Amanda has a drinking problem. She asks the patient if he drinks. The patient replies, "Not really." Amanda does not explore the answer any further.

Answers by the patient that seem to provoke another question are significant. All denying-type answers or evasive answers cause the alert health professional to question the integrity of the answer. Asking another question, such as "What do you mean by…" often will produce a revealing response. For instance, asking "What do you mean when you say you only drink beer?" may elicit the reply, "Well, I never touch whiskey. I used to, but I don't anymore." Here the message from the patient is, I can't be an alcoholic because I have stopped the hard stuff. The professional might think just the opposite. This is not proof positive, but it provides a clue on which to focus. Many substance abusers are skilled at misrepresenting their consumption and have no problem blatantly denying their use until they are caught by the law or a toxicology screen of their urine.

The alcoholic patient who admits to having a drinking problem is uncommon, possibly because there is a stigma attached to it and denial is part of the disease. Most will deny that they have a problem, so you must depend on other clues. A history of domestic violence, car accidents, and certainly DUI arrests is most revealing. *Look back at the case study of Jack. The arrests and probably the advice of his lawyer are what bring him in for treatment.*

The following are some of those social, economic, and physical consequences of alcoholism:

- Marital problems, divorce, separation.
- Impotence, sexual problems, sexual abuse.
- Being arrested for drunken driving.
- Violence or emotional or physical abuse.
- Being laid off, losing a job, not doing well at work, not getting along with the boss.
- Bankruptcy, business failure.
- Difficulties with the children, poor school performance.

Another common tool is the **CAGE** mnemonic: Have you ever felt (1) you should *Cut* down your drinking, (2) *Annoyed* by others' comments about your drinking, (3) *Guilty* about your drinking, (4) you needed an *Eye* opener (drink on rising in the morning)? Even one positive answer is significant.

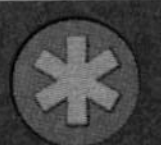

Key Point

CAGE Acronym for key words in the following questions: "Have you ever felt: (1) you should *Cut* down your drinking, (2) *Annoyed* by others' comments about your drinking, (3) *Guilty* about your drinking, (4) you needed an *Eye* opener (drink on rising in the morning)?" One positive answer is significant.

Psychologic Effects of Alcoholism

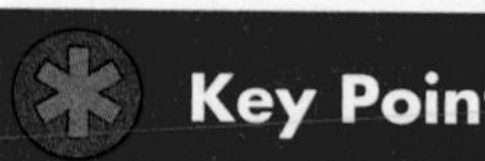

Key Point

Emotional augmentation over-response to normal stress and events.

Defensiveness is another common trait of alcoholics. **Emotional augmentation** refers to an over-response to normal stress and events of everyday life with a lowered threshold for action if a person is concerned about something. For example, a man on the run from the police may think that every phone call or knock on the door is the police. Likewise, when drinking, an alcoholic husband may react with more than usual anger to any comments by his wife. Emotional augmentation seems to be provoked by alcohol. The wife, upset by the anger, may respond with even more anger. A vicious circle can be set up unless the nondrinker learns to moderate her responses. That may sound easy, but in practice is very difficult, and families of alcoholics are encouraged to attend Al-Anon meetings, a sister group of AA that believes that alcoholism is a family disease. *In the case study of Jack do you note any possible emotional augmentation?*

A major effect of alcoholism is that alcohol dominates the alcoholic's life. Thoughts of when, where, and how to get more booze take precedence over everything else, including family, business, economic concerns, and health. Alcohol is more important than food, family, friends, and even self-respect.

The psychologic changes that occur in alcoholism have been divided into first-, second- and third-order symptoms.

First-order symptoms are neuropsychologic disturbances caused by drinking in a person prone to dependence. Examples include loss of control, blackouts (memory defects during drinking), anguish, and emotional augmentation.

Second-order symptoms represent the psychologic reactions of the patient to first-order symptoms. Examples include denial, rationalization, deterioration of self-image, depression, and regression to more childlike behavior (for example, dependent and self-centered behavior). Also, someone who is drunk most of the time between the ages of 20 and 40 will not possess the emotional maturity of a 40-year-old if he or she sobers up at 40. Maturity will be delayed and will be more like that of a 20-year-old.

Third-order symptoms are those that result from the interpretations of friends, therapists, and society. The symptoms include shame, guilt, and conflict from the idea that psychologic defects rather than addiction cause alcoholism. This belief, in turn, leads to primitive behavior by the alcoholic, either against himself or herself or against others, including hostility. Yet alcoholics may *seek* negative labels from friends and provoke fights with their spouses to have an excuse for taking their next drink.

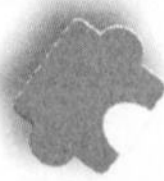

Physical Effects of Alcoholism

There are numerous physical effects of alcoholism. They include:

- A red face and neck.
- A high incidence of cancer of the gastrointestinal tract, pancreas, liver, stomach, head, neck, lungs (because of associated smoking), and bladder.
- Pneumonia.

- Cirrhosis (a serious, progressive scarring of liver tissue).
- Heart disease, especially heart failure and atrial fibrillation.
- Neuropathy (nerves stop working, causing distortion of sensation in the legs, impotence, or imbalance).
- Inflammation of the intestines with vomiting, diarrhea, and internal hemorrhage; also acute pancreatitis, acute hepatitis, and gastritis.
- Trauma from accidents.

Approximately 30 percent of fatal car accidents and more than 30 percent of fatal pedestrian accidents are associated with alcohol. Alcohol plays a role in heart disease, certain cancers, pneumonia, and cirrhosis of the liver. Cirrhosis develops in approximately 10–20 percent of alcoholics. Drownings, fatal fires (usually from cigarettes), and fatal industrial accidents also have a high association with alcohol. And fatal accidents are only the tip of the iceberg.

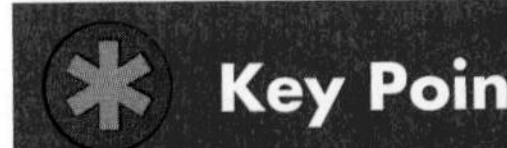

Fetal alcohol syndrome learning and cognitive disabilities and congenital abnormalities in babies of mothers who drink excessively during pregnancy.

Fetal alcohol syndrome occurs in babies of mothers who drink excessively during pregnancy. The syndrome occurs in up to 30 percent of the babies of alcoholic mothers. The effects of the syndrome include learning and cognitive disabilities and congenital abnormalities.

Suicide and homicide are also common occurrences among alcoholics.

Alcoholics may also suffer from Wernicke-Korsakoff's syndrome. Wernicke's syndrome is a confusional state accompanied by double vision and unsteady gait. It is caused by thiamine deficiency, common in alcoholics. If not treated, it may cause persistent memory loss called *Korsakoff's syndrome*.

Withdrawal from alcohol produces another set of physical effects. The best known is delirium tremens, or DTs, which only occurs in about 5 percent of alcoholics, making it quite uncommon. However, the DTs carry a significant mortality. The usual withdrawal syndrome consists of signs of autonomic hyperactivity (fast pulse, high blood pressure, sweating, and fever), anxiety, insomnia, tremor (the shakes), incoordination, and myoclonus (muscle jerking). Some alcoholics develop epileptic seizures (rum fits), hallucinations, delusions, confusion, or delirium upon withdrawal.

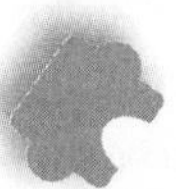

Treatment of Alcoholism

There are many schools of thought on how to treat alcoholism. Some health professionals tell patients to stop drinking because of the threat to physical health and prescribe drugs to help their patients stop. Some encourage alcoholics to talk about their problems. Others work chiefly to try to motivate the patient to enter a treatment program. Professionals in some inpatient treatment centers think that alcoholics need to be coerced (that is, forced) into treatment and that they will become motivated during but not before treatment. Often the spouse and family will precipitate a crisis, forcing the patient to enter the program. Some suggest AA. Motivational interviewing is increasingly being used (see Chapter 9). These varying approaches hold one goal in common: to get the alcoholic off alcohol.

It is because physicians are left to identify alcoholics that so many go untreated. The identification of alcoholism should also be the concern of psychologists, mental health workers, counselors, social workers, physician's assistants, and nurses. Most spouses know whether their partners have drinking problems. Some deny it because they also have a drinking problem, are afraid of the spouse, or fear the stigma should the problem be out in the open. Some health workers may deny it because the patient is middle class, is likable, or is an upstanding member of the community. Or the health worker may have a drinking problem, too.

It can feel intrusive or embarrassing to ask a patient about drinking. Sometimes a patient will react negatively or say something like, "Are you accusing me of being an alcoholic?" A good response would be, "No, I was just wondering whether alcohol had ever been a problem for you." It is all too easy to fall into the trap of glossing over the subject.

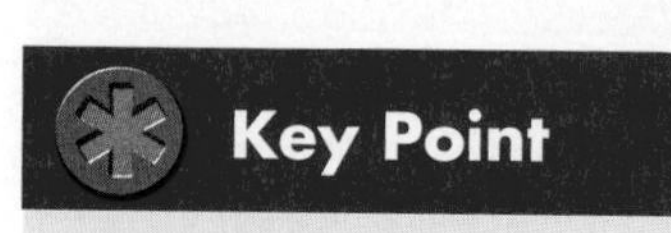

Treatments of alcoholism MI, CBT, AA, individual and group therapy, medication.

The old model of treatment of alcoholism and alcohol problems was one of stigma and disease. The client's reaction was often denial. This model did not address problem drinkers, and coercive treatments alienated many. Current **treatments of alcoholism** are:

- Motivational interviewing using Transtheoretical Model of Change (see Chapter 9).
- Individual and group therapy.
- Cognitive behavioral therapy.
- AA.
- Medication.

Therapy for Alcoholism

Psychotherapy today treats alcoholism but also the associated mental health problems. Alcoholics even off alcohol have two and a half times as much depression, three times as much panic disorder, a higher incidence of anxiety, and four times as much drug abuse as other clients. This dual treatment for mental health and chemical dependency is called *co-occurring treatment.*

Intensive psychotherapy without substance abuse consideration frequently brings too many anxieties to the surface too rapidly. This may cause the alcoholic to start drinking again or exacerbates the drinking. Instead, what is often used is supportive psychotherapy that involves "here and now" approaches such as Gestalt therapy, psychodrama, or transactional analysis. These approaches explore why the patient drinks, the consequences of past drinking, and the consequences of continued drinking. They focus on denial and the role of alcohol in preventing psychologic wellness.

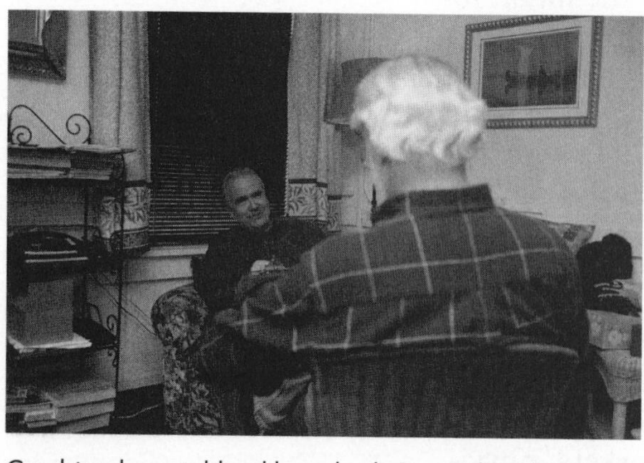

Combined mental health and substance disorders may require multiple treatment methods.

Alcoholic patients may already be receiving psychotherapy for an underlying personality disorder, but the therapist may not be aware of the extent of their drinking. As mentioned earlier, it is classic for those with bipolar disorders to remain undiagnosed and to self-medicate with alcohol.

An alcoholic patient can be both angry and dependent at the same time. If a health professional shows anger with a patient, the patient may have an excuse to drink again. The alcoholic uses anger as an excuse. Psychoanalytic thinking has likened the alcoholic to an infant. Alcoholics are still seeking the security of the bottle and may have immature or arrested personalities. A surprising number of alcoholics remain psychologically dependent on their mothers, and their developmental level may be stalled at the age in which they first began serious drinking. Individualized counseling with a drug and alcohol counselor is often beneficial, as are group meetings.

If an alcoholic's social network consists mainly of other alcoholics or addicts, the therapies we have discussed so far will be of little help. An alcoholic in this situation needs motivation not only to stop drinking but also to change his social network. He needs a place to live and money to live on. Initially, he may be on welfare, but eventually he will need a job and perhaps some education to perform that job. A halfway house, for example, may provide the new community that such a patient needs. AA urges the alcoholic to change "people, places, and things" to get away from the culture of drinking.

Alcoholics Anonymous

Group therapy creates a group or social network that is anti-alcohol rather than pro-alcohol. AA is a special example of group therapy but is managed by peers (all members are themselves alcoholics) rather than health professionals. AA was started in 1935 by an alcoholic stockbroker, Bill Wilson, and an alcoholic physician, Dr. Robert Smith. Bill Wilson became "the face of AA" whereas Dr. Smith believed in anonymity and humility, that the AA member should seek no recognition for good deeds. This philosophy remains a strong value in AA today. The only requirement for membership is a desire to stay sober and help other alcoholics achieve sobriety. AA also insists that the alcoholic accept the fact that she or he is an alcoholic. Other aspects of AA include:

- The motto "one day at a time." This motto encourages the alcoholic to think of staying sober only for today. The motto discourages the alcoholic from starting to drink again because, although the thought of staying sober forever is too hard to accept, for today it is possible.
- Invoking the help of a higher being, not for the sake of a religious conversion but as a way of appealing to a higher, spiritual force.
- Discouraging what the group calls "stinking thinking," or the tendency of alcoholics to use denial, rationalization, or blame to explain things.
- A 12-step program to sobriety that takes members through 12 levels as they recover. Emphasis is placed on attending meetings, a higher power, and finding and using a sponsor. Narcotics Anonymous uses the same 12-step program to achieve abstinence and maintain recovery.
- The well known Serenity Prayer: God grant me the serenity to accept the things I cannot change, courage to change the things I can, and the wisdom to know the difference.

AA has a spiritual side to it. For patients with strong religious beliefs, spiritual help may be instrumental in motivating them to stop drinking. They trust their lives to a higher power.

Al-Anon, the sister organization for partners or families of alcoholics, talks about the three Cs: you didn't *cause* it, you can't *control* it, and you can't *cure* it. As David Sheff says in his book *Beautiful Boy,* "To varying degrees we have spent years accepting and rationalizing behavior in our loved ones that we would never tolerate in anyone else."

Alateen is a similar organization for the children of alcoholics. Adult Children of Alcoholics (ACOA) is a group that supports the grown children of alcoholics, who generally continue to feel the pain of their upbringing.

Moderation Management (MM)

Key Point

Moderation Management (MM) movement for problem drinkers similar to AA for alcoholics.

Moderation Management (MM) is a movement that started in the early 1990s. It offers self-help for problem drinkers, not those who have the most severe problems. The person begins with 30 days of abstinence, and then drinks according to a number of rules; for example, not more than 4 drinks a day or 14 drinks a week for men (3 and 9 respectively for women). MM has zero tolerance for drinking and driving. For the problem drinker, alcohol use is a learned behavior and has become a habit. MM teaches responsibility, empowerment, and moderation.

For the alcoholic, however, the disease holds him or her powerless. Only total abstinence can truly help an alcoholic, although harm reduction exemplified in the rules of MM hold merit if they work to truly reduce harm. The danger occurs when people with alcoholism believe that they can do some drinking (a form of "stinking thinking") and end up in trouble again.

Once an alcoholic has stopped drinking, it may take six months to two years for his or her personality and anxiety level to return to normal. He or she then has to deal with the damage that the alcoholism caused. Problem drinkers may try Moderation Management (MM) first, but if that is unsuccessful, MM may be a stepping stone to AA.

Cognitive Behavioral Therapy

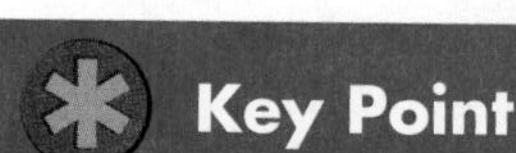

Key Point

Cognitive behavioral therapy (CBT) therapy that deals with thought processes, beliefs, and behavioral responses to influence problematic emotions or behaviors.

Cognitive behavioral therapy (CBT) is used for relapse prevention: The patient learns to identify and correct problematic behavior, explores the positives and negatives of use, and identifies and anticipates high-risk

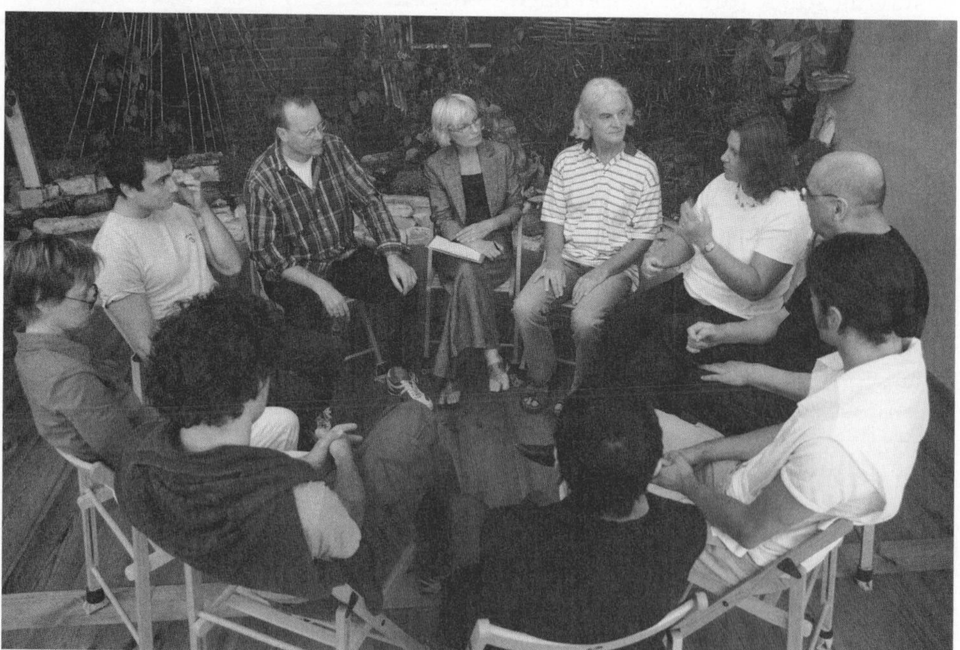

Group therapy may deal with thoughts, beliefs, and behaviors.

situations. CBT is also used to help adolescents control the stimulus that leads to drug use and control feelings and thoughts leading to the urge to obtain the drug. "Priming" refers to a simple slip, but there comes a "choice point" when the user has the opportunity to decide whether the primed brain is going to progress to an orgy of drug use. Cues associated with previous drug use like smell, visual cues, music, and sex are also important to recognize and avoid. Once the addict is primed or presented with a cue, he or she might call his or her sponsor or counselor or work out at the gym as alternative ways of coping.

Drug Treatment of Alcoholism

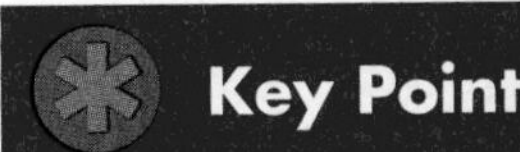

Medications for alcoholism vitamins, Antabuse, Revia, Campral, and Topamax.

Using sedatives during acute withdrawal is common in hospitals. Sedatives diminish withdrawal symptoms like agitation, insomnia, hallucinations, and tremor. Giving sedatives to an outpatient is a two-edged sword, however. On the one hand, sedatives may reduce withdrawal symptoms, make life more comfortable, and help the alcoholic sleep. On the other hand, the alcoholic may become addicted to sedatives, which is known as *sedativism*. Further, taking sedatives clouds thinking and can interfere with vigilance in staying sober. Sedatives also can mask the issues that the alcoholic must deal with in order to stay sober. And sedativism is particularly a problem because of *cross-tolerance*, meaning that tolerance to the sedatives may have occurred as a result of alcohol abuse even though this sedative was never before used by the patient. In other words, within a group of drugs, tolerance may develop to another drug without a history of use of the second drug. Thus the most successful treatment for alcoholics avoids all medications with addictive properties, and the person in recovery must be vigilant to avoid these medications even when facing surgery and/or dealing with pain. In fact, health professionals should suspect a potential relapse when a client in recovery is "med-seeking." This person should receive immediate treatment, call his or her sponsor, and return to meetings.

Vitamins are commonly used for alcoholics. Wernicke-Korsakoff's syndrome, one of the serious complications of alcoholism, can be prevented by administering thiamine and vitamin B1. Alcoholics frequently obtain most of their calories from alcohol. A diet that is deficient in certain vitamins accounts for some of the physical effects of alcohol.

Disulfiram—trade name Antabuse—is a medication that causes no symptoms when taken alone but causes severe side effects when taken with alcohol. Patients, who drink while taking Antabuse feel flushed, turn red as though they will explode, and feel very nauseated. Although Antabuse therapy is appropriate for some patients, it does not cure alcoholism. It simply makes patients feel terrible if they drink (a form of behavior modification that focuses on punishment). If a patient is feeling desperate enough for a drink, she or he may simply wait for the last Antabuse to wear off before drinking.

Another drug, Naltrexone—trade name Revia—blocks the pleasurable effect of alcohol, which may also help some clients.

Acamprosate—trade name Campral—blocks some receptors while activating other receptors in the brain, helping patients with alcohol dependence to have a decrease in cravings.

Topiramate—trade name Topamax—is a seizure medicine that has been shown to increase abstinence rates in alcoholics.

Some psychiatrists prescribe antidepressants if they think a patient is suffering from both alcoholism and depression, but all mood-altering medications are a risk in treatment for substance abuse.

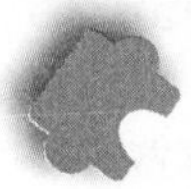

Classifications and Statistics on Addictive Drugs

The general principles of addiction are similar for both alcohol and other addictive drugs.

Substance abuse: significant distress, manifested by three of the following: a failure to fulfill school, work, or parenting obligations; hazardous use (e.g., driving); recurrent substance-related legal problems (e.g., DUI); or continued substance use despite persistent or recurrent social or interpersonal problems.

Substance dependence: significant distress manifested by three of the following: tolerance; withdrawal; increasing consumption; desire to quit; excessive time spent on abuse; fewer social, occupational or recreational activities; or continued use despite knowing physiologic and psychologic effects.

Substance use disorder: includes substance abuse and, more seriously, substance dependence.

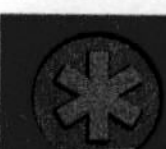

Key Points

Substance abuse significant distress, with three of the following: failure to fulfill school, work, or parenting obligations; hazardous use (e.g. driving); recurrent substance-related legal problems (e.g., DUI); continued substance use despite persistent or recurrent social or interpersonal problems.

Substance dependence significant distress, with three of the following: tolerance; withdrawal; increasing consumption; desire to quit; excessive time spent on abuse; less social, occupational, or recreational activities; continued use despite psychological or physical effects.

Substance use disorder a disorder that includes substance abuse and, more seriously, substance dependence.

Addiction depends on many factors, and addictiveness varies from drug to drug. The so called "gateway drugs" like cannabis and alcohol escalate drug risk taking as they relax inhibitions. Users are more likely to take greater risks under their influence. Recently, prescription drugs such as Ritalin have been found to be "gateway" for teenagers who learn to misuse their prescriptions to get high.

Alcohol and heroin are two different extremes of addictive drugs. Heroin kills a large number of addicts early on. By contrast, alcohol claims a smaller proportion of addicts early on and claims them much later. However, during a long period of alcoholism, much harm can be done to the family and others.

Cannabis (marijuana), cocaine, and some hallucinogenic drugs used to be referred to as "recreational drugs"; however, this is obviously a euphemism, as they are really addictive substances. What may seem to start out as recreation rapidly becomes dependent.

Low doses of sedatives and hypnotics promote relaxation; high doses induce confusion or sleep; even higher doses may produce coma, and, if enough is consumed, death may result from paralysis of the breathing muscles as controlled by the lower brainstem. Sedatives and hypnotics include alcohol, the anti-anxiety agents, and a wide variety of other drugs.

Any combination of the sedatives and hypnotics has the potential to be lethal. This is called the **additive effect**. Drinking combined with taking diazepam (Valium) or a barbiturate puts the user at a high-level dose because of the combined effect of these drugs. The additive effect accounts for many accidental deaths each year from overdose. Sometimes the overdose is an active suicidal act that results from the depression and despair common in addiction.

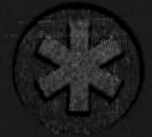

Key Point

Additive effect the cumulative effect of sedatives (e.g., alcohol, benzodiazepines, barbiturates, sleeping pills, inhalants, anesthetics).

Substances: Category and Name	Examples of *Commercial* and Street Names	DEA Schedule*/ How Administered**	*Intoxication Effects*/Potential Health Consequences
Cannabinoids			
hashish	boom, chronic, gangster, hash, hash oil, hemp	I/swallowed, smoked	*euphoria, slowed thinking and reaction time, confusion, impaired balance and coordination*/cough, frequent respiratory infections; impaired memory and learning; increased heart rate, anxiety; panic attacks; tolerance, addiction
marijuana	blunt, dope, ganja, grass, herb, joints, Mary Jane, pot, reefer, sinsemilla, skunk, weed	I/swallowed, smoked	
Depressants			
barbiturates	*Amytal, Nembutal, Seconal, Phenobarbital:* barbs, reds, red birds, phennies, tooies, yellows, yellow jackets	II, III, V/injected, swallowed	*reduced anxiety; feeling of well-being; lowered inhibitions; slowed pulse and breathing; lowered blood pressure; poor concentration/* fatigue; confusion; impaired coordination, memory, judgment; addiction; respiratory depression and arrest; death *Also, for barbiturates—sedation, drowsiness*/depression, unusual excitement, fever, irritability, poor judgment, slurred speech, dizziness, life-threatening withdrawal *for benzodiazepines—sedation, drowsiness*/dizziness *for flunitrazepam*—visual and gastrointestinal disturbances, urinary retention, memory loss for the time under the drug's effects *for GHB*—drowsiness, nausea/vomiting, headache, loss of consciousness, loss of reflexes, seizures, coma, death *for methaqualone—euphoria/* depression, poor reflexes, slurred speech, coma
benzodiazepines (other than flunitrazepam)	*Ativan, Halcion, Librium, Valium, Xanax:* candy, downers, sleeping pills, tranks	IV/swallowed, injected	
flunitrazepam***	*Rohypnol:* forget-me pill, Mexican Valium, R2, Roche, roofies, roofinol, rope, rophies	IV/swallowed, snorted	
GHB***	*gamma- hydroxybutyrate:* G, Georgia home boy, grievous bodily harm, liquid ecstasy	I/swallowed	
methaqualone	*Quaalude, Sopor, Parest:* ludes, mandrex, quad, quay	I/injected, swallowed	
Dissociative Anesthetics			
ketamine	*Ketalar SV:* cat Valiums, K, Special K, vitamin K	III/injected, snorted, smoked	*increased heart rate and blood pressure, impaired motor function/* memory loss; numbness; nausea/vomiting *Also, for ketamine—at high doses, delirium, depression, respiratory depression and arrest* *for PCP and analogs—possible decrease in blood pressure and heart rate, panic, aggression, violence*/loss of appetite, depression
PCP and analogs	*phencyclidine;* angel dust, boat, hog, love boat, peace pill	I, II/injected, swallowed, smoked	

(continued)

Hallucinogens			
LSD	*lysergic acid diethylamide:* acid, blotter, boomers, cubes, microdot, yellow sunshines	I/swallowed, absorbed through mouth tissues	*altered states of perception and feeling; nausea;* persisting perception disorder (flashbacks) *Also, Also for LSD and mescaline—increased body temperature, heart rate, blood pressure; loss of appetite, sleeplessness, numbness, weakness, tremors* *for LSD—persistent mental disorders* *for psilocybin—nervousness, paranoia*
mescaline	buttons, cactus, mesc, peyote	I/swallowed, smoked	
psilocybin	magic mushroom, purple passion, shrooms	I/swallowed	
LSD	*lysergic acid diethylamide:* acid, blotter, boomers, cubes, microdot, yellow sunshines	I/swallowed, absorbed through mouth tissues	
Opioids and Morphine Derivatives			
codeine	*Empirin with Codeine, Fiorinal with Codeine, Robitussin A-C, Tylenol with Codeine:* Captain Cody, schoolboy; (with glutethimide) doors & fours, loads, pancakes and syrup	II, III, IV, V/injected, swallowed	*pain relief, euphoria, drowsiness/*nausea, constipation, confusion, sedation, respiratory depression and arrest, tolerance, addiction, unconsciousness, coma, death *Also, for codeine—less analgesia, sedation, and respiratory depression than morphine* *for heroin—staggering gait*
fentanyl and fentanyl analogs	*Actiq, Duragesic, Sublimaze:* Apache, China girl, China white, dance fever, friend, goodfella, jackpot, murder 8, TNT, Tango and Cash	I, II/injected, smoked, snorted	
heroin	*diacetylmorphine:* brown sugar, dope, H, horse, junk, skag, skunk, smack, white horse	I/injected, smoked, snorted	
morphine	*Roxanol, Duramorph:* M, Miss Emma, monkey, white stuff	II, III/injected, swallowed, smoked	
opium	*laudanum, paregoric:* big O, black stuff, block, gum, hop	II, III, V/swallowed, smoked	
oxycodone HCL	*Oxycontin:* Oxy, O.C., killer	II/swallowed, snorted, injected	
hydrocodone bitartrate, acetaminophen	*Vicodin:* vike, Watson-387	II/swallowed	
Stimulants			
amphetamine	*Biphetamine, Dexedrine:* bennies, black beauties, crosses, hearts, LA turnaround, speed, truck drivers, uppers	II/injected, swallowed, smoked, snorted	*increased heart rate, blood pressure, metabolism; feelings of exhilaration, energy, increased mental alertness/*rapid or irregular heart beat; reduced appetite, weight loss, heart failure, nervousness, insomnia *Also, for amphetamine—rapid breathing/*tremor, loss of coordination; irritability, anxiousness, restlessness, delirium, panic, paranoia, impulsive behavior, aggressiveness, tolerance, addiction, psychosis
cocaine	*Cocaine hydrochloride:* blow, bump, C, candy, Charlie, coke, crack, flake, rock, snow, toot	II/injected, smoked, snorted	
MDMA (methylenedioxy-methamphetamine)	Adam, clarity, ecstasy, Eve, lover's speed, peace, STP, X, XTC	I/swallowed	
methamphetamine	*Desoxyn:* chalk, crank, crystal, fire, glass, go fast, ice, meth, speed	II/injected, swallowed, smoked, snorted	

(continued)

methylphenidate (safe and effective for treatment of ADHD)	*Ritalin:* JIF, MPH, R-ball, Skippy, the smart drug, vitamin R	II/injected, swallowed, snorted	*for cocaine—increased temperature/*chest pain, respiratory failure, nausea, abdominal pain, strokes, seizures, headaches, malnutrition, panic attacks *for MDMA—mild* *hallucinogenic effects, increased tactile sensitivity, empathic feelings/* impaired memory and learning, hyperthermia, cardiac toxicity, renal failure, liver toxicity *for methamphetamine—aggression, violence, psychotic behavior/* memory loss, cardiac and neurological damage; impaired memory and learning, tolerance, addiction *for nicotine*—additional effects attributable to tobacco exposure; adverse pregnancy outcomes; chronic lung disease, cardiovascular disease, stroke, cancer, tolerance, addiction
nicotine	cigarettes, cigars, smokeless tobacco, snuff, spit tobacco, bidis, chew	not scheduled/smoked, snorted, taken in snuff and spit tobacco	
Other Compounds			
anabolic steroids	*Anadrol, Oxandrin, Durabolin, Depo-Testosterone, Equipoise:* roids, juice	III/injected, swallowed, applied to skin	*no intoxication effects/*hypertension, blood clotting and cholesterol changes, liver cysts and cancer, kidney cancer, hostility and aggression, acne; in adolescents, premature stoppage of growth; in males, prostate cancer, reduced sperm production, shrunken testicles, breast enlargement; in females, menstrual irregularities, development of beard and other masculine characteristics
Dextromethorphan (DXM)	*Found in some cough and cold medications; Robotripping, Robo, Triple C*	not scheduled/swallowed	*Dissociative effects, distorted visual perceptions to complete dissociative effects/*for effects at higher doses see 'dissociative anesthetics'
inhalants	*Solvents (paint thinners, gasoline, glues), gases (butane, propane, aerosol propellants, nitrous oxide), nitrites (isoamyl, isobutyl, cyclohexyl):* laughing gas, poppers, snappers, whippets	not scheduled/inhaled through nose or mouth	*stimulation, loss of inhibition; headache; nausea or vomiting; slurred speech, loss of motor coordination; wheezing/*unconsciousness, cramps, weight loss, muscle weakness, depression, memory impairment, damage to cardiovascular and nervous systems, sudden death

Source: National Institute of Drug Abuse

**Schedule I and II drugs have a high potential for abuse. They require greater storage security and have a quota on manufacturing, among other restrictions. Schedule I drugs are available for research only and have no approved medical use; Schedule II drugs are available only by prescription (unrefillable) and require a form for ordering. Schedule III and IV drugs are available by prescription, may have five refills in 6 months, and may be ordered orally. Some Schedule V drugs are available over the counter.*

***Taking drugs by injection can increase the risk of infection through needle contamination with staphylococci, HIV, hepatitis, and other organisms.*

****Associated with sexual assaults.*

Please study the following table, taken from the National Institute on Drug Abuse, which lists commonly abused drugs: cannabinoids, depressants, dissociative anesthetics, hallucinogens, opioids, stimulants, and others.

In addition to the review of illicit drug use (see next section), The Substance Abuse and Mental Health Services Administration (SAMSHA) reported in 2006 that misuse of prescription drugs exceeds the combined use of *all* street drugs except marijuana. This phenomenon is possible because prescription drugs are so available, quality controlled, and easy to steal. Further, desperate addicts will find ways to gain access to methadone, suboxone, and any other medications with a street value so that they may sell what they do not use. Medical personnel must always be vigilant to protect against drug-seeking behavior among addicts.

Key Points

Statistics on drug abuse 8 percent of Americans used illicit drugs in last month, and 9 percent are drug or alcohol dependent. Abuse twice as common in males as females.

Polysubstance abuse use of two or more different substances of abuse—very common. Alcohol, marijuana, sedatives, opioids and cocaine are top five.

Statistics on Drug Abuse

In 2007 8 percent of the U.S. population over 12, or 20 million people, used illicit drugs within the last 30 days when surveyed, and 9 percent were classified as substance-dependent (including alcohol). Of these 17 percent abused drugs alone, 14 percent abused drugs and alcohol, and 67 percent abused alcohol alone. In 2007, 12.5 percent of males over 12 and 5.7 percent of females had a substance abuse disorder (see oas.samhsa.gov for more details). Many drug takers use more than one drug; this is called **polysubstance abuse**. The following details "drug use in the last month for Americans over the age of 12:"

- Marijuana 14.4 million (5.8 percent)
- Sedatives 6.9 million (2.8 percent)
- Opioids 5.2 million (2.1 percent)
- Cocaine 2.1 million (0.8 percent)
- Hallucinogens 1 million (0.4 percent)
- Methamphetamine 500,000 (0.2 percent)

Attitudes regarding drug use are important. In 2007 90 percent of 12- to 17-year-olds felt their parents would strongly disapprove of trying marijuana, and they were less likely to try because they knew their parents disapproved. Eighty-three percent disapproved of peers using marijuana. Of substance abusers, only 6.4 percent felt they needed treatment.

How does addiction start? In 2007, 14.5 percent of 12- to 17-year-olds were approached by drug pushers. Thirteen percent of people over the age of 18 who first used marijuana before age 14 were substance abusers. By contrast, only 2.7 percent of those who first used marijuana when they were older than 18 became substance abusers. The drug most used first by people over age 12 was marijuana (56 percent), followed by opioids (19 percent), inhalants (11 percent), sedatives (8 percent), stimulants (4 percent), hallucinogens (2 percent), and cocaine (1 percent). These drugs and the prescriptions of others are easily available.

The reasons given for trying drugs were curiosity, peer pressure, and feeling a need to have a life experience. But once drugs are started, self-control can fizzle as brain function changes as a direct result of the drug.

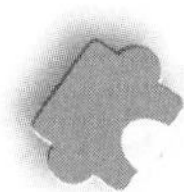

Effects of Substance Abuse

Mental Effects

Drug abuse is associated with anxiety and depression. People may use drugs to numb their symptoms, but the abuse often compounds their problems and prevents their getting proper treatment. Stimulants increase anxiety, especially panic disorder, and exacerbate insomnia. Alcohol, sedatives, and opioids numb depression for a few hours but over weeks cause depression. Hallucinogens and stimulants may precipitate psychoses. Drug abuse is associated with unemployment, imprisonment, family disharmony, cognitive dysfunction, poor decision making, financial loss, and sex that would otherwise not have occurred.

Physical Effects

Sex that would not otherwise occur may be associated with human immunodeficiency virus (HIV), hepatitis B and C, sexually transmitted diseases, and sexual assault. Intravenous drug abuse may be associated with HIV, hepatitis, and *Staphylococcal endocarditis* (fatal inflammation of the heart valves related to intravenous drug use). Drug abuse is highly correlated with smoking and alcohol, which are both also health risks. Overdoses may lead to seizures, respiratory depression, pneumonia, confusion, coma, and death. Cocaine may cause heart attacks and strokes. Drugs may also cause fetal impairment, auto accidents, suicide, and violence.

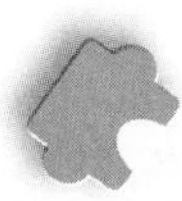

Medical Use of Marijuana and Legalization Issues

Medical use of marijuana is currently permitted in 13 states: Alaska, California, Colorado, Hawaii, Maine, Michigan, Montana, Nevada, New Mexico, Oregon, Rhode Island, Vermont, and Washington. Generally this means that these states have decriminalized the state penalties for use, possession, and cultivation of marijuana by patients who possess written documentation from a physician that their health might benefit from its medical use. Arizona also allows physicians to prescribe marijuana under limited circumstances, and Maryland allows "medical use" as a defense in court.

In most of these states, this right to written permission is open enough, with many ailments being covered, that some experts believe it will lead to decriminalization for all. Others, especially in California as it faces mounting deficits, see legalization as a way for states to capture tax revenues that would spin off from the legal sale of this drug. Such economic forces are very persuasive, but the risk of allowing yet another harmful substance to be legal is a great concern to those in health care and those trying to raise healthy kids in impoverished neighborhoods. It should also be noted that the need for Marijuana Anonymous (a 12-step program like AA) has increased in states that have legalized medical use of marijuana.

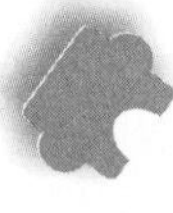

Prevention and Treatment of Substance Abuse

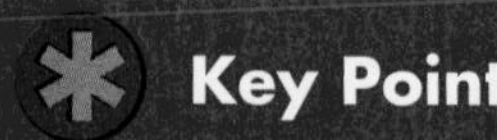

ONDCP Office of National Drug Control Policy.

The Office of National Drug Control Policy (**ONDCP**) gives grants to schools for drug testing and for education of teachers, parents, and students, and it runs the National Youth Anti-Drug Media campaign. The ONDCP also promotes drug-free communities, workplaces, and prisons.

School-based random student drug testing has been used in over 4,000 schools nationwide. It helps students defy peer pressure and provides early intervention for "at risk" students. The programs use a public health approach to decrease community addiction rates. The U.S. Supreme Court upheld the constitutionality of random student drug testing in 1995 and 2002.

Risk factors for drug abuse are:

- Substance-abusing peers or parents
- Absent or problem parents
- Poor parental discipline
- Permissive parents
- Student absenteeism
- Access to prescriptions
- Aggressive behavior in adolescents
- Poor social skills
- Poor academic performance
- Transition periods in adolescent life
- Early drug use

Method of drug administration is also a potent risk factor. Smoking, snorting, or intravenous injection lead to greater addictive potential because of the sudden bolus effect to the brain creating a sudden rush of pleasure.

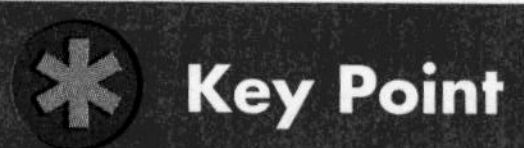

DARE Drug Abuse Resistance Education.

The national **DARE** program, or Drug Abuse Resistance Education, is active all over America. These prevention programs are aimed at parents, teachers, and adolescents. They stress peer relationships, parental relationships, academic support, self-assertiveness, and drug-resistance skills. Programs are more effective in multiple than single settings: school, church, clubs, sport programs, and media. Sometimes particular drugs become popular within specific communities, and this can be targeted.

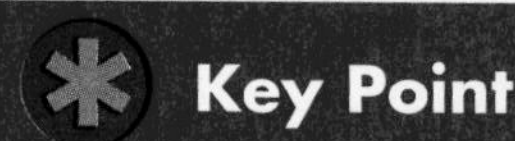

Treating addiction detoxification, psychological treatment, medications.

In **treating addiction**, first detoxification must take place. Successful long-term treatment cannot take place while the patient is still using the drug. Withdrawal may cause physical or psychologic symptoms. This may require in-patient hospitalization and in-patient treatment. Detoxification has little effect on long-term treatment but must still occur first. It is the period of getting over physical withdrawal when an addict stops a drug and may require medical management for health safety.

Medications may be used for ongoing management (e.g., methadone or suboxone for opioid abuse). But most treatment is psychologic.

The ONDCP lists the following facts about drug abuse treatment:

- No single treatment works for all people.
- Treatment needs to be readily available.
- Effective treatment attends to multiple needs of people, not just their drug use.

- The patient may need several other services.
- Treatment must be continued long enough; usually more than three months.
- Individual, group, and behavioral treatment are important.
- Co-occurring mental health issues should be treated, and medication may be needed.
- Treatment need not be voluntary to be effective.
- The patient should be monitored continuously during treatment.
- The patient may need checking for HIV, hepatitis, tuberculosis, and sexually transmitted diseases.

Psychologic Treatment

Psychologic treatment uses motivational interviewing, which is discussed in Chapter 9, CBT reviewed under treatments for alcohol, group, individual, and multiple approach models. Narcotics Anonymous (NA) is the 12-step program derived from its fellow program, AA, which addresses the needs of those addicted to drugs. It functions as AA does, and many of its members use AA meetings interchangeably with NA on the basis of meeting availability. These meetings are especially important to assist those in recovery to maintain their abstinence.

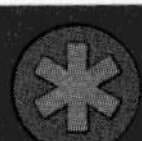
Key Point

Psychologic treatment motivational interviewing; CBT; group and family, individual, and multiple approach models.

Group therapy is used with the addict, family, peers, and other drug users. Individual therapy may involve supportive psychotherapy and individual drug counseling. The Matrix Model, in which the therapist is teacher and coach developing a positive Rogerian relationship and using that relationship to change behavior, also uses many therapies in combination. There should be continuous drug testing of the urine with consequences for relapse. Some programs use tokens or money rewards (e.g., for drug-free urine).

Pharmacologic Treatment

While the addict is being treated for chemical dependency, co-occurring mental health issues should also be checked for and treated. Pharmacologic treatment includes treatment of opioid addictions with methadone or suboxone. Several medications may help alcoholics, as discussed earlier, but hallucinogens and stimulants at present are not treatable with medications.

Methadone, when given at the right level, will eliminate the physical cravings for heroin. Suboxone does the same thing with the added benefit that suboxone users become ill if they attempt to mix suboxone with heroin. However, addicts learn to skip a dose when social cravings are strong, and then they appear to be using suboxone but actually are still addicted to the illicit substance. Conscientious treatment programs will do frequent urine toxicology screens to determine whether prescribed or street drugs are in their patients' systems.

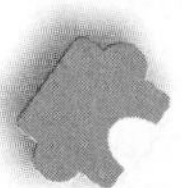

Smoking

Smoking is the single largest cause of preventable death and ill health in the United States today. It is the most common addiction, and it is an enormous problem. Twenty-one percent of Americans smoked in 2006. Nicotine is highly addictive.

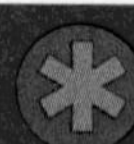

Key Point

Tobacco dependence continued consumption of tobacco, which the patient cannot control despite significant physical, economic, or social side effects. Smoking is the single largest preventable cause of death—438,000 deaths a year in United States.

Tobacco dependence is a continued consumption of tobacco, which the patient cannot control, despite significant physical, economic, or social side effects. One difference between tobacco dependence and alcoholism is that the economic consequences for smoking are not immediately apparent (except for spending about $2,000 a year for a one-pack-a-day habit). Also, the physical side effects of smoking, such as health problems like cancer, heart attacks, and emphysema, are usually serious later in life. Often at this late stage the patient's perception is "If I'm going to die from cancer, at least don't take my cigarettes away." Smokers do not perceive future physical problems as a reason not to smoke. It is tragic that smoking-related cancers do attack some individuals in their early 30s, and these often result in death.

The social consequences of smoking—pressure from peers, having to go to smoking areas, and higher insurance rates—remain the largest reason why people do not smoke. However, in a society in which about one-fifth of the citizens smoke, it is difficult to say it is unacceptable behavior. Unlike drug abuse, it is a legal act. The attitude that smoking is acceptable behavior is the reason that smoking is not perceived as a significant addiction like heroin.

The Physical Effects of Smoking

Key Point

Adverse effects of tobacco carbon monoxide, nicotine, tar, passive smoking.

Withdrawal from smoking causes craving, anxiety, insomnia, impaired attention, a preoccupation with the actions associated with smoking, headaches, and gastrointestinal disturbances. Research shows that even when people smoke low-nicotine cigarettes, they smoke to maintain their serum nicotine levels. They do this by increasing the number of cigarettes they smoke or by stopping up the filter holes to raise the nicotine concentrations of the smoke they inhale. There can be no doubt that nicotine is a psychoactive substance.

Cigarettes exert their adverse effects in four main ways:

- Through carbon monoxide levels, which accelerate arteriosclerosis (hardening of the arteries), which can cause heart attacks, strokes, and gangrene.
- Through nicotine, which, via its psychoactive effects, reinforces and habituates the user to smoking.
- Through irritants in tar that may cause chronic lung disease (emphysema and bronchitis or cancer).
- Through passive smoking, for example, standing in the same room with someone who is smoking. The health of the babies of pregnant smokers also is jeopardized through passive smoking.

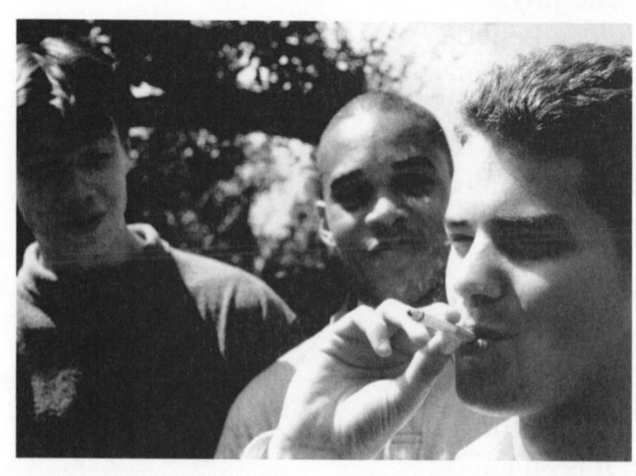

Young people experiment with smoking but will take 14 years off their lives if they become addicted to cigarettes.

There are some two million deaths in the United States each year. Of these deaths, approximately 438,000 are caused directly by smoking. In other words, tobacco causes almost one in five deaths in the United States. Half of all Americans who continue to smoke will die from smoking-related diseases. Thirty percent of deaths from cancer and 90 percent of deaths from chronic lung disease are caused directly by smoking. On top of this are

About 438,000 U.S. deaths attributable each year to cigarette smoking*

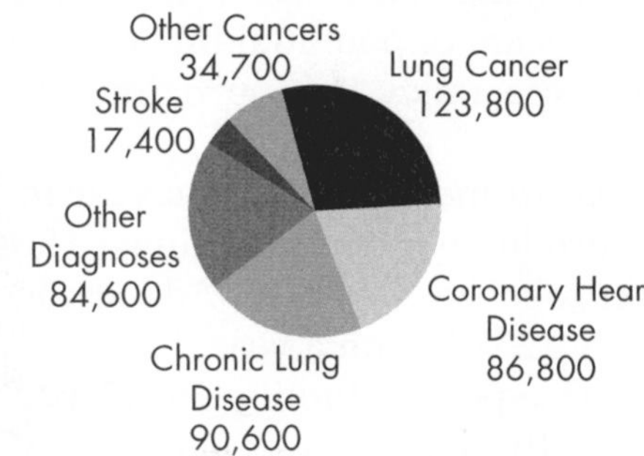

Source: CDC SAMMEC, MMWR 2005; Vol. 54, No. 25:625–8.

the smoking-related deaths from heart disease, strokes (smokers have a 20–50 percent greater incidence of stroke than nonsmokers), gangrene (over 90 percent of gangrene victims either smoke or have diabetes), aortic aneurysm, and peptic ulcers. Lung cancer risk is 23 times greater in male smokers than in lifelong nonsmokers.

Cancers with a proven higher incidence in smokers include cancer of the lip, tongue, tonsil, mouth, head, neck, larynx, lung, esophagus, bladder, kidney, pancreas, stomach, and cervix. In addition, smoking accelerates facial wrinkling, periodontal (gum) disease, risk of death from being on the contraceptive pill, stillbirth, and neonatal (newborn) death.

For every one of those 438,000 people who die every year from smoking, there are many more who suffer (patients on respirators, persons repeatedly admitted with pneumonia, and those who are chronically short of breath). Eight and a half million people suffer from chronic smoking-related conditions like COPD and heart disease. Statistically, each cigarette a person smokes shortens the smoker's life by five minutes.

Passive smoking involves sidestream smoke and mainstream smoke. Sidestream smoke comes from the end of the cigarette and constitutes 85 percent of a room's pollution. Sidestream smoke contains 10–15 percent carbon monoxide. (This percentage is the amount present in the smoke itself, not in the room.) Mainstream smoke is smoke that has been exhaled by the smoker; it accounts for the other 15 percent of a room's pollution. Such smoke contains only 5 percent carbon monoxide.

Passive smoking may affect the fetus by causing low birthweight (200 grams less on the average). Some of the many consequences of low birthweight include neonatal death, stillbirth, and intellectual handicap (math performance has been proven to be lower in primary school children whose mothers smoked during pregnancy).

The children of smokers have more bronchitis, pneumonia, asthma (70 percent more hospitalizations for asthma), and middle ear problems than the children of nonsmokers, are shorter in stature, and have a higher incidence of sudden infant death syndrome. Women whose husbands smoke get 10–20 percent more cancer of the lung. In terms of health risk, spending eight hours at work with people who smoke is probably equivalent to smoking several cigarettes a day, which is why increasingly more work and public places do not permit smoking.

Economic Effects of Smoking

Key Point

Smoking effects average loss of 14 years' life expectancy in smokers; average cost in United States $257 billion a year.

In the United States, smoking causes 3.3 million years of potential life lost in men and 2.2 million years of potential life lost in women. Smoking, on average, reduces life expectancy by approximately 14 years (American Cancer Society 2008).

Smoking costs the consumer $76 billion a year in health costs and $92 billion a year in lost productivity and earnings. Those who smoke spend $90 billion a year on tobacco products. Added together, smoking costs America approximately $257 billion a year. This amounts to $842 per capita or, for an *average* five-person family, $4213 per year. Who pays this money? All citizens pay through a lower standard of living because of increased health costs and decreased productivity. Employee health premiums also share the burden of the smoker with all insured members. For each pack of cigarettes sold in 1999, $3.45 was spent on medical care due to smoking and $3.73 was lost in productivity, for a total cost to society of $7.18 per pack (American Cancer Society 2008).

Why Do People Smoke?

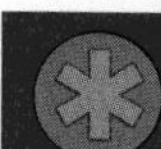

Key Point

Why kids smoke media pressure, peer approval, addiction, weight control, ritual.

According to the American Cancer Society (2005 figures), in the United States, 21 percent of people smoke. Ninety percent of those who smoke would like not to smoke. Perhaps part of the reason is that the social effects of smoking are unpleasant. One study showed that smoking is the number one turnoff in blind dates, coming in ahead of obesity. Friends may not invite the smoker home. In restaurants, nearby diners may ask the smoker to put out his cigarette. Spouses may apply pressure, and so may children. Insurance premiums will be less for nonsmokers and this is true for life insurance, fire, health, auto, homeowner, and disability policies.

Despite all these reasons, people continue to smoke. It should be obvious that people in this circumstance are not just "being sociable" or exhibiting normal behavior. No, they are addicted to smoking.

Social pressure, particularly from teenage or young adult peers, is a common reason to start smoking. Teenagers are told by their peers and by cigarette advertisements that smoking is adult and sexy, normal and fun. With a teenager's intense desire for peer approval and conformity, it is not difficult to see how smoking starts. Cigarette smoking fell from 42 percent in 1965 to 21 percent in 2006. However 32 percent of male students and 25 percent of female students in high school said they had smoked within the last month, suggesting that smoking is still felt to be "cool."

Gradually, secondary psychologic factors become important. The individual becomes conditioned by the smell and taste of cigarettes and by the stimulation of smoke at the back of the throat (called bronchial eroticism). Keeping their weight down is another reason some cite for smoking. In fact, the vast majority who cite this reason are smokers who quit smoking for a time but started again because they gained so much weight. The physical activity of smoking offers a ritual that carries with it a sense of security. Some smokers even describe smoking as "like a friend." The inhaling and exhaling may be comforting.

However, when the pharmacologic effects begin, what started as a social act becomes an addiction. Continuing to smoke reinforces the habit, and the smoker avoids withdrawal symptoms by taking more nicotine.

Helping Clients Stop Smoking

Identifying the smoker, of course, is easy. But there is no use telling a smoker that her habit is dirty and causes lung cancer. Her response is sure to be something like, "Maybe it's not clean, but it's not illegal, and I enjoy it" or "I won't get lung cancer; only one in eight gets lung cancer" (which amounts to playing Russian roulette).

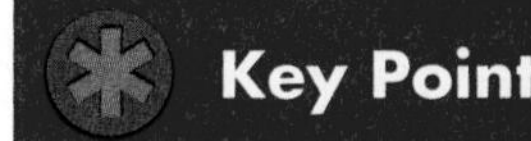

Helping clients stop smoking focusing on health interaction at hand and using it to push client to stop. Use your authority and your relationship.

As with the alcoholic, the health practitioner needs to confront smokers with the most pertinent reasons why they are suffering physically, economically, or socially. Begin by identifying health areas that should be of concern to a patient; explore anything remotely connected with smoking that may have a psychologic value to a client. A common way to present health problems is to go over with the smoker:

- Lung function tests or chest X-rays that show evidence of emphysema.
- A chest computed tomography scan showing nodules that need follow-up in case they are lung cancer.
- Histories in the patient's own family or friends of any disease connected with smoking (for example, cancer of the lung).
- Risk factors for heart disease, for example, a borderline blood pressure or cholesterol level, or a family history of heart disease.
- Morbidity associated with chronic lung disease.
- Incidence of low back pain (smoking doubles the chances of low back pain).

The health practitioner can also discuss with the young how it is a turn-off with dates, causes wrinkles, and may mean the physician won't prescribe a contraceptive pill.

Hospital nurses, exercise physiologists, nurse practitioners, physical therapists, respiratory technicians, or dietitians may all demonstrate the presence of a real physical problem or concern. Say, for example, that during contact with a patient, the topic of smoking has not come up, but the patient's breath reveals that he smokes. At this point, ask if he has ever thought he would like to be able to give up smoking. If there is even a glimmer of interest, ask whether he would like to stop smoking now. Explain that the risks are real and that the longer a person smokes the more these risks increase. If the patient agrees, a discussion may begin even if it includes a referral.

Like the alcoholic, the smoker finds it difficult to quit. A few will quit because of the advice of a health professional. A well-timed question may come when outside factors are also encouraging the smoker to quit. A health professional may offer that last little push the smoker needs. Remember that the patient needs to be sold on the idea. Most patients have been pressured by their spouses, children, friends, or workmates. They already are at least a little afraid of the consequences, and they have been exposed to at least a little of the social antagonism toward smoking. The section "Transtheoretical Model of Change" in Chapter 9 discusses gauging when the patient is ready to change and how to deal with each stage.

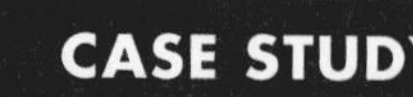

CASE STUDY 8-3

Mary, a 22- year-old mother with asthma, is being treated in the emergency room by a respiratory therapist. The two of them strike up a conversation about a common friend. The therapist then asks whether she is going to have another child. Mary says she has one child and plans on having another three. The therapist turns the conversation to Mary's smoking. She asks if she is ready to quit. Mary says she has thought about it but is not sure that she could quit right now, as she has so much stress in her life with her new baby. The therapist tells Mary that she understands but that asthmatics need to stop smoking because it worsens their asthma. In addition, she tells her that she should not smoke in pregnancy and should give it up before she becomes pregnant again. She gives Mary literature about asthma and smoking in pregnancy. She also gives Mary a smoking hotline card and says that when she is ready, she should call the number on the card. She also suggests that, if Mary feels that stress reduction would help her stop smoking, she could refer her to someone.

Specific techniques for stopping smoking include the following:

- Smoking cessation clinics. Patients who find it extremely difficult to quit are good candidates for this approach. Clinics involve combinations of lectures, money deposits refundable only after a period of abstinence, aversion therapy designed to make smoking seem less appealing (for example, having to smoke five cigarettes an hour for two hours or having to smoke while holding a cigarette between the little and ring fingers), and desensitization (for example, timed regular cigarettes regardless of urge to smoke). Initial success rates are around 23–90 percent, but fall to 20–40 percent after one year. Most smokers need more than one try before they succeed.
- Literature. Literature offers the self-motivated patient various techniques to try alone (e.g., cold turkey and progressive reduction).
- Nicotine replacements. Patches, gum, or inhalers ease withdrawal but result in a six-month quit rate of only 7 percent.
- Bupropion—brand name Zyban—has a 15 percent quit rate after one year versus 10 percent for placebo.
- Varenicline—brand name Chantix—has a 23 percent quit rate after one year versus 10 percent for placebo. However, a greatly increased incidence of suicide has been linked to this medication, and it may soon be removed from the market.
- Counseling with drugs. Counseling markedly increases quit rates (e.g., Zyban with counseling has a one-year quit rate of 30 percent versus 15 percent for Zyban alone.
- Hypnotherapy, acupuncture, progressive filters. Anecdotal evidence exists for these modalities, and they may be used if more scientifically documented treatments fail or are rejected by the patient.

Some enlightened companies offer financial incentives to employees who quit smoking. Smoking employees cost the employer more in absenteeism, lost productivity, higher insurance premiums, and maintenance costs. Aware of the $1,400 per employee cost of smoking, a company may offer smokers something like $1,000 to stop smoking for, say, a year. In the long run and for long-term employees, such a policy saves money.

Smoking prevention is equally important. Among students who are exposed to smoking prevention teaching, the smoking rate is 15–50 percent less than among those who are not exposed. An incentive to present to young people for never smoking is that the children of smoking parents are very likely to copy their parents. A person who smokes jeopardizes not only his own future but also the futures of his children.

Health care providers must think constructively about approaching this subject. Since smoking is the number one preventable cause of ill health and death in the United States, health professionals need to be vigorously antismoking. However, be careful to maintain a professional attitude, not discriminatory and prejudiced, as such efforts will be counterproductive. The patient will sense antagonism, through words or body language, and deny, rationalize, and avoid.

Those wishing to quit smoking may use one of the following resources for information on how to quit:

- Local pharmacist
- Personal physician
- American Cancer Society, Inc. 1599 Clifton Road NE, Atlanta, GA 30329–4251, 1–800-ACS-2345, www.cancer.org
- www.smokefree.gov/
- www.cdc.gov/tobacco/quit_smoking/index.htm

Summary

This chapter discussed the problem of addiction, referred to as substance abuse or chemical dependency, and smoking. It defined addiction, dependence, habituation, and tolerance and cited the addict's need to continue the substance abuse as stronger than the social and physical consequences that are the effect of using alcohol or other drugs. The causes of alcoholism include the strong likelihood of a biological predisposition to addiction; the psychologic response to alcohol common to most abusers, such as using alcohol to mask other psychological problems, including social phobia; and the response to peer pressure for substance misuse; as well as the cultural links to abuse that may also be hereditary. Patient responses may be used to determine a patient's diagnosis, along with a history of the patient's arrests, domestic life, and job history.

The psychologic effects of alcoholism include emotional augmentation; blackouts; denial in the face of problems; depression; deterioration of self-image; and finally, internal conflict, shame, and guilt. The physical effects of alcoholism include a red face, higher incidence of certain cancers, cirrhosis of the liver, heart disease, neuropathy, pneumonia, intestinal disorders. and trauma from accidents. Fetal alcohol syndrome occurs in babies of mothers who drink excessively during pregnancy. The physical effect of the DTs, which are part of the withdrawal syndrome and cause shaking, are sweating, insomnia, stomach pain and even death. Treatments for alcoholism include motivational interviewing, cognitive behavioral therapy, individual and group therapy, AA, and medication.

The chapter then focused on the classifications of addictive drugs other than alcohol and pointed out the current problem of the extensive misuse of prescription drugs exceeding all street drug use except marijuana. A discussion of neurotransmitters and the limbic system or reward center of the brain aids in the understanding of why drugs are so addictive. The mental and physical effects of substance abuse include an initial numbness, followed by depression in those who use alcohol, sedatives, and opioids. Stimulant drugs increase anxiety, especially panic disorders, and exacerbate insomnia whereas hallucinogens and some stimulants may precipitate psychoses. Drug abuse is also associated with many secondary diseases such as HIV, hepatitis B and C, seizures, and heart disease. This section also reviewed the 13 states which now offer medical use of marijuana and discussed the issues related to legalization of marijuana.

The prevention and treatment of substance abuse include approaches to youth who have never tried drugs and efforts to target at-risk students to help prevent drug use. Detoxification is necessary when a person moves away from many substances, and multiple treatment strategies must be offered to assist the addict in getting off drugs and staying off them. Narcotics Anonymous helps these addicts just as AA assists the alcoholic. Methadone and suboxone are two pharmacologic treatments that assist the opioid addict (heroin) from relapsing if properly used.

Smoking is the most common preventable cause of death in the United States today. The consequences of smoking can be highly lethal to both the smoker and those around them. Smokers give up on average 14 years of life for their habit and suffer many ailments and risk the health of infants exposed to smoke. Smoking costs the American consumer $76 billion dollars a year in health costs and $92 billion in lost productivity and earnings. Most smokers would like to quit but, as addictive as nicotine is, need encouragement from health professionals as well as family and friends. Clients should be encouraged to attend smoking cessation programs, perhaps hypnotherapy or acupuncture clinics, review literature, use a nicotine patch or gum to help with the addiction, or try other medications and counseling.

Chapter Review

Key Term Review

Addiction: Physical and/or psychologic dependence on a substance (often leading to drug-seeking behavior).

Additive effect: Sedatives (e.g., alcohol, benzodiazepines, barbiturates, sleeping pills, inhalants, anesthetics), all of which may have a cumulative effect.

Alcoholics Anonymous (AA): Informal meeting society for recovering alcoholics wanting to achieve and maintain sobriety. The organization uses a 12-step program to help people stay off alcohol and believes that complete abstention is the only way.

Alcoholism: Chronic consumption of alcohol that continues despite significant interference with a person's physical, economic, or social health.

CAGE: Alcoholism assessment, the name of which is an acronym for key words in the following questions: "Have you ever felt: (1) you should *Cut* down your drinking, (2) *Annoyed* by others' comments about your drinking, (3) *Guilty* about your drinking, (4) you needed an *Eye* opener (drink on rising in the morning)?" Even one positive answer is significant.

Cognitive behavioral therapy (CBT): Psychotherapeutic approach that deals with thought processes, beliefs, and responses to influence problematic emotions or behaviors.

DARE: Drug Abuse Resistance Education.

Downregulation: Decrease in number of receptors (e.g., for dopamine) on surface of cell, making it less sensitive to further stimulation (e.g., by dopamine).

Emotional augmentation: An over-response to normal stress and events of everyday life with a lowered threshold for action.

Fetal alcohol syndrome: A syndrome that occurs in babies of mothers who drink excessively during pregnancy.

Moderation Management (MM): Organization that believes that problem drinkers can continue to drink in a controlled fashion, but, if they fail, suggests AA.

Neurotransmitter: Chemical substances released from nerve endings to stimulate other nerves.

ONDCP: Office of National Drug Control Policy.

Physical dependence: Physiologic need for a substance, resulting in a withdrawal syndrome when substance is ended.

Polysubstance abuse: Use of two or more different substances of abuse, a very common problem.

Problem drinkers: Drinkers who have high alcohol consumption but may stop of their own volition without medical treatment, peer group support, or a spiritual awakening. May progress to alcoholism.

Psychologic dependence: Addiction to a substance leading to a psychologic withdrawal.

Psychologic treatment: Motivational interviewing; CBT; group and family, individual, and multiple approach models.

Substance abuse: Significant distress, manifest by three of the following: failure to fulfill school, work, or parenting obligations; hazardous use (e.g., while driving); recurrent substance-related legal problems (e.g., DUI); or continued substance use despite persistent or recurrent social or interpersonal problems.

Substance dependence: Significant distress manifested by three of the following: tolerance; withdrawal; increasing consumption; desire to quit; excessive time spent on abuse; fewer social, occupational, or recreational activities; or continued use despite knowing physiologic and psychologic effects.

Substance use disorder: A disorder that includes substance abuse and, more seriously, substance dependence.

Tobacco dependence: Continued consumption of tobacco that the patient cannot control, despite significant physical, economic, or social side effects.

Treating addiction: Detoxification, psychologic treatment, medications.

Treatments of alcoholism: Motivational interviewing, CBT, AA, individual and group therapy, medication.

Chapter Review Questions

1. What are the essential aspects of the definition of alcoholism, and what makes diagnosis difficult?
2. List cultural and occupational associations with alcoholism.
3. List the physical consequences of alcoholism.
4. List the diseases associated with smoking.
5. How much does smoking cost society, and what percentage of men and women still smoke?
6. What is the difference between physical dependence, tolerance, and psychologic dependence?
7. What is fetal alcohol syndrome?
8. What is the difference between substance abuse, substance dependence, and substance use disorder?
9. List risk factors for drug abuse.

Case Study Critical Thinking Questions

1. Present convincing arguments that the father in Case Study 8-1 of Jack is also a substance abuser.
2. In Case Study 8-2, why did the emergency room nurse back off asking further questions about the patient's drinking?
3. In Case Study 8-3, give three reasons why the respiratory therapist managed Mary well.

References

1. Angeles, Steve. "Schwarzenegger Opens Debate on Legalizing Marijuana." *North American News Bureau,* May 8, 2009.
2. Cancer Fact and Figures 2008. American Cancer Society.
3. Cheever, S. *My Name Is Bill.* NY: Simon and Shuster, 2004.
4. Cook, C. H., Hallwood, P. M., Thomson, A. D. "B Vitamin Deficiency and Neuropsychiatric Syndromes in Alcohol Misuse." *Oxford Journals* 33(4):317–336; 1998.
5. Dingfelder, S. "The Military's War on Stigma." *Monit Psychol* 40(6):52–55; 2009.
6. Fielding, J. E. *Smoking, Health Effects and Control.* American Cancer Society, 1986.
7. Frank, D. and Bill, W. *The Annotated AA Handbook.* New York: Frank D. Barricade Books, 1996.
8. http://medicalmarijuana.procon.org
9. *Results from the 2007 National Survey on Drug Use and Health: National Findings,* (NSDUH Series H-34, DHHS Publication No. SMA 08–4343). Rockville, MD, http://oas.samhsa.gov
10. www.drug-rehabs.com
11. Kishline, A. *Moderate Drinking.* New York: Crown Publishers, Inc., 1994.
12. Klein, J. "*Why Legalizing Marijuana Makes Sense*." *Time,* April 02, 2009.
13. Lankenau, S. E., et al. "Prevalence and Patterns of Prescription Drug Misuse among Young Ketamine Injectors." *J Drug Issues* 37(3):717–736; 2007.
14. Manchikanti, L. "Prescription Drug Abuse: What is being done to address this new drug epidemic." *Pain Physician* 9(4):287–321; 2006.
15. Mendelson, J. R., Mello, N. K. *The Diagnosis and Treatment of Alcoholism.* New York: McGraw-Hill, 1985.
16. *Twelve Steps and Twelve Traditions.* New York: Alcoholics Anonymous World Services, Inc., 1981.
17. *The Smoking Digest.* Bethesda, MD: National Cancer Institute and National Institutes of Health, published yearly.
18. Sheff, D. *Beautiful Boy*. Boston: Houghton Mifflin, 2008.
19. Smoking www.nlm.nih.gov/medlineplus/smoking
20. Treatment of Alcoholism www.mayoclinic.com/health/alcoholism/DS00340/DSECTION=treatments-and-drugs
21. Commonly Abused Drugs from National Institute of Drug Abuse www.drugabuse.gov/DrugPages/DrugsofAbuse.html

Additional Readings

1. *Alcoholism.* Seattle, WA: Madrona Publishers, Inc., 1981.
2. http://en.wikipedia.org/wiki/Medical_cannabis
3. On Wernicke-Korsakoff syndrome. www.nim.nih.gov/medlineplus/ency/article/000771.htm.
4. www.medicinal-marijuana.com
5. Milan, J. R. Ketcham, K. *Under the Influence. A Guide to the Myths and Realities.*
6. www.aa.org/ Alcoholics Anonymous
7. www.cancer.org American Cancer Society
8. www.moderation.org Moderation Management
9. www.ncadd.org National Council on Alcoholism and Drug Dependence
10. www.drugabuse.gov Principles of Drug Addiction Treatment: A Research-based Guide
11. www.samhsa.gov Substance Abuse and Mental Health Services Administration
12. www.dea.gov Drug Enforcement Administration
13. www.niaaa.nih.gov National Institute on Alcohol abuse and Alcoholism
14. www.nimh.nih.gov National institute of Mental Health
15. www.whitehousedrugploicy.gov Office of National Drug Control Policy (ONDCP)
16. www.asam.org American Society of Addiction Medicine

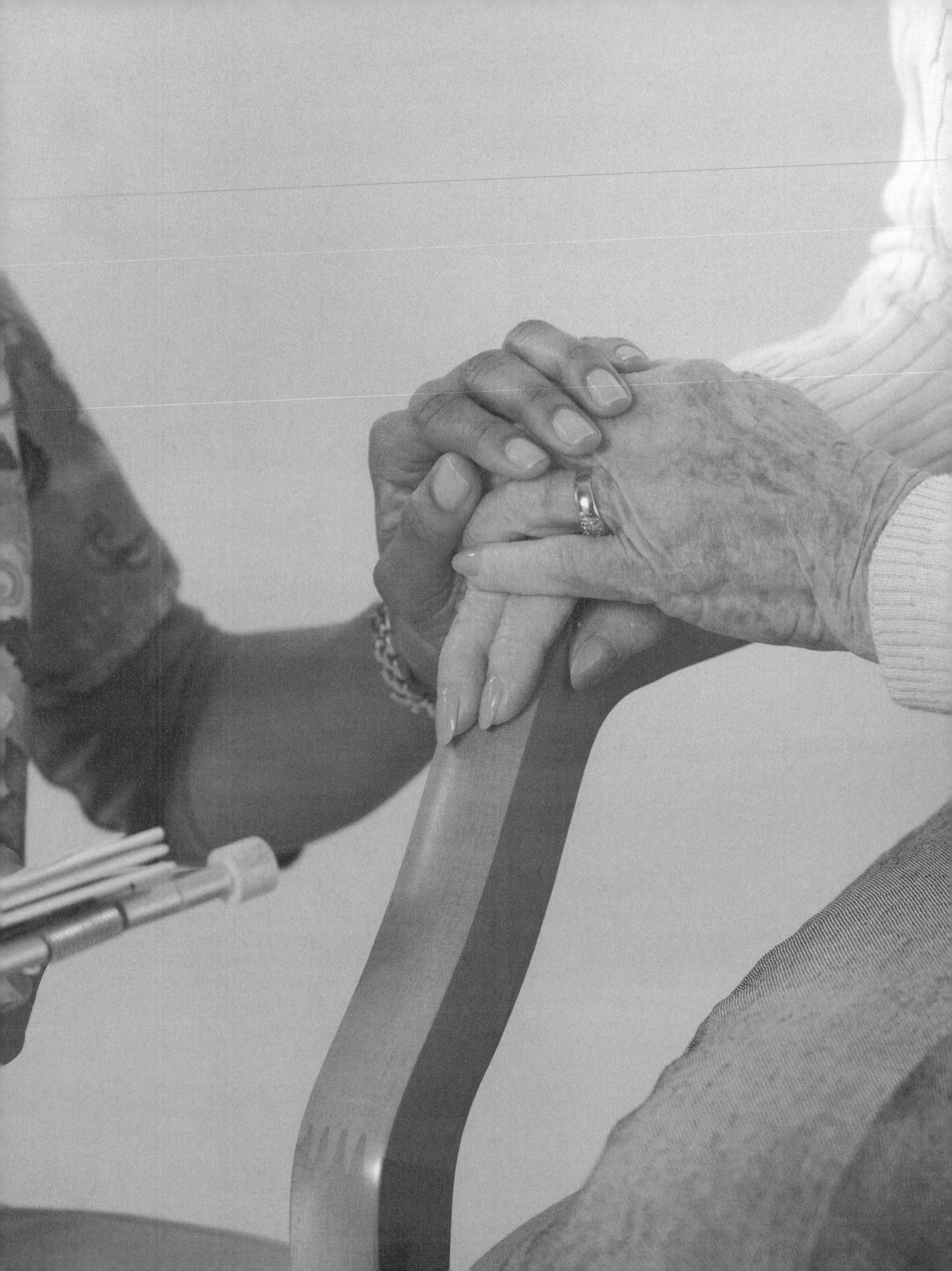

The Role of Counseling in Prevention

Learning Outcomes

After reading this chapter, you should be able to:

9.1 Explain counseling and how it evolves from communication skills and list careers which rely on counseling skills.

9.2 Differentiate between genetic programming, environmental conditions, and lifestyle factors and the role of counseling in each.

9.3 Synthesize genetic programming, environmental conditions, and lifestyle factors while examining the health issues of obesity and metabolic syndrome.

9.4 Describe the impact of genetic, environmental, and lifestyle factors on mental health.

9.5 Demonstrate an understanding of the motivation strategy called AIM.

9.6 Understand the transtheoretical model of change and its technique called motivational interviewing.

Key Terms

- Awareness, information, and motivation (AIM)
- Aerobic exercise
- Amniocentesis
- Antagonists
- Appraisal-focused coping
- Body mass index (BMI)
- Contingency management
- Cognitive dissonance
- Emotion-focused coping
- Environmental conditions
- Etiology
- Food pyramid
- Genetic counseling
- Genetic programming
- Influencing response
- Leading response
- Lifestyle factors
- Metabolic syndrome
- Motivation
- Motivational interviewing (MI)
- Obesity
- Overweight
- Primary prevention
- Problem-focused coping
- Secondary prevention
- Sedentary
- Self-efficacy
- Stress
- Token economy
- Transtheoretical model of change (TTM)
- Visceral fat

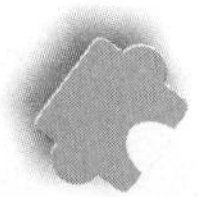

Defining Counseling

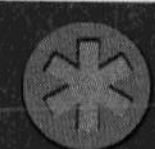

Key Point

In this chapter both the term "patient" and "client" are used. Most health professionals think in terms of a patient–professional relationship, but the context of preventive thinking somewhat alters this relationship: the customer of preventive health care may be well. The word "patient" denotes a loss of wellness and is not as appropriate.

Good counselors begin with the good communications skill described in the first two chapters of this text. A counselor must first comprehend what the client or patient is concerned about and does so by observing body language, paraphrasing, and empathizing. In fact, the very acts of paraphrasing and conveying empathy are the key tools for many types of counseling (recall the Rogerian model in Chapter 3).

Using simple but well-practiced skills, a health professional will be able to access serious client concerns and influence the client's response to these issues. Further, in a preventive model, when a disease or problem has either not yet surfaced (**primary prevention**) or is still highly treatable to prevent advanced complications (**secondary prevention**), counseling may play a major role in helping the client.

The use of communication skills used to lead the client is referred to as a **leading response**, with the communication moving in a direction guided by the health professional (as opposed to a "continuing response," which elicits more of strictly what is on the client's mind). According to Danish (1980), there are three types of leading responses: (1) questions; which as discussed earlier, are best kept open-ended to gain the most information from the client but in any case the person who asks the question leads the conversation; (2) advice giving, which health professionals are often required to provide and which should be done in a clear, simple, specific, and realistic manner; and (3) **influencing responses**, which are used to encourage or discourage behavior the client mentions (e.g., "What a great idea!" or "Let's think about how that might turn out in case there is a better way for you to get your boss's attention").

Leading responses should be used only when the health professional already understands what the client's concerns and needs are, in other words, after the health professional has listened and paraphrased and can empathize with the client. Only then is it safe to make a leading response other than a very basic question to clarify the speaker's intent.

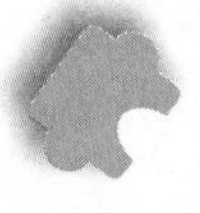

Genes, Environmental Conditions, and Lifestyle Factors

When we become unwell, the source of our problem can be traced to one or more of the following: genetic programming, environmental conditions, or lifestyle factors.

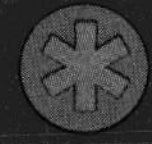

Key Points

Genetic programming inherited characteristics carried by our genes.

Environmental conditions the world around us.

Many diseases, or weaknesses that predispose us to disease, are inherited (i.e., **genetic programming**). Heart disease, high blood pressure, diabetes, and many lesser known conditions are at least in part inherited. Those with a familial risk of colon cancer make up 20 percent of all patients with this cancer. There is also the BRCA gene, which is linked to many cases of breast cancer. Findings such as this make a fairly convincing argument that cancer also can be genetically determined.

Other diseases can be caused by **environmental conditions** in the world around us. The quality of the air and water are among the most obvious concerns. Noise pollution and overcrowding also influence the potential for disease. Concern is growing for causes of permanent damage to the environment; strong protests against dependence on oil and the concern over the disposal of hazardous wastes are evidence of the value people place on protecting the environment. Some scientists believe it is already too late to prevent damage from the thinning of the ozone layer. Without sufficient ozone protection from the sun's ultraviolet rays, there will be many more victims of skin cancer.

Other major environmental concerns were voiced about the tragedies at Love Canal and at Woburn, Massachusetts, where children playing on a former hazardous dump site have been the victims of a high number of leukemias. In 1986, Chernobyl, U.S.S.R., was the site of the world's largest nuclear power accident. Thousands of Russians were affected, and vegetation and animal life throughout Europe were contaminated. The world may not yet know all of the consequences of this catastrophe. The varied uses of asbestos have resulted in health problems for many. Certainly there is convincing evidence that the environment brings about a significant proportion of today's diseases.

Most of the diseases people have can be at least partially traced to their **lifestyle factors**. As discussed in Chapter 8, cigarette smoking is the largest preventable cause of death in the United States today. Drinking alcohol; abusing other drugs; having high fat, high salt, and high sugar diets; and leading **sedentary** (inactive) lives are all detrimental to health. Lifestyle issues also include sleep, watching television, playing video games, and coping with stress. Some lifestyles even involve direct and overt assaults on health. Two examples would be race car drivers and teenagers who frequently get involved in street fights.

The public has become increasingly convinced of the importance of healthy lifestyles: jogging, walking, cycling, and other forms of aerobic exercise. At the same time, sales of red meat have decreased, indicating another change in lifestyle among Americans. The incidence of heart disease has also been declining in recent years. This decline probably is due to the combined effect of less smoking, better eating, more exercise, and more aggressive treatment of blood pressure and serum cholesterol. Vitamin D deficiency has been linked even in Western societies to an increased incidence of heart disease, cancer, and fractures, and such knowledge has led to an increased use of Vitamin D.

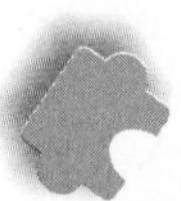

Prevention and Counseling

Genetic View

Genetic counseling can have a direct impact on disease prevention. In its earliest days, genetic counseling was primarily limited to working with couples who had already produced a child with a genetically linked birth defect. Such counseling provided information to the couples about their chances of subsequently having a healthy offspring. Couples then weighed this information against their desire to have more children or their ability to cope with another child with a disability and made an informed decision. These decisions generally were made before conceiving another child.

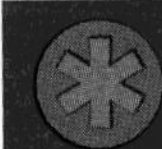

Key Point

Genetic counselor professional who assesses genetic risk and presents the statistics in a cogent way to the individual.

Amniocentesis became available to the general public about 30 years ago. This test is an invasive procedure that involves removing amniotic fluid from the pregnant woman. The needle of a syringe is directed through the abdominal wall into the fluid that surrounds the growing baby. This fluid contains both maternal and fetal cells. When these cells are cultured, the existence of certain genetic diseases can be determined. Most prominent among these diseases are Down syndrome and spina bifida. Amniocentesis is now recommended for women who are expecting to deliver after the age of 37 or who have a family history of these abnormalities. It can also be used to detect a number of other diseases.

Counseling initially plays a role in informing a couple about amniocentesis. The risks and benefits must be carefully explained to prospective users. (Amniocentesis itself may cause miscarriage.) Encouraging a couple to have this test may prevent the birth of a child who could not be accepted by the couple and whose quality of life would be severely limited. If a fetus should test positive for one of these problems, counseling would then play a key role in determining the final outcome of the pregnancy.

It must be noted that all counseling and health care needs to be sensitive to the religious and cultural values of the client/couple. For many people abortion means "taking a life," and, no matter what the circumstances, this is viewed as a "sinful act." Clients who believe this will not choose abortion no matter what the finding is from the medical tests, and they should not be pushed to consider acting against their beliefs nor should health professionals be required to counsel clients in matters that are against their own religious convictions.

Further, neither Down syndrome nor spina bifida affects each child the same way. That is, some Down syndrome children are only mildly developmentally delayed and have the potential for nearly normal lives whereas others suffer severe cognitive impairment, severely shortened lives, and a host of physiological limitations. Parents need to know what they are up against. In all likelihood, what will their baby be like? What, if any, chance does their baby have of being close to normal? What community and medical support will be available? What decisions do most people in their position make? What impact does a Down syndrome baby have on the rest of the family? (The impact of a Down syndrome baby on the family is usually enormous. Sometimes it is helpful for the couple to meet a parent with a Down syndrome child.)

The health professional who counsels such a couple must help them to deal with the answers to these questions. Many of the answers are not easy to face. Most couples faced with a positive test for Down syndrome choose to have an abortion. It is not necessarily true that couples who would not consider abortion do not elect to have the test initially. Some couples may test in order to prepare themselves. Others test without allowing themselves to think about a negative outcome until it is reality. In any event, a health practitioner with good counseling skills can play a valuable role in assisting the couple to make the decision that is best for their family.

Genetic counseling may best be used for preventive strategies. A large number of genetic diseases might be decreased or postponed through counseling that ties in lifestyle issues. For example, people with a strong family history of cancer or heart disease are facing more risk than the average person if they choose to smoke. Those with diabetes in their families

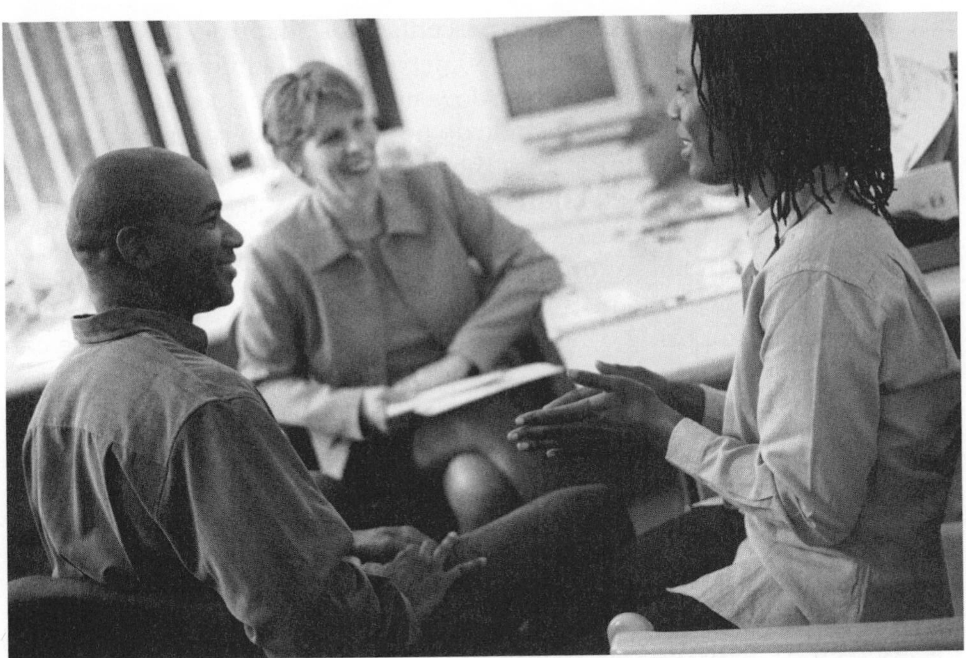

Genetic counseling helps a couple to weigh risk factors.

might postpone the onset of the disease by limiting weight gain. Many diseases have known risk factors that the health care provider will seek out and examine.

Once the genetic factors are clear, the health professional looks at environmental conditions. Is this man exposed to any substance that has the potential for causing heart disease? Since he comes from a family with such a high incidence of heart disease, this question should focus especially on any environmental conditions he might hold in common with his afflicted ancestors. For example, the health worker should take a close look at the work environment if the man works in the same place as his great-grandfather and all the deceased male members of his family.

Lifestyle factors may offer the greatest potential for increased longevity. A man who is at high genetic risk for heart disease can do much to control his risk if he avoids becoming overweight, avoids cigarettes, limits his use of alcohol, controls high blood pressure, gets 20–30 minutes of aerobic exercise four times a week, lowers his cholesterol and sodium intake through diet, and realistically controls the stress in his daily life. **Aerobic exercise** involves moving without great resistance while making the heart muscle work; walking, jogging, and swimming are examples. Anaerobic exercise involves significant resistance; weight lifting and rowing are examples. Controlling stress is discussed later in this chapter.

The examples in the previous paragraphs illustrate that a person who is primarily at risk for a disease via one pathway can prevent or postpone that disease through attention to the other pathways (avoiding suspect chemicals in the work environment and adopting a lifestyle that includes diet, exercise, limiting abusive substances, and medical control of blood pressure when needed).

Genetic counseling can serve to prevent health problems in two additional ways. First, genetic counseling can help people live with impending health problems or determine their need for doing so. Some genetic diseases, for instance, strike a high percentage of offspring. An example is Huntington's disease, which affects 50 percent of all children born to one affected parent. Because the disease does not become evident until the victim is already 30–50 years old, people do not know for certain that they are carrying the disease until it strikes them. And usually it strikes *after* they have already had their own children, setting up a new generation of potential victims. However, there are now tests to determine whether a person will be a victim of Huntington's. A genetic counselor or counseling health professional can help the person who is living under this threat to know what the future will bring. Understanding what the future will be like can help Huntington's victims make decisions about parenting.

Living and waiting for the symptoms of such a disease to begin sounds like torture. Yet many of those who could now have the test and know their fate refuse to do so. They continue to wish to live in hope rather than face a possible horrible truth. They also continue to bear children, believing it is their right and the real meaning of life. Although such responses are understandable, they place an obvious burden on the genetic counselor, who not only is unable to help the individual but also sees the problem extending into future generations. Again, the family's religious beliefs may be guiding them.

Second, genetic counseling can help individuals accept themselves. Many people have been victims of social pressure to become perfect. Especially victimized are the overweight. People who are naturally overweight as a result of hereditary factors need to understand the reasons for their heaviness. Torturous diets and expensive fads will never offer good health to a person who is genetically programmed to be overweight. The only thing that weight reduction regimens do for such people is make them anxious and doubtful of their self-worth. Counseling must inform and support those who are fighting against heredity for, except in small modified instances, they can never win. Precisely determining hereditary factors for obesity may not yet exist, but a tendency to be overweight can be predicted if we look at our relatives. And although a person who might have been programmed to be overweight may still have a good deal of influence over how high that weight actually rises, the struggle to be thin is a losing battle.)

Environmental Conditions

The field of genetic programming has a developed role for genetic counselors, but this is lacking for the environment, that is, there is no environmental counselor per se. Health or sanitation officers, environmental engineers, occupational health clinic personnel, company nurses, solid and hazardous waste disposal experts, and employees of the Occupational Safety and Health Agency (OSHA) probably fill the most recognizable roles in this category. Certainly, environmental protection agencies and groups rely on the expertise of these trained specialists. Allied health professionals play roles in their related fields as environmental counselors when they provide information on lead paint, asbestos, and proper use, disposal, and storage of hazardous chemicals. All too often, however, private citizens have been the ones who have smoked out major environmental hazards.

The chemicals that seeped into the ground at Love Canal, New York, until the mid-1970s; the environmental damage that Agent Orange did in

Vietnam; the toxins that may have led to Gulf War syndrome; and the chemicals that are leaking into wells all over this country are part of the potential legacy of death for generations to come. Yet in most of these situations, the government, the chemical plants, and the gas and manufacturing companies have not come forward to admit responsibility for long-term environmental damage. Indeed, they seem rather to hide and bluff their way through accusations of wrong until they are forced to correct a chemical horror.

Union Carbide is one of the companies that has had to take some responsibility for its actions. When Carbide's insecticide gas dioxin was accidentally emitted into the atmosphere of Bhopal, India, 2,000 persons died instantly and thousands of others were permanently injured. Yet, even in the face of this catastrophe, Virginians who live near a similar Union Carbide plant in the United States have been told that such a tragedy could never happen to them.

It took decades and hundreds of hours of litigation before asbestos was declared carcinogenic, even though the asbestos workers who were dying from lung cancer in great numbers were certain of it. To some companies and groups, avoiding financial liability appears to be more significant than saving human lives.

Health professionals may need to use counseling skills to alert individuals to dangers in the environment.

Lifestyle Factors

Why can Bill eat enormous quantities of food and never gain weight while Craig watches his diet constantly and still gains? Why can Ellen work two jobs and then go out dancing and drinking while Marcia has trouble feeling well-rested after eight hours of sleep? Chances are that genetic programming is a key factor if age is held constant. But what would happen to Marcia if she had to work both of Ellen's jobs? What would happen to Ellen if she had to get eight hours of sleep every night? Chances are these alterations in lifestyle would bring about dramatic changes in each person's physical and mental health.

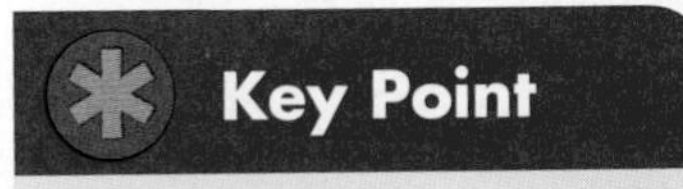

Lifestyle factors how we choose to live.

Lifestyle involves a high element of choice, and most of the advice or counseling health professionals give revolves around lifestyle factors. As already noted, the course of diseases may be altered or postponed by a healthy lifestyle.

In an agrarian society, rigorous exercise was a part of daily life. Even city folks got regular exercise before the automobile was introduced. Today's sedentary lifestyle is blamed for high disease risk. Every period in history has offered unique risk factors, however. One hundred years ago there was a high death rate that resulted from the complications of burning (people relied on wood), childbirth, farm accidents, and communicable diseases.

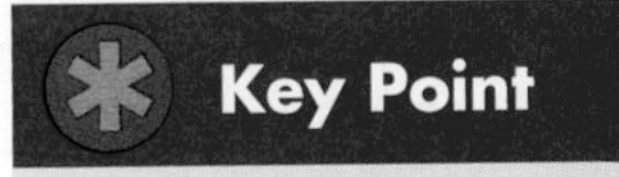

AIM awareness, information, and motivation: three keys to health counseling.

The role of counseling for prevention relies on making the client aware of the risk factors that exist today, providing the client with information that will permit a change to take place, and actively working to motivate the client to adopt a healthier lifestyle. This strategy, called **awareness, information, and motivation (AIM)**, is described in the last section of this chapter.

Table 9.1 Lifestyle Factors that Influence Health Risk

Amount of sleep	Use of leisure time
Marital status	Hobbies and interests
Number of family members	Occupation
Attitude toward health care	Living environment
Exercise	Smoking
Job stress	Number of sexual partners
Eating habits	Use of caffeine
Drinking habits	Religious beliefs and practices
Use of recreational drugs	Hours on the road

Table 9.1 lists some of the risk factors that influence health in today's society.

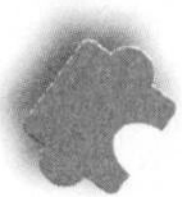

Metabolic Syndrome

A serious epidemic in the western world is obesity. Current U.S. data from the National Health and Nutrition Examination survey (NHANES 2001–2004) show 64 million Americans are obese and another 74 million are overweight. Predictions are that in 2015 40 percent of adult Americans and 25 percent of American children will be obese. One-third of Americans are obese; 33 percent are women and 29 million, or 30 percent, are men.

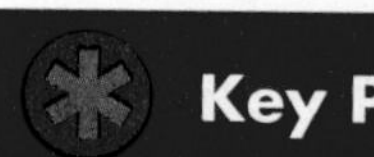

Key Points

BMI worldwide obesity scale, which divides weight in kilograms by height in meters squared.

Overweight BMI 25 to 30;

Obese BMI over 30;

Morbid Obesity BMI over 40;

Super-obese BMI over 50.

Obesity is measured by **body mass index (BMI)**, which, according to the National Institutes of Health (NIH), is an index of weight adjusted for the height of the individual. It is calculated by dividing a person's weight in kilograms by height in meters squared. NIH and the American Dietetic Association then have similar formulas to convert to pounds.

Underweight is a BMI of less than 18.5, normal is 18.5 to 25, **overweight** is 25 to 30, obese is over 30, extreme or morbid obesity is over 40, and super-obese is over 50. The World Health Organization recommends this definition of overweight.

The primary associations of obesity are:

- Heart disease, especially coronary artery disease, heart failure, and stroke.
- Cancer of the breast, colon, uterus, prostate, kidney, esophagus, and gallbladder.
- Metabolic syndrome—the biggest preventable cause of death after smoking.
- Hypertension, hypercholesterolemia, and diabetes.
- Osteoarthritis, especially of knees and back.

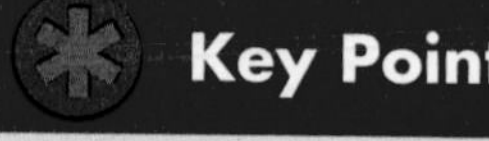

Key Point

Metabolic syndrome syndrome defined by three of the following: high cholesterol, high blood pressure, high fasting blood sugar, and obesity.

The chief morbidity (illness) and mortality (death) that result from obesity comes from metabolic syndrome, which is the greatest current cause of cardiovascular disease. **Metabolic syndrome**, also called insulin

Body Mass Index Table

	Normal						Overweight					Obese										Extreme Obesity														
BMI	**19**	**20**	**21**	**22**	**23**	**24**	**25**	**26**	**27**	**28**	**29**	**30**	**31**	**32**	**33**	**34**	**35**	**36**	**37**	**38**	**39**	**40**	**41**	**42**	**43**	**44**	**45**	**46**	**47**	**48**	**49**	**50**	**51**	**52**	**53**	**54**
Height (inches)	Body Weight (pounds)																																			
58	91	96	100	105	110	115	119	124	129	134	138	143	148	153	158	162	167	172	177	181	186	191	196	201	205	210	215	220	224	229	234	239	244	248	253	258
59	94	99	104	109	114	119	124	128	133	138	143	148	153	158	163	168	173	178	183	188	193	198	203	208	212	217	222	227	232	237	242	247	252	257	262	267
60	97	102	107	112	118	123	128	133	138	143	148	153	158	163	168	174	179	184	189	194	199	204	209	215	220	225	230	235	240	245	250	255	261	266	271	276
61	100	106	111	116	122	127	132	137	143	148	153	158	164	169	174	180	185	190	195	201	206	211	217	222	227	232	238	243	248	254	259	264	269	275	280	285
62	104	109	115	120	126	131	136	142	147	153	158	164	169	175	180	186	191	196	202	207	213	218	224	229	235	240	246	251	256	262	267	273	278	284	289	295
63	107	113	118	124	130	135	141	146	152	158	163	169	175	180	186	191	197	203	208	214	220	225	231	237	242	248	254	259	265	270	278	282	287	293	299	304
64	110	116	122	128	134	140	145	151	157	163	169	174	180	186	192	197	204	209	215	221	227	232	238	244	250	256	262	267	273	279	285	291	296	302	308	314
65	114	120	126	132	138	144	150	156	162	168	174	180	186	192	198	204	210	216	222	228	234	240	246	252	258	264	270	276	282	288	294	300	306	312	318	324
66	118	124	130	136	142	148	155	161	167	173	179	186	192	198	204	210	216	223	229	235	241	247	253	260	266	272	278	284	291	297	303	309	315	322	328	334
67	121	127	134	140	146	153	159	166	172	178	185	191	198	204	211	217	223	230	236	242	249	255	261	268	274	280	287	293	299	306	312	319	325	331	338	344
68	125	131	138	144	151	158	164	171	177	184	190	197	203	210	216	223	230	236	243	249	256	262	269	276	282	289	295	302	308	315	322	328	335	341	348	354
69	128	135	142	149	155	162	169	176	182	189	196	203	209	216	223	230	236	243	250	257	263	270	277	284	291	297	304	311	318	324	331	338	345	351	358	365
70	132	139	146	153	160	167	174	181	188	195	202	209	216	222	229	236	243	250	257	264	271	278	285	292	299	306	313	320	327	334	341	348	355	362	369	376
71	136	143	150	157	165	172	179	186	193	200	208	215	222	229	236	243	250	257	265	272	279	286	293	301	308	315	322	329	338	343	351	358	365	372	379	386
72	140	147	154	162	169	177	184	191	199	206	213	221	228	235	242	250	258	265	272	279	287	294	302	309	316	324	331	338	346	353	361	368	375	383	390	397
73	144	151	159	166	174	182	189	197	204	212	219	227	235	242	250	257	265	272	280	288	295	302	310	318	325	333	340	348	355	363	371	378	386	393	401	408
74	148	155	163	171	179	186	194	202	210	218	225	233	241	249	256	264	272	280	287	295	303	311	319	326	334	342	350	358	365	373	381	389	396	404	412	420
75	152	160	168	176	184	192	200	208	216	224	232	240	248	256	264	272	279	287	295	303	311	319	327	335	343	351	359	367	375	383	391	399	407	415	423	431
76	156	164	172	180	189	197	205	213	221	230	238	246	254	263	271	279	287	295	304	312	320	328	336	344	353	361	369	377	385	394	402	410	418	426	435	443

Source: Adapted from Clinical Guidelines on the identification, Evaluation, and Treatment of Overweight and Obesity in Adults. The Evidence Report.

resistance or "syndrome X," is a complex syndrome defined by three of the following five factors:

- High cholesterol.
- High blood sugars.
- High blood pressure.
- Maximum girth over 35 inches for women, or 40 inches for men.
- BMI over 30.

Key Point

Visceral fat fat in and around organs, especially intraperitoneal—liver, kidneys, omentum, mesentery and bowels—but also the heart. Opposite of subcutaneous and intramuscular fat which is less metabolically active.

Inactivity, Western diet, genetics, and aging lead to increased **visceral fat**. This, in turn, causes chemicals to be made that lead to high blood pressure, insulin resistance with elevated fasting blood sugars, low high-density lipoprotein, high triglycerides, and inflammation that increases the chance of blood clots forming on the cholesterol deposits in the arteries. Metabolic syndrome doubles mortality in men and quintuples mortality in women. Visceral fat makes you pot-bellied or apple-shaped whereas subcutaneous fat makes you pear-shaped (fat around buttocks and thighs).

In the 1950s about 50 percent of Americans smoked, and smoking was the major cause of heart disease. Now, thanks to public education, only 21 percent of Americans smoke, and the major cause of heart disease has shifted to the metabolic syndrome.

A number of strategies have been helpful in maintaining weight loss in people for whom weight is a problem. Health professionals must employ their knowledge and counseling and motivational skills to assist clients in the difficult challenge of weight loss and maintenance.

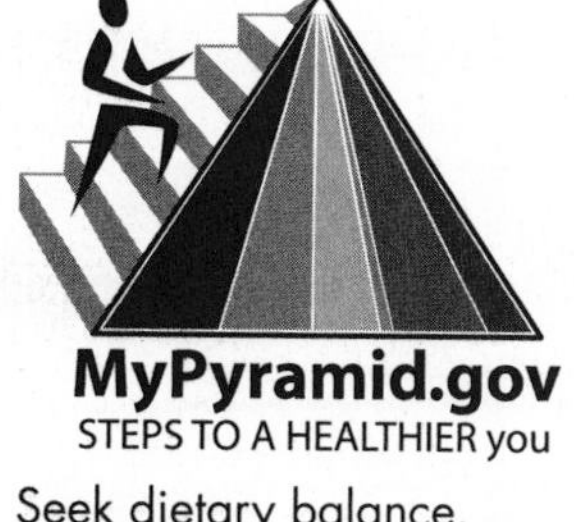

Seek dietary balance.

Health professionals also have to be cognizant of eating disorders and the promotion of healthy eating and physical activity rather than "dieting." Public health measures in children are school exercise programs, removing soda and candy machines from schools, changing school nutrition programs, and establishing good dietary and exercise behaviors in childhood. In adults public health measures include pregnancy counseling (excessive weight gain during pregnancy is very common in previously obese women), focusing on women (who typically do household food shopping and preparation), and promoting the **food pyramid** (an educational tool of dietary balances) and exercise.

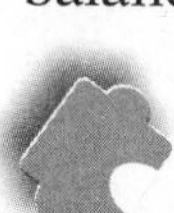

Counseling and Mental Health

Considerations of genetics, environment, and lifestyle are also meaningful when we focus on what influences mental health.

Genetic Considerations

Determining the relationship of heredity to mental health is not an easy task. Mental illness has multiple causes, physiological and otherwise. There are now, and will continue to be, more tests demonstrating how our genes have resulted in emotional illnesses. Evidence already exists, for example, of a tendency toward alcoholism in many families. Environmental and lifestyle factors figure prominently in disease onset as they may trigger what is genetically programmed.

Genetic links to mental illness are difficult to determine because of the overlap of environmental factors. Consider this example:

CASE STUDY 9-1

Young Tom has been raised in the presence of chronic alcohol abuse. Every time his mom and dad are unhappy, they open a bottle to drown their sorrows. There are few days when they do not turn to alcohol.

When Tom enters high school, his life isn't going smoothly. He finds his schoolwork difficult, he is tired of his part-time job, and his teachers are unsympathetic. His friends think it is great fun to get drunk in the restrooms and then go to class. Soon drinking becomes a way of life for Tom.

Did Tom learn to drink because his mom and dad demonstrated that "booze" was the best way to cope? Are his friends primarily responsible for Tom's problems? Did he inherit a program for alcoholism that was physically determined to take effect as soon as he took his first drink? Or are there other considerations that must be examined?

Schizophrenia has been the subject of much **etiological** research (research that looks for causes). One major question has been whether a schizophrenic who has one or two schizophrenic parents inherits the condition or develops mental illness because of her or his environment. For many years the hazards of being raised by mentally disturbed people were believed to be the cause of second-generation mental illness.

Then a reasonably large sample of twins and siblings was studied. These children had at least one schizophrenic parent. Half of them were raised by or around the schizophrenic; the other half were raised in homes free of any clear signs of mental illness. However, the incidence of second-generation schizophrenia remained consistent. That is, the children of one schizophrenic had a higher incidence (10 percent) of schizophrenia than did the population as a whole (1 percent). Further, whether they were raised with their family of origin or in a schizophrenia-free environment, the percentage of victims remained the same. Finally, there was a higher incidence of schizophrenia among the children who had two schizophrenic parents than among those who had only one schizophrenic parent. This study makes a fairly convincing case for the influence of heredity on some forms of mental illness. Of course, schizophrenia emerges in families with no *known* previous history of schizophrenia. Also, even when both parents are schizophrenic, not all offspring are similarly afflicted. These exceptions may indicate that heredity alone is not a sufficient explanation.

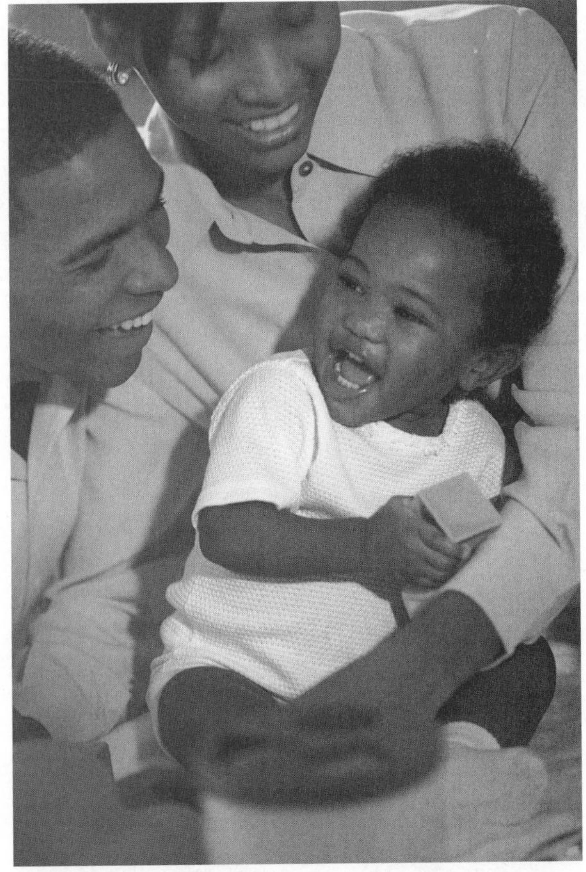

This child is likely to be healthy if mom and dad are healthy.

How does such information help when counseling for prevention? Well, just as the potential victims of heart disease, diabetes, or cancer might wish to understand their risk factors, so do the potential victims of alcoholism, schizophrenia, and manic depression. Taken to the healthy extreme, the child of alcoholics who wishes to be certain of never becoming alcoholic might never drink alcohol. Or the cautious individual with an alcoholic background would be alert to possible signs within herself so that she could seek treatment before a problem got out of hand.

The children of schizophrenics and manic depressives might recognize a need for lifelong medication if they fall victim to their heredity. Awareness and information are essential to accepting the need for prolonged medication. In many cases the medication may allow for near-normal functioning. In the past, victims of these afflictions tended to deny their mental illness and self-medicate with alcohol, which always leads to disastrous consequences that take a heavy toll on both victims and their families.

The more aware a person is about a genetic tendency for mental illness, the more effective counseling may be in other areas. For example, people who are at high risk for mental illness would do well to learn good coping strategies for stress, choose an occupation that best accommodates their individual needs, and develop the kind of support groups that will most promote their ability to function.

Environmental Conditions

The possibility of an environmental link to mental illness focuses on the notion that mental illness can be "learned" through repeated exposure to a mentally ill parent. The relationship of a disturbed environment to the onset of illness has been fairly well accepted by mental health experts. Patients with all degrees of psychological impairment are virtually *expected* to reveal a traumatic past. A difficult family life, blaming problems on mother, and complaints of having received no love are common revelations in psychotherapy. Few people would argue that an abused child has no reason for emotional difficulties. The degree of emotional difficulty appears to depend on the severity of abuse. The book *Sybil* revealed a life of maternal torture of a child. As a defense against this brutality, Sybil developed some 17 separate and distinct personalities, most of whom did not know one another (this is a dissociative disorder). Closing her life off in little boxes and separating from them was the only way Sybil survived. Yet years later, when she was no longer being tortured, continued psychotherapy freed her enough so that she became nearly normal and could face life with just one personality.

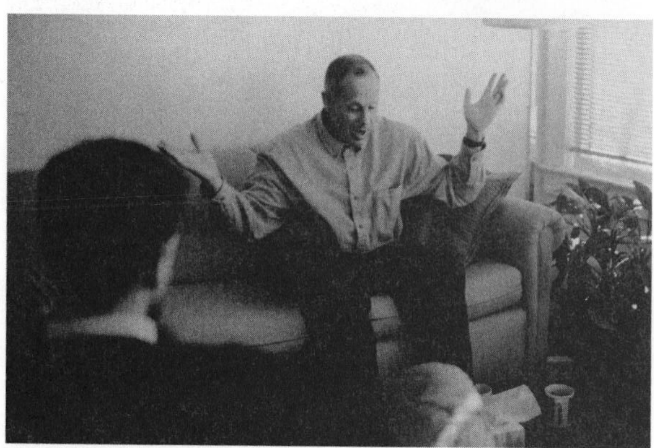

Seek counseling to learn better coping strategies.

If mental illness is learned as a response to environmental stress, it may be unlearned when the stress is eliminated or reduced. Unfortunately, many people do not see their own responses to stress as inappropriate or have never learned appropriate coping strategies. Abused children tend to abuse their own children. One reason is a psychological phenomenon that makes those who were the passive victims of an act need to repeat that act on someone else. Children who were helpless in the face of abuse may get "revenge" through their own children.

Other abused children truly have "learned" that the only way to control children is with harsh physical punishment. They have probably also learned that kids are good punching bags for handling frustrations. No one demonstrated any other options for coping with stress. A boss tells them off at work, and they hurry home to punish somebody.

Still other abused children react differently. Perhaps they had at least one significant adult role model who was not brutal, or perhaps they have a special inner awareness. In any case, they recognize fully that they themselves were misused by their parents. Further, they are determined not to treat their own children as they were treated. Such individuals struggle to make good the wish not to repeat history. If they have dealt with their anger and other psychological scars, it is possible that they will not abuse their kids. But, if they have difficulty coping with life in general and if they refuse the notion of psychotherapy, they are likely to repeat the pattern of child abuse.

An essential point here is that early recognition of potential emotional problems warrants early treatment. Counseling that helps the young adult resolve parental conflicts and close off the past prevents that individual from perpetuating the abuse. "Fix yourself before you have your kids so your kids will have a better chance" is a good slogan for counseling prevention.

Environmental considerations for mental health can also be broad in scope. For example, overcrowding and noise pollution have their own impact on mental health. Studies with rats have shown that overcrowding can make animals paranoid. Competition for space and guarding against and fearing neighbors are all part of paranoia. We can easily transfer this knowledge from rats to human beings. Just think of the number of locks most inner city people have on their doors. The kind of trust that is the norm in a rural community has been totally conditioned out of those who live in large urban areas. Finding an environment that offers enough stimulation to be energizing without generating unmanageable stress is an important consideration for good mental health.

Social and familial support during illness is also an environmental consideration. As discussed in the final section of this chapter, such support is the cornerstone of motivation.

Lifestyle Factors

Stress is undoubtedly the most significant word in our lifestyle vocabulary. It is a sense of outside pressure leading to discomfort. Some people cannot be happy until the stress goes out of their lives. Others accept stress as natural, cope with it well, and even thrive on reasonable amounts of it (called normal stress or eustress). How many times have you heard people say that they work better under pressure? However, the hands of a potter must apply just the correct amount of pressure for a piece of art; too much pressure and the pot collapses. Stress, anxiety, and depression are generally considered negative feelings. To a great extent they have common roots. Certainly no human being goes through life without experiencing some degree of these emotional states. What is important to understand is how and why these feelings become mental illness or serious problems.

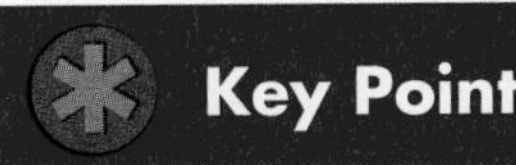

Stress external forces that lead to distress.

One aspect of stress or social pressure is the all-consuming quest for perfection. Those who accept the notion that being thin is essential—and most who do are females between 12 and 24 years old—will take any drug that will help them lose weight. Speed, cocaine, ipecac, diuretics, and laxatives have all been abused by people who want to be thin.

Lifestyle affects mental as well as physical health. Symptoms can be the cause or the effect of lifestyle problems. For example, sleeplessness often indicates emotional disturbance. And if sleeplessness occurs for a prolonged period of time, it can also lead to physical health problems. A lifestyle that pushes a person to "party" or work with little rest sets the stage for both mental and physical health to deteriorate.

An individual who feels stressed can choose either a good coping strategy or a poor one. Good coping strategies would be physical exercise as a release for stress or simply dealing directly with the source of the problem. Examples of poor coping would be denying that anything is wrong, calling in sick to "punish" the boss, or overusing alcohol or other drugs.

Poor coping usually comes from a sense of inadequacy or a loss of self-efficacy (belief in self). People may say to themselves "Oh, I can't handle this" or "I'll show them if they think they can put me down."

Balance or harmony probably provides the individual with the best chance for good mental health: a balance between work and play; a sense of freedom yet a sense of responsibility; meaningful connections with other human beings especially in primary relationships; and, above all, a belief in one's own basic goodness.

Coping Styles

According to Lazarus and Folkman (1984) coping styles may be viewed as **appraisal-focused coping, problem-focused coping**, and **emotion-focused coping**. (1) Appraisal-focused strategies occur when the person modifies the way he or she thinks, for example, by employing denial or distancing themselves from the problem. People may alter the way they think about a problem by altering their goals and values, such as by seeing the humor in a situation. (2) The problem-focused style deals with the cause of the problem. For example, a person learns more about his or her diagnosis and learns new skills to cope with a disease even if he or she must rearrange his or her life around the illness. (3) The emotion-focused style involves releasing pent-up emotions, distracting oneself, managing hostile feelings, meditating, or using systematic relaxation procedures, for example, to handle the stressor.

Day and Livingstone (2003) and Matud (2004) suggest that women use more emotion-focused coping then do men, who tend to use more problem-focused. They speculate that emotion-focused is not as effective and may cause more psychologic stress, postulating that this is why women report more stress, anxiety, and depression. However, in 2009, the American Psychological Association (APA) published results of a survey that for the first time found the number of middle-aged men reporting stress related to money, job stability, and work had surpassed that of women.

Review the coping skills at the top of the next page. Plug other stressors into the center square. For instance, try pressure to take drugs, pressure to smoke, pressure to have sex, or financial pressure. Then list poor and good ways of coping with these stressors.

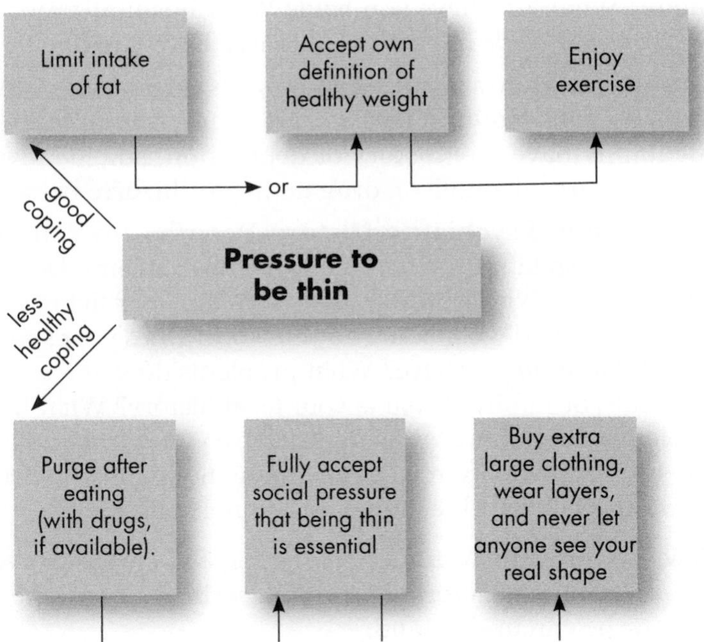

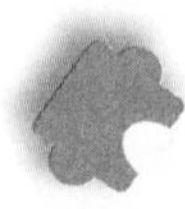

Motivational Strategies for Prevention: AIM

Earlier in this chapter we mentioned a counseling strategy called AIM (awareness, information, and motivation). This strategy relies on the basic scientific knowledge that all health care relies on. How it differs significantly is in its emphasis on motivation. Although health practitioner knowledge is essential to providing service, it is not sufficient. In fact, the health professional who has only knowledge will fail. Counseling skills are a necessary part of success: learn *what* will motivate clients and then learn *how* to motivate them.

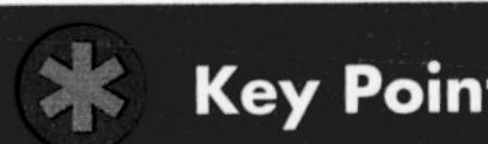

AIM awareness, information, and motivation as tools for health counseling.

Counseling, of course, is a scientific process, and no counselor needs to be more of a scientist than does the health care provider who counsels toward prevention. AIM relies on a scientific process to analyze significant aspects of each individual client. The awareness and information aspects of this process depend on a thorough understanding of the client's genetic, environmental, and lifestyle factors.

Awareness

As scientists, health professionals are aware of the underlying causes of many diseases. Knowledge of risk factors must be transmitted to our clients in language that they understand.

Begin with the client's history. Using the counseling model described in Chapters 1 and 2 with open-ended questions whenever possible, seek the following information:

Previous History. Where did you grow up? What did your parents do? Where did you go to school? How well did you do in school socially and intellectually? What jobs have you held? What hospitalizations and operations have you had? What serious diseases have you had?

Family History. How many brothers and sisters do you have? What serious diseases do your siblings, parents, children, or grandparents have? Does your family have any history of depression, suicide, overweight, high blood pressure, alcoholism, drug taking, or bizarre behavior?

Personal, Social, and Psychiatric History. Describe any counseling you have had or any hospitalization for mental health problems. Do you smoke, drink, or take drugs? Where do you live? What are your living conditions? Where do you work and what hours do you work? Does your spouse work? How many children do you have? What problems do you have with your children, friends, or family? What is your legal history? What financial or sexual problems do you have? Who do you have your primary relationship with? How much do you exercise? How many hours do you drive a day? What causes stress in your life? What do you normally eat?

This review is to provide awareness of the most likely threats to this client's wellness. These risk factors are then described to the client in language that she or he can understand.

Ideally, several health practitioners would act as a team to study the client's family disease/health profile carefully. The same care, of course, would be given to the client's health status. The review of the client's history would focus intensely on lifestyle factors including diet and exercise.

Conveying findings back to the client is a crucial point and one that is often ignored in ordinary health care settings. Many health professionals, especially physicians, take a thorough family history, but few convey anything to the client. For example, a physician may see several overlapping medical problems in close relatives. These problems might make the physician think the client is a good candidate for a stroke. But, unless the client has *developed* stroke risk factors, it is unlikely that the physician will mention the risk. One justification for this approach is to not frighten someone about symptoms they may never develop. But the point of preventive counseling is to tell the client *before* symptoms develop.

This issue comes down to regarding the patient as responsible for the patient's health. If the health professional is ultimately responsible for the patient's health, then a traditional medical model—gathering important information about each client and using it when or if necessary—is followed.

The preventive model, however, places responsibility for the patient's health *on the patient*. Information regarding the patient's family background, current health status, and future forecasts are to be given to the patient/client. Then the client can decide how seriously to take this information.

A healthy 30-year-old who is told he has a relatively high risk factor for heart attack may, in fact, want to ignore this threat until symptoms develop. But what if he doesn't? What if he conscientiously wants to modify his diet and increase his exercise because he is now aware of this particular risk to him? This client may know what the risk factors for heart attack are. He may even see a pattern within his own family. But, until a health professional works with him as an individual while looking at all his familial risk factors, he may not see his own destiny. *Awareness* spells out for a healthy client what he or she needs to be most aware of.

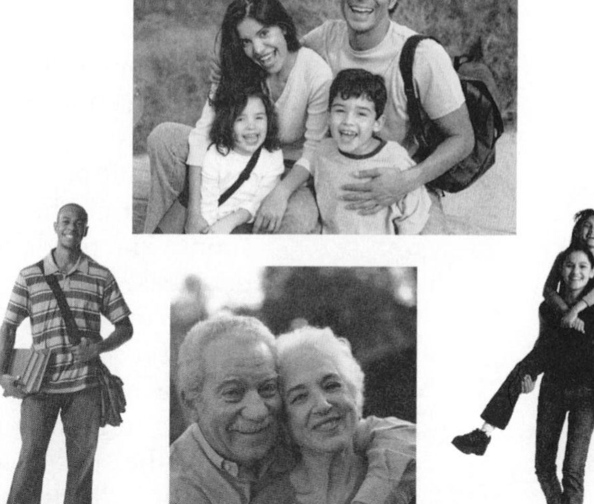

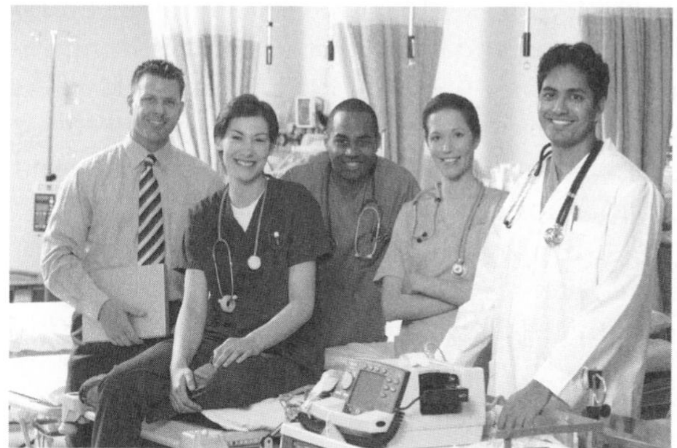

Individual, Optimal Health Care

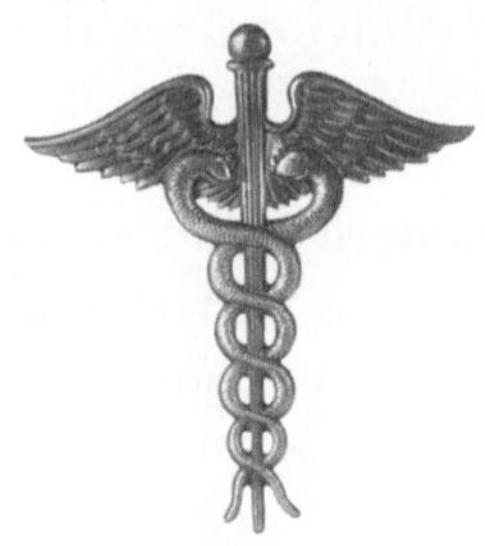

Members of the health care team must determine what will motivate individuals.

Information

The reason health professionals study long hours, read extensively, and conduct research is to broaden their information base. Health professionals also consult with one another to further increase the scope of their information base. Giving appropriate information follows awareness in the responsible counseling process. The client who is told that she is at risk for a heart attack also needs to be told what she can do about that risk. Awareness alone would be cruel. Awareness coupled with information allows the client to see both the problem and its potential solution. To be optimally helpful, the health practitioner must convey enough information and the right information. Handing the person at high risk a pamphlet on how to avoid heart attack might be helpful, but it is insufficient. Rather, the prevention counselor needs to delve into the client's current lifestyle. Holding up a model of perfection and advising the client to mimic it is too easy for the health professional and is destined to fail with the client.

The helpful health care provider needs to know what constraints the client faces in trying to change her behavior and so improve her health. If, for example, exercise is highly important for this client, the health provider needs to explore what gets in the way of exercising. How does this client stop herself from getting exercise? Chances are that she will say she does not have time to exercise. Traditionally, the health practitioner would go through the client's daily schedule with her and help her see how she could budget the exercise in. This might still be helpful, but with in-depth information, precisely helpful advice can be offered with the motivational interviewing techniques described in the final section of this chapter.

The health professional might first ask what exercising means to the client. Does it perhaps mean jogging five miles followed by a shower and a change of clothes? What if the client could gain all the conditioning response she needs for a healthy body from four 20–30 minute brisk walks per week? Doesn't that free up time? Doesn't it also eliminate the need for showering and changing clothes, thus allowing more flexibility? And doesn't it sound like a small sacrifice for continued good health?

Information follows awareness. It provides the client with options for helping to maintain health in the face of risk. Also, since it takes into account the special needs of the individual client, it is the *best information* for that individual.

Motivation

In the past, awareness, especially in the face of developing health problems, was believed to be a sufficient motivational force to get people to change their behavior. Health professionals believed that if people knew they would become increasingly unwell unless they followed certain instructions, they would surely do what they should. Information that approached the client at his or her own level or took particular needs into account was seen as a further advance (see more under motivational interviewing later in this chapter). Maybe everyone couldn't keep his or her weight at the right level for optimal health, but couldn't everyone adjust his or her diet to reduce high fats or heavy salts? The answer was—and is—*no*. Even together, awareness and information have left a tremendous gap in compliance. That gap is called motivation.

Motivation can be defined as an inner drive that forces the individual toward action. If survival is instinctive, the quest for wellness would appear to be motivational in and of itself. But the vast history of patient noncompliance tells us we must look beyond awareness of risks.

We usually assume that individuals who seek health care are at least somewhat motivated. But from the outside, it is difficult to know how motivated a patient is. A real understanding of motivation can only be gained on an individual basis. That is, what motivates one individual to act may in fact stop another from acting. Consider this example.

CASE STUDY 9-2

Joan Ku has cared for her invalid mother-in-law for seven years. She finds the daily tasks of caring for her mother-in-law to be tedious, difficult, boring, and generally unrewarding.

When Joan is then diagnosed as having high blood pressure, her physician prescribes exercise, diet changes, and rest, and mentions that Joan may have to both take medication and change her lifestyle if she cannot lower her blood pressure through these methods. If Joan believes that prolonged high blood pressure may lead to the removal of her mother-in-law from her home, what is she likely to be motivated to do?

This example may seem contrived, but it is a reasonable example of what actually happens. Recall our discussion of illness behavior in Chapter 4. For some individuals and families, the illness itself becomes rewarding. And if illness is a reward, then wellness is a punishment. If you are a student of logic, this becomes the only plausible explanation for noncompliance. That is, *the disease itself is rewarding*. Further, the *patient finds some aspect of compliance more difficult than the problem itself*.

Behavior Modification

A basic key to behavior modification is determining what the reward is. A classic example is the child who wants parental attention. Little Jesse's parents are often too busy and preoccupied with other matters to pay much attention to him. So Jesse throws his dinner on the kitchen floor. His parents, who do not like to have food wasted and their meals disrupted, spank him. Has Jesse been punished or rewarded? If you think he has been punished, recall what he was trying to get. Bear in mind, too, that rewarding negative behavior only serves to increase it.

Health professionals who want to motivate a patient are frequently successful when they find the right reward to modify the patient's behavior. But the key to success lies in distinguishing punishment from reward. Here is another example.

CASE STUDY 9-3

Gretchen, 37, is married and has two adolescent children. Gretchen has a long history of frequent hospitalizations because of anorexia nervosa. At times she has held her own emotionally and done well enough with her weight to be out of danger. Then, virtually overnight, she falls apart emotionally and drops 15 pounds in a matter of days. When this happens, Gretchen must be hospitalized.

This pattern, which Gretchen has repeated for 10 years, has the health professionals who care for her baffled. They reason that a woman who wants to get well and enjoy her young family will struggle hard to keep her weight up and avoid hospitalization. They see time with her family as Gretchen's reward for good eating.

But what has been the reward for Gretchen? Hospitalization has been the reward. Peace and quiet have been the reward. Time away from a demanding, hectic, often unpleasant family life has been the reward. This reward has motivated Gretchen to starve herself. Years before, Gretchen learned that people did not bother her or expect too much from her when she was ill, especially when she was in the hospital. She is no longer on a bizarre quest for thinness. She now uses anorexia to cope with too much environmental stress. She starves to gain her reward: a peaceful environment.

Once hospitalization is determined to be Gretchen's goal, her anorexia is virtually cured. All the health professional had to do was promise Gretchen that she could be hospitalized upon request. Anytime the stress became too much for Gretchen she could be hospitalized—without weight loss.

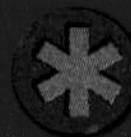

Key Points

Contingency management specific rewards given or withheld contingent or dependent upon specific behavioral changes.

Token economy usually, in-patient reward tokens for desirable behaviors which patient can use for desirable commodity—a form of behavior modification.

Instead of having to starve herself, Gretchen could be rewarded at a normal weight.

Motivation may make use of **contingency-management** procedures and token economies as these strategies are often successful in changing or modifying behaviors by the immediate rewards they offer. With contingency-management systems, patients frequently are required to deposit money. Contingent upon attending group sessions or changing a behavior, the patient gets the money back. In one particularly affluent group, participants were paid $250 for every five pounds they lost. This system frequently works, at least in the short run, because most people feel rewarded when they earn money and punished when they lose it.

A **token economy**, which is generally used with an inpatient population, is even more individually tailored. Tokens are given as rewards for adopting desirable behaviors. The patient can then exchange tokens for a privilege or desirable commodity. For example, the patient who earns two tokens for cleaning his room each day may, after five days, exchange them for a privilege like smoking alone on the hospital grounds, which costs 10 tokens. This is a more sophisticated form of behavior modification than contingency management because the tokens are exchanged for a reward of the patient's choosing. If a specific reward such as smoking rights were offered for good behavior, some patients would not consider this a reward. Tokens allow everyone to choose what will be rewarding to them.

Cognitive Dissonance

Key Point

Cognitive dissonance seeking of harmony by the human mind in making choices, which involves rationalizing the advantages to the choice made.

Theories other than behavior modification influence thinking on motivation. One such important theory is the theory of **cognitive dissonance**. According to this theory, the human mind is always seeking to simplify and reconcile information. The mind is seeking a state of harmony or consonance. Consider the example of trying to decide which of two products to buy. While struggling to decide between product X and product Y, a person's mind is in a state of disharmony or dissonance. Once product Y is purchased, the mind focuses on all its good characteristics. This is rationalization that the right product was bought. Further, the flaws in product X come to mind as justification for not having bought it. This allows the mind to return to a state of harmony. It also helps to explain why many individuals have fierce brand loyalty.

Transferred to motivational theory, cognitive dissonance explains something about campaigns waged to change human behavior. Fear is a tactic often used by those who want to encourage people to quit smoking. Many clearly link smoking with cancer. But most smokers will deny the truthfulness of this link. They will say that they do not fear cancer. People who have a tremendous fear of cancer will most likely have quit smoking on their own or will never have smoked because tremendous fear creates a state of dissonance. To overcome this fear, those who are concerned about cancer cannot smoke or the dissonance would be too great.

For those who do smoke, a cancer fear campaign simply increases their resistance. They cannot both smoke and live in fear, so they deny the message of the campaign. They may even increase their smoking to prove to themselves that they are not afraid. This then returns them to a state of harmony, regardless of what it does to their lungs. In this example, what is expected to be the motivator—fear—actually prevents the smoker from making any positive health change.

Antagonists to Motivation

A final concept essential to understanding motivational theory is the concept of **antagonists** to motivation. To understand this idea, look at the victims of chronic illness. (An antagonist is something that opposes something else.)

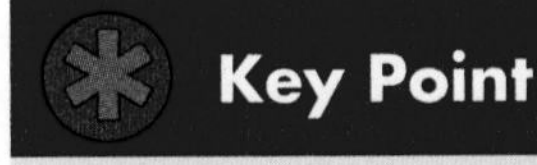

Antagonists to motivation things that work against client motivation.

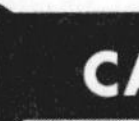

CASE STUDY 9-4

Initially, Jaime, a diabetic patient, seemed highly motivated to comply with his diet, exercise, and insulin regimens. Frequently, however, he suffered mild insulin reactions because of the tight control he kept. When he complained about these reactions, the health care provider assured him that they were a necessary part of good management and promised he would learn to better adjust his insulin and activity to reduce the number of reactions. But insulin reactions continued to make Jaime feel frail and unwell.

Jaime then realized that the limitations of his diet had made him somewhat of a social burden. He was no longer invited out to dinner very often, which was demoralizing. Jaime decided to take his chances on what the future might bring and go ahead and run his life with higher blood sugars. To a certain point his physical feelings improved along with his social life. (Note: The authors are not suggesting his actions are healthy.)

The physical discomfort of insulin reactions (weakness, sweating, racing heart, shaking and possible loss of consciousness) coupled with some social limitations felt like punishment to this patient. If he believed his compliance was resulting in punishment, then he would not continue to comply.

Compliance

Not enough work has been done in the area of motivation and compliance. Recent work suggests that screening may yield a profile of patients who are most likely to comply with preventive regimens. Perhaps by concentrating efforts on patients who are most likely to succeed there will be an increased number of successes and a cost benefit to society.

Screening for success involves evaluating for risk factors, individual skills, history, social factors and attitude. The profile for a successful patient is many-faceted. Genetic, environmental, and lifestyle factors must be evaluated. The individual's commitment to success or change is imperative. Finally, the individual's history of successes, ability to comprehend a complex problem, and ability to treat himself or herself must be evaluated.

Generally, a patient who has family responsibilities and support is a good candidate for success. Getting or staying well because there are people who need and love you appears to be a good motivator. Patients in midlife generally comply best. Adolescent patients quickly tire of or ignore protocols aimed at a distant gain when they are asked to make sacrifices in the present. Other older patients comply well because the threat of physical illness is so near.

Good mental health and at least average intelligence are also important to success. But the factor that is the most difficult to measure and predict—inner motivation—is undoubtedly the key ingredient for success.

Although the principle of screening may be supportable, applying it is not. In practice, few programs would turn a candidate away because she or he appeared to be a poor risk. The ethical dilemma raised is, given limited resources, do we have the right to give less time to people because they are likely to waste it and give that time to someone who is likely to make good use of it? Better motivational interviewing skills can assist those who are yet to fully contemplate a behavior change.

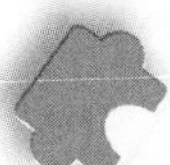

Transtheoretical Model of Change

A major current approach to treatment uses the **transtheoretical model of change (TTM).**

Categories of Change

The transtheoretical model of change recognizes that behavioral change goes through stages and divides people into six categories:

- *Pre-contemplation:* "I don't have a problem" or "I drink but I'm not an alcoholic." The client feels the health issue is a nonissue. The appropriate management is informational only as the patient is in denial (e.g., "You have cirrhosis; if you continue to drink you will halve your life expectancy; if you ever decide you need any help please call me or see me, I am available at any time.")
- *Contemplation:* "Maybe I'll change someday." The client thinks about changing but is ambivalent. "I can do it by myself." The appropriate management is to get the patient to list the pros and cons, for example, "I have cirrhosis; if I continue to drink I may halve my life expectancy and my wife is going to leave me and I already have been convicted of driving under the influence twice." The provider should follow this admission by: "Then do you think you should stop drinking? Would you see me again?" This stage may last months or years.
- *Recognition/Preparation:* "I've got to do something." The client is ready for change. The appropriate management is heavily supportive. "I absolutely agree; have you thought about attending an AA meeting?" The provider might arrange an appointment with an alcohol counselor, show the client a list of local AA meetings, or call the client at home or see him or her again. Goal setting, preparation, and motivation are key.
- *Action:* "I'm doing it!" The client has stopped drinking and is attending AA. Less support is needed, but the provider should reinforce and support the changes that have already been made; and plan with the patient what may go wrong and how to handle set-backs and barriers. It is best to have a plan in place to problem-solve solutions to potential slips.

- *Maintenance:* "I did it!" The client has not drunk for a year. The habit has changed, hopefully permanently.
- *Relapse:* "I fell off the wagon." At any time a person on maintenance may relapse into contemplation or recognition/preparation. The provider should ask: "How did you feel when you were sober? Do you want to stop again?"

This model offers progress through the stages by implementing a series of 10 processes of change that involve pretesting clients; expressing confidence, uncovering discrepancies, expressing empathy, and rolling with resistance—actions tailored to the client's stage. In fact, the model rests heavily on the health professional making appropriate interventions for each stage or level. For example, it was found that an intensive action-maintenance–oriented approach was highly successful with clients who were at the action stage for smoking cessation, but this approach failed miserably for those who were in the precontemplation or contemplation stages (Ockene, Ockene, and Kristellar, 1988). All clients used to be treated as though they were in the recognition stage, thus leading to inappropriate management. Treatment must be targeted to the stage of TTM. Be brief, give feedback on personal risk, reinforce that responsibility for change is the patient's, give the patient a menu of alternatives, use empathy as a counseling style, and encourage self-sufficiency. Remember that denial is a defense, *not* a character issue.

Motivational Interviewing

Motivational interviewing (MI) is based on TTM (Prochaska & DiClemente, 1983; Prochaska & Velicer, 1997) and is currently the most popular stage model in health psychology. This is because (1) the stages and their corresponding responses are somewhat measurable, lending themselves to be used as "evidence-based," that is, clinicians may indicate some measures of success or statistics to demonstrate the effectiveness of treatment (grant-making agencies and taxpayers' groups increasingly insist on proof of the efficacy of treatment), and (2) the stages allow application over a broad spectrum of health issues such as smoking cessation, weight control, substance abuse control, condom use, and other pro-health behaviors such as mammography.

Motivational interviewing is a client-based technique similar to Rogerian counseling except that the counselor is also trying to influence the client to change. Motivational interviewing uses four principles:

1. Empathy: This was discussed in Chapter 2.
2. Develop discrepancies: "If this is how you want your life to be, why do you spend your evenings drinking when you want to do other things?"
3. Roll with resistance: If a client says, "I'm not going to AA," the counselor will not even ask why not but will just explore other avenues. The counselor will not take this as something pathological about the client but rather human nature.
4. Support **self-efficacy**: "OK, I understand you don't want to see the doctor now; if you want a referral later let me know."

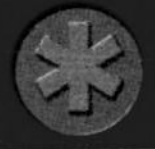

Key Points

Motivational interviewing (MI) specific technique using nondirective and empathic eliciting style to motivate client or to use client's own motivation to change, pushing the client to articulate ambivalence.

Transtheoretical model of change (TTM) a model that divides people into six categories: precontemplation, contemplation, recognition/preparation, action, maintenance, and relapse.

Summary

This chapter began with a definition of counseling and demonstrated the evolution of communication skills into good counseling techniques by introducing the influencing response. Health-related occupations that are based on counseling skills were also reviewed. Both mental health and physical health were discussed in terms of risk factors that counseling may mediate with emphasis on a preventive model. Risk factors were viewed in three major categories: genetic programming, environmental conditions, and lifestyle factors. The preventive model places the patient or client in the position of responsibility for his or her own wellness.

The final section of this chapter reviewed motivational strategies. First it reviewed AIM, which stands for awareness, information, and motivation and is based on:

- Analyzing the client sufficiently to know what actually constitutes a reward for him or her.
- Behavior modification techniques like contingency management and token economies.
- The theory of cognitive dissonance, which shows us that denial is used to avoid conflict. Sometimes this denial gets in the way of motivation.

It also discussed transtheoretical model of change (TTM) and the application of the TTM model, which is known as motivational interviewing and is the most widely used approach to motivation currently in use. MI focuses on:

- Stages of change: precontemplative, contemplative, preparation, action, and maintenance.
- Interventions needed to correspond to these stages.

MI helps predict success and helps with health behaviors. It has the advantage of being measurable.

Chapter Review

Key Term Review

Awareness, information, and motivation (AIM): Counseling technique using awareness, information, and motivation as tools.

Aerobic exercise: Use of large muscle groups that increases oxygen flow.

Amniocentesis: Medical procedure in which amniotic fluid is removed from abdomen of pregnant women. Tests run on this fluid indicate certain health characteristics of the fetus.

Antagonists: Opponents, against good.

Appraisal-focused coping: Altering the value or view of stress, for example, using humor to cope.

Body Mass Index (BMI): A number that expresses degree of body fat.

Contingency management: Specific rewards given or withheld contingent or dependent upon specific behavioral changes.

Cognitive dissonance: The seeking of harmony by the human mind in making choices and the consequent rationalization of the advantages of the choice made.

Emotion-focused coping: Coping of a stressed individual, who tries to "let his or her feelings out" or use relaxation techniques to cope with stress rather than attempt to directly change the stress object.

Environmental conditions: The world around us.

Etiology: Cause.

Food pyramid: Food guide that shows the consumer how much of each food group is advised.

Genetic counseling: The assessment of genetic risk by a professional and presentation of the statistics in a cogent way to the individual.

Genetic programming: Inherited characteristics carried by our genes.

Influencing response: Response that influences the action the client may take.

Leading response: Communication skills by the health professional used to lead the client. May include advice giving, questioning, and influencing.

Lifestyle factors: How we choose to live.

Metabolic syndrome: Generally, the combined occurrence of any three of the following in one individual: obesity, diabetes, high cholesterol, and high blood pressure.

Motivation: Drive toward a particular action.

Motivational interviewing (MI): Specific technique using a nondirective and an empathic eliciting style to motivate client. MI uses client's own motivation to change and pushes the client to articulate ambivalence.

Obesity: BMI over 30.

Overweight: BMI over 25.

Primary prevention: Action taken to prevent or delay the onset of a disease.

Problem-focused coping: Learning more about the stressor and then taking direct action to cope with the stress (e.g., changing lifestyle to cope with a disease or quitting a problematic job).

Secondary prevention: Action taken to delay or prevent complications once a disease process has begun.

Sedentary: Inactive.

Self-efficacy: Belief in self.

Stress: External forces that lead to distress.

Token economy: Usually, in-patient reward tokens for desirable behaviors that patient can use for desirable commodity—a form of behavior modification.

Transtheoretical model of change (TTM): A model that divides people into six categories: precontemplation, contemplation, recognition/preparation, action, maintenance, and relapse.

Visceral fat: Fat in and around organs, especially intraperitoneal—liver, kidneys, omentum, mesentery and bowels—but also the heart.

Chapter Review Questions

1. Compare the risk factors of an agrarian society to our current risk factors. Which society had (has) the longest life expectancy? Try looking at these risk factors by gender differences between agrarian and today.
2. Discuss the difficulties of motivating an AIDS victim to comply with safe sex practices.
3. Your client is putting on weight. You know both her parents had diabetes and her father died of a heart attack aged 39. How would you address the situation?
4. After reading this chapter you calculate your BMI is 32. Would you take any action based on this?
5. On the basis of our discussion in this chapter, what do you think causes mental illness?

Case Study Critical Thinking Questions

1. Review Case Study 9-1. What is the risk of Tom becoming an alcoholic?
2. Please review Case Study 9-2. How may diseases be rewarding? Do you personally associate any comforts with illness? Look up the term "Munchausen syndrome by proxy" and see what understanding you might have of this difficult psychiatric syndrome.
3. If a person looks for rewards in illness behavior, as in Case Studies 9-2 and 9-3, what might this be saying about him or her? Describe the coping styles his or her behavior indicates and outline better ways he or she might handle stress.
4. Review Case Study 9-4. How may health professionals intervene to return this man to a level of safer compliance? Will victims of chronic health problems make extensive sacrifices in the present to avoid a possible punishment in the future? (These expectations are part of prevention, but successes are limited.)

References

1. American Dietetic Association: www.eatright.org
2. Auchincloss, Louis. *Sybil.* Boston: Houghton Mifflin, 1952.
3. Danish, S., D'Augelli, A. R., Hauer, A. L. *Helping Skills: A Basic Training Program.* New York: Human Sciences Press, 1980.
4. Day, A., Livingston, H. Gender differences in perceptions of stressors and utilization of social support among university students. *Can J of Beh Sci* 35:73–83; 2003.
5. Harr, J. *A Civil Action*. NY: Vintage, 1996.
6. Harris Interactive. "The Recession is Stressing Men more than Women." APA Stress in America Survey. *Monit Psych* 40:7; 2009.
7. Lazarus, R., Folkman, S. *Stress, Appraisal and Coping.* New York: Springer, 1984.
8. Lethbridge-Cejku, M., Vickerie, J. "Summary Health Statistics for U.S. Adults." National Health Interview Survey, 2003, National Center for Health Statistics. *Vital Health Stat* 10(225), 2005.
9. Lynch, H., de la Chapelle, A. "Hereditary Colorectal Cancer." *New Engl J Med* 348:919–932; 2003.
10. Matud, M. "Gender Differences in Stress and Coping Styles." *Pers Indiv Differ* 37:1401–1415; 2004.
11. Miller, W. R., Rollnick, S. *Motivational Interviewing: Preparing People for Change*. New York: Guilford Press, 2002.
12. Mokdad, A., et al. "Prevalence of Obesity, Diabetes, and Obesity-Related Health Risk Factors." 2001. *J Amer Med Assoc* 289(1):76–79; 2003.
13. National Center for Health Statistics. "Chartbook on Trends in the Health of Americans." *Health, United States 2006*. Hyattsville, MD: Public Health Service, 2006.
14. Ockene, J., Ockene, I., Kristellar, J. "Assessing the Stages of Change and Decision-Making." *The Coronary Artery Smoking Intervention Study*: Worcester MA: National Heart, Lung and Blood Institute, 1988.
15. Prochaska, J., DiClemente, C. "Stages and Processes of Self-Change of Smoking: Toward an Integrative Model of Change." *J Consult Clin Psych*51:390–395; 1983.
16. Prochaska, J., Norcross, J., DiClemente, C. *Changing for Good: A Revolutionary Six-Stage Program for Overcoming Bad Habits and Moving Your Life Positively Forward.* New York: Avon Books Inc, 1994.
17. Prochaska, J., Velicer, W. "The Transtheoretical Model of Health Behavior Change." *Am J Health Promotion* 12:38–48; 1997.
18. Reich, Charles A. *The Greening of America: How the Youth Revolution Is Trying to Make America Livable.* NewYork: Random House, 1970.
19. Rumania et al. "Population-Based Prevention of Obesity." *J Am Heart Assoc* 118:428–464; 2008.
20. Sue, D. W. Sue, D. *Counseling the Culturally Different,* 2nd ed. New York: Wiley, 1990.
21. Weiss, M., Weiss, F. *Living beyond Breast Cancer.* New York: Times Books, 1997.
22. Winstons, M. "AIDS and a Duty to Protect." *Hastings Center Report.* Feb 1987, 22–23.
23. *Obesity: Preventing and Managing the Global Epidemic.* Report of a World Health Organization Consultation on Obesity, Geneva, 3–5 June, 1997. World Health Organization, Geneva, 1998.
24. www.cancer.gov/cancertopics/factsheet/risk/brca
25. www.nhlbi.nih.gov/guidelines/obesity/ob_dlns.htm
26. www.pyramid.com

Additional Readings

1. Carter, Rosalynn. *Helping Someone with Mental Illness.* New York: Times Books, 1998.
2. Green, Hannah. *I Never Promised You a Rose Garden.* New York: Holt, Rinehart & Winston, 1964.
3. Kuczmarski R., Flegal K. "Criteria for the Definition of Overweight in Transition: Background and Recommendations for the United States." *Am J Clin Nutr* 72:1074–1081; 2000.
4. "Physical Status: The use and Interpretation of Anthropometry." Report of a World Health Organization Expert Committee, Series 854. World Health Organization, Geneva, 1995.
5. Shute, N. *On the Beach.* New York: W. Morrow, 1957.

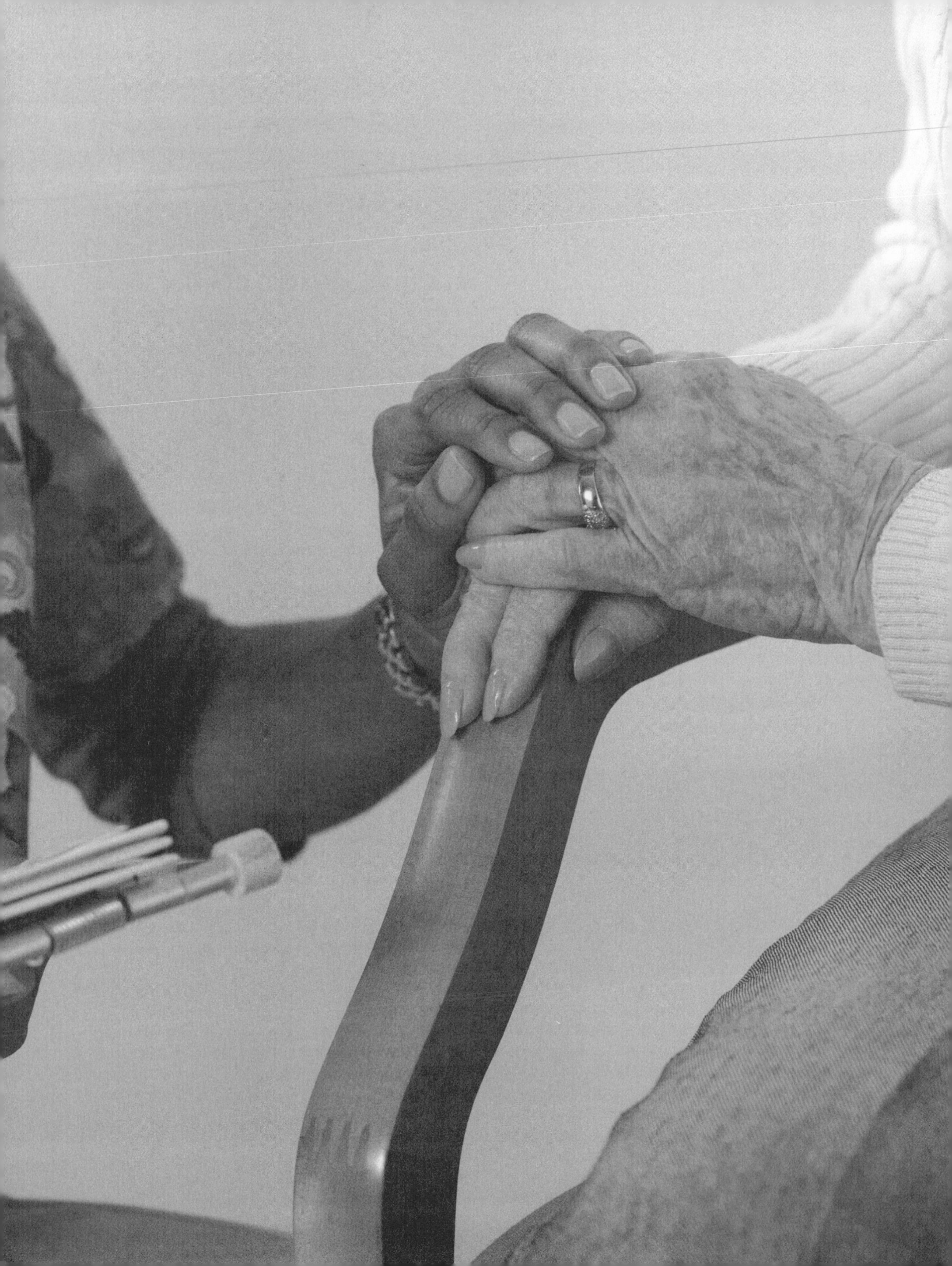

Interdisciplinary Communication

Learning Outcomes

After reading this chapter, you should be able to:

10.1 Understand changing roles in health care.
10.2 Differentiate between inter- and intradisciplinary communications.
10.3 Identify multiple definitions of your role.
10.4 Discuss the difference in roles of consultant, collaborator, and referral source.
10.5 Understand the use of the word "network."
10.6 Explain the relationship between allied health professionals and physicians.
10.7 Describe personality conflicts and turf issues.
10.8 Evaluate the importance of networking.
10.9 Describe different types of interdisciplinary communication.
10.10 Explain how teams function and what makes one successful.
10.11 Describe examples of health care teams.
10.12 Differentiate between team leader and case manager.
10.13 Understand the different components of health information technology.
10.14 Explain where America is going in the future with health information technology.
10.15 Discuss advantages and disadvantages of health information technology.

Key Terms

Acronym
Case conference
Case manager
Collaborators
Computerized physician order entry (CPOE)
Consultant
Crisis intervention
Electronic health record (EHR)
e-prescribe
Formal network
Health
Health information technology (HIT)
Hospice
Informal network
Interdisciplinary communication
Interoperability
Intradisciplinary communication
Legacy
Networking
Picture archiving and communication system (PACS)
Referral source
Role
Task focus
Team leader
Turf

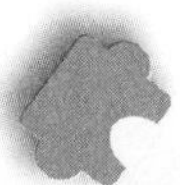

Changing Roles

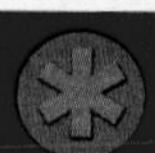

Key Point

Role all behaviors expected from a person who occupies a particular position and status.

A **role** can be defined as all the behaviors expected from a person who occupies a particular position and status in a social pattern. What is expected from health professionals requires examination of changing roles, communication roles, who defines the roles, and the specific roles of consultant, collaborator, and referral source.

The role of yesteryear is not the role of today. Society changes, technology changes, the law changes, and allied health professionals change. The advent of amniocentesis, for example, changed the genetic counselor's role dramatically. In certain states, the nurse midwife is prohibited by law from independent practice. But, when the law changes, so does the role of the nurse midwife.

Most health professionals are expanding their roles. Podiatrists, for example, are moving away from the foot and more toward the body mechanics involved with walking and running. They now meet the needs of a society that is interested in jogging.

Health care providers are becoming increasingly involved in management. In recent times, nurses may have been heavily involved in one-on-one patient care, personal care, psychological support, and surgical aftercare. Now they face a different world. Pharmacists also have seen their roles change. The complexities of modern pharmacology make drug dispensing to hospitalized patients a specialized and critical task.

Because lawsuits are so common in our society, health care providers spend a lot of time on documentation. It is now common to find many kinds of specialists in hospitals, for example, pediatric physical therapists, respiratory therapists, occupational therapists, rehabilitation therapists, and cardiac rehabilitation therapists. New changes in society have even created a need for new professionals, such as medical records specialists and coding specialists.

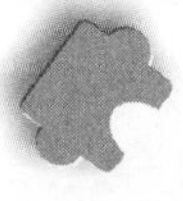

Inter- and Intradisciplinary Communication

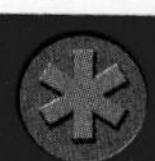

Key Point

Intradisciplinary communication communication between members of the same health specialty.

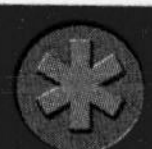

Key Point

Interdisciplinary communication communication between members of different health specialties

Communication within a team is dealt with later in this chapter. The topic here is one-on-one communication. An important aspect of the role in such communication is to know to whom you are talking.

Intradisciplinary communication is communication between members of the same health specialty, for example, when one physical therapist speaks to another.

Interdisciplinary communication is communication between different health practitioners, for example, when a dietitian speaks to an occupational therapist. The language spoken and the roles assumed are affected by whether communication is occurring with someone who works within your own discipline and your relative positions within the hierarchy of command.

It is important that technical terms and abbreviations be kept as simple as possible so that different professionals can understand each other. For example if a physical therapist says "independent in ambulation," does that mean the patient walks without the help of another person, or does it mean without the help of a walking aid, or does it mean both?

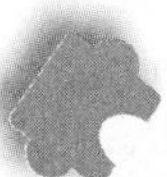

Who Defines the Role?

Roles are defined by the patient, the job description, professional specialty training, your own perception, or liability.

Patients usually prefer to get to know one person well and relate to that person for their health needs. But health care is a highly specialized field with multiple areas of expertise, so one health care provider cannot always possess the necessary expertise. Health practitioners must be able to assess when it would be in their patients' best interest for other experts to be involved. Here you yourself will be defining your role. Sometimes the health professional defines the role; sometimes it is defined by the patient; and sometimes roles will be added by pure chance or circumstance.

CASE STUDY 10-1

Jack, a physical therapist in private practice, is seeing a patient, Jim Harbor, for neck pain. Jim, a 55-year-old male, asks Jack about back pain, which he has had for 20 years. Jack wonders if it would be appropriate to refer Jim to a physician. What if Jim turned out to have cancer of the spine? Jim then asks Jack to treat his back as well. Later Jim mentions that his mother has just died from leukemia. Jim is having sleepless nights and spends 10 minutes talking about it. Jack must use his own judgment about a mental health referral. He may be the only access point the patient has to the health care system. Referral probably should be made only if Jack thinks the grief reaction is becoming pathologic. On the other hand, Jack thinks that maybe he should enquire about Jim's relationship with his primary care physician and whether he has spoken to his physician about his back or his sleepless nights.

Sometimes the patient defines your role by talking about psychologic problems because you are the health practitioner she or he feels comfortable with or because you just happen to be there at the right time. For this reason, all health care workers need to be aware of crisis intervention therapy.

Crisis intervention involves brief counseling, typically for a few weeks, to resolve a major crisis in a patient's life. Such therapy focuses on environmental modification and decision making rather than on deep psychologic issues. Crisis intervention therapy is usually used when the patient's premorbid personality is relatively healthy and when the patient can understand the maladaptive responses that may have been involved in the crisis. Not every situation warrants this type of intervention. The health care provider needs to explore the situation sufficiently to judge whether such brief intervention would be appropriate.

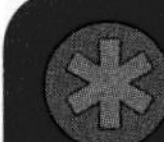

Key Point

Crisis intervention brief therapy to resolve a major crisis in a patient's life.

Who else defines your role? Frequently a hospital or clinic has written job descriptions for its employees. Applicants often see a written job description before they are employed. Obviously the health professional in private practice is in a far better position to define his or her own role and has more latitude than does a health professional employed by an organization. But a written job description need not contradict professional activities and ethics within a chosen field.

Professional perception is an important determinant in defining roles. What is the scope of the specialty? How does your specialty fit in with other specialties? What have people in your specialty done historically? Your perceptions after training and while in practice will further mold your own role definition. What are the potentialities of your specialty? What do you feel most comfortable doing? How do you see yourself best relating to other specialties? What meaningful role expansion do you perceive? What are your time constraints?

One further important determinant is liability, which imposes legal restraints on roles. These are the sorts of issues in which liability may determine roles. Whereas, for example, obstetric nurses are permitted to deliver babies in some states, in other states it is illegal. When should one refer? How much testing should be done? How much documentation is necessary? How much explaining is appropriate for each patient? What if the hospital tells you to do something you do not feel comfortable doing? Also, the length of treatment or hospital stay may not be within the health professional's role to decide, as it should be, but may be dictated by insurance companies often referred to as "third-party payers."

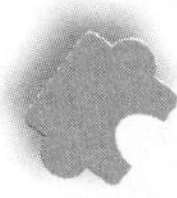

Roles of Consultant, Collaborator, and Referral Sources

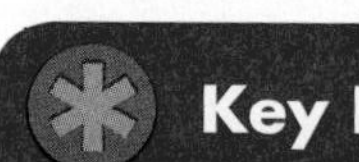

Key Point

Consultant temporary adviser on current problems.

A **consultant** usually acts as a temporary adviser on current problems. The consultant does not necessarily need to see the patient. Scheduling problems in an X-ray department, for instance, could be discussed with an organizational consultant either from the outside or inside of the institution. If changes are needed or departments must share time, the outside consultant is seen as more objective—not making choices based on favorites. An outside consultant such as an ergonomic expert might also make recommendations that would be seen as objective and therefore are more easily accepted. If the recommendations were rejected, the outside consultant would be unlikely to experience any role conflicts.

Alternatively, an inside consultant, for instance the chief of the school of X-ray technology, might be asked for an opinion. This person would be more likely than an outside person to know the personalities involved, to understand the subtleties of how the department functions and to understand the workings of the X-ray department. But it would be harder to reject this person's opinions because they would be the opinions of an insider and a leader.

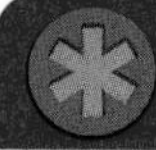

Key Point

Collaborators two or more people working together toward a common end.

Collaborators are two or more people working together to a common end. They may share or even exchange roles. For example a physical therapist and an occupational therapist may discuss with each other and help each other in the rehabilitation of a stroke patient. There is give and take in the relationship.

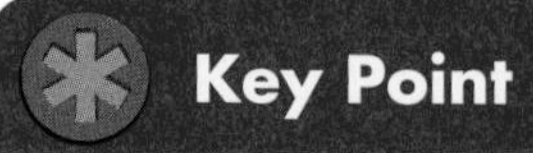

Key Point

Referral source another person to supply information or care for the patient.

A **referral source** is someone the health professional turns to for material information or to transfer patient care. An example would be a physical therapist referring a patient to a speech therapist for swallowing problems after a stroke. A referral source is not an adviser and may play a continuing role, which is the opposite of the consultant role. However, patient care profits when referral sources collaborate.

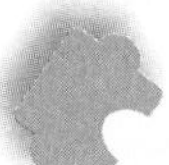

Formal and Informal Teams/Networks

Health care is provided by health care teams that may either be apparent or hidden.

When a person is admitted to the hospital, the health team is apparent. The physical therapist, medical technologist, phlebotomist, X-ray technician, surgeon, and primary care physician are all on site and all appear at the bedside.

But when a person visits a dentist's office, the team is hidden. The dentist may refer a dental problem to a dental technician, hygienist, periodontist, endodontist, or another specialist or may discuss a problem with a medical doctor. He or she may even admit a patient to the hospital, for example, for anesthesia. The patient is therefore using a hidden network that the dentist can activate at any time.

Almost all health care professionals are part of a network. (Communicating with other network members provides a good opportunity to use communication skills.) If the health care team is apparent and obvious, it is called a **formal network** or *formal team.* Teams may come together physically, as in a patient care conference, for example. Team members relate to each other through defined relationships, in an organized structure. Networking takes place by rules and procedures. Or teams may never actually come together but use, for instance, the patient's hospital chart for communication between team members. Such an arrangement may be called an **informal network** or *informal team.*

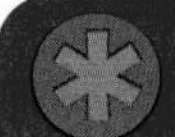

Key Points

Formal network team that is apparent and obvious, assembled for exchange through defined relationships in an organized structure.

Informal network team that is hidden, with no set rules or procedures to follow and no permanent structure.

Types of Networks

Sharing roles in health care may be carried out in a number of ways, as illustrated in the diagram on network structures.

A pyramid, the last example in the diagram on network structures, is also a team, but it emphasizes a hierarchy with a formal pecking order. As a health care provider, you should ideally know the area of expertise and role of each person in a pyramid or team and should use each person to the best advantage for each of your patients. Unfortunately, resentments, jealousy, and other human emotions often create conflict within a network.

CASE STUDY 10-2

Esther has severe peripheral vascular disease, and the surgeon has spoken to her about amputation of her right leg. At the same time the surgeon orders passive range of motion exercises on both legs as Esther will not get out of bed. The physical therapist has conflicting feelings. She does not see any point in performing passive range of motion exercises on a leg that is about to be amputated. Should she simply carry out the order blindly? Should she speak with the surgeon and risk a confrontation? Should she check with other physical therapists in the department?

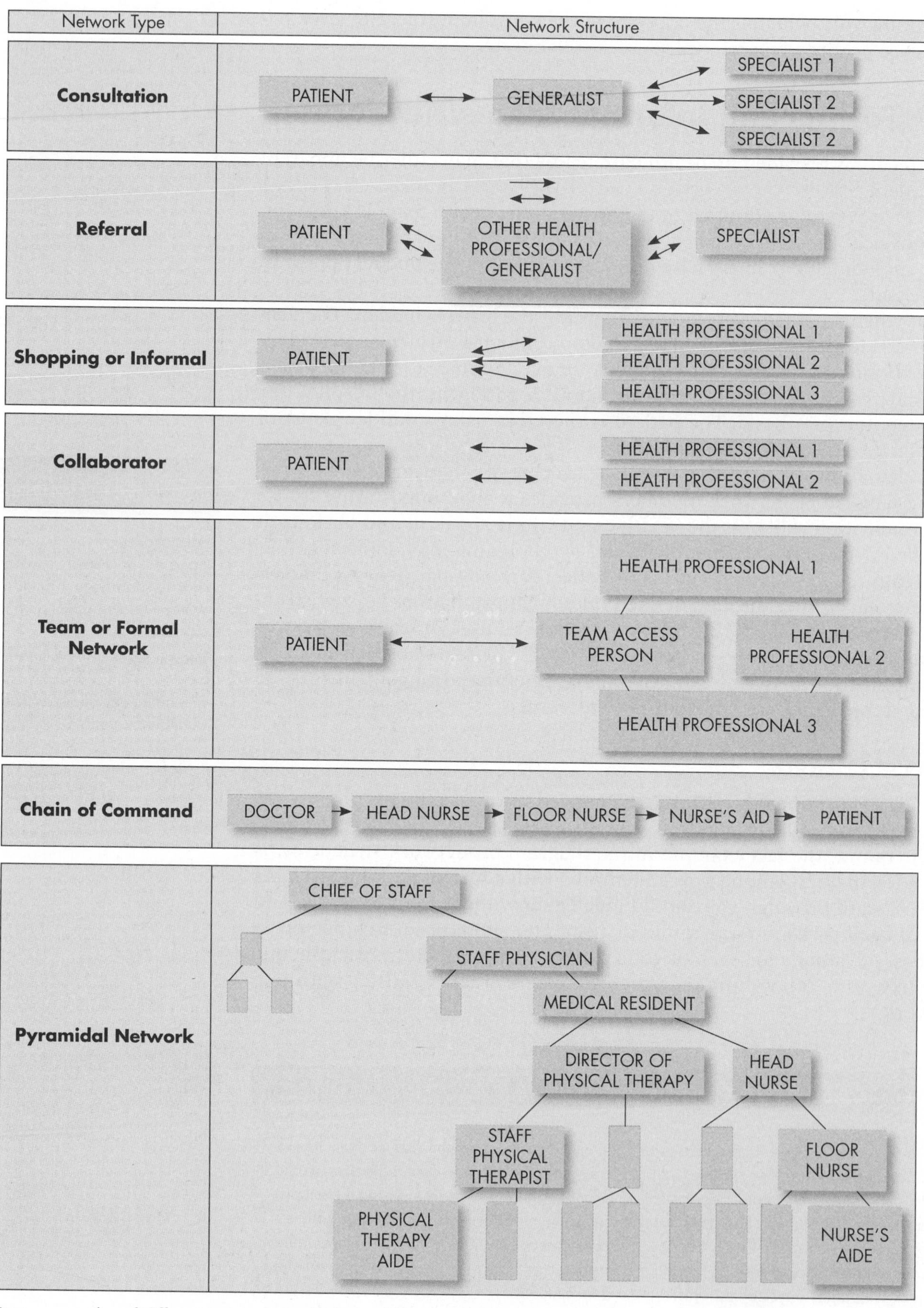

Some examples of different networks and relationships in health care.

Sharing Expertise vs. Sharing the Burden

The reasons for referral, collaboration, consultation, or networking are many. Usually the reason should be that referral or consultation is best thing for the patient physically, psychologically, and financially. Sometimes, however, referral is made for the professional's psychologic benefit; this is called passing the buck. At other times a referral may be made for the patient's psychologic benefit. Before such a referral is made, the professional involved needs to examine why the patient requires it, what might be done about it, and whether he or she can realistically do anything about the situation. After this exercise, the professional may find that, if a referral is necessary, it may be to a social or mental health worker rather than to a dietitian or physician or physical therapist.

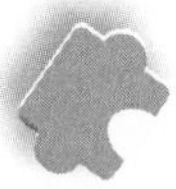

Relationship of Allied Health Professionals to Physicians

How do allied health professionals relate to physicians? How autonomous are the health professionals? The answer depends on where the health professional is on the continuum of technician to professional. An electrocardiogram (EKG) technician takes an EKG when the physician directs. A psychologist, who is on the other end of the continuum, can be an independent professional.

Autonomy is more likely if:

- The professional has a complex expertise.
- The professional is licensed by the state legislature or is an independent practitioner.
- The professional is separately reimbursed by third-party payers.
- The professional is not wholly dependent on the physician for liability.

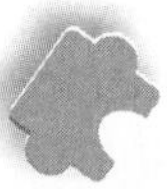

Personality Conflicts and Turf Issues

Personality conflicts are inevitable. Some health professionals are authoritarian, some are casual, some are unprofessional, some are biased, and others are ineffectual. Even though health professionals strive to set themselves apart from ordinary human failing, they are still human. Each of us must examine our own strengths and weaknesses and try to discuss conflicts sensitively and professionally.

Turf refers to territorial rights within an area of expertise. If health professionals step outside their area of expertise, they are in danger of stepping on the toes of other health professionals. Someone will be offended. Be particularly sensitive about turf issues until acquiring knowledge of a network in a particular locale. Take on a role that is consistent with your specialty and tread lightly outside that area until you know the ground better. Alternatively, discuss turf issues with others within your network or with an outside mentor. Recall how it feels when someone steps on *your* turf. Problems occur when multiple specialties have overlapping areas, when the roles may be blurred or shared. Sharing may be hard and turf is not clear-cut.

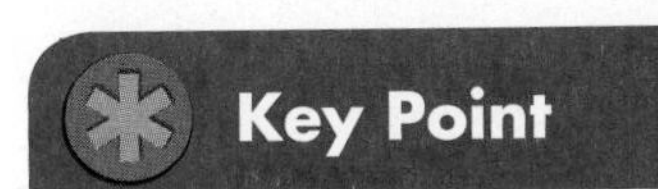

Turf territorial rights within an area of expertise.

The most effective way to deal with turf issues, as well as all issues of both formal and informal networks, is to use good communication skills. Focusing on the needs of peers, paraphrasing, and establishing a rapport help functioning and work enjoyment.

Position of the Student in Shared Roles

Although students may feel awkward, they actually have an advantage. As nonexperts, students have just come from the patient's world. They can generally assume a role of patient advocate and confidante much more easily than a teacher can. They may have much more time to spend with the patient. They may be regarded by the patient as someone who is half health professional and half friend. In assuming this role, students are creating a stepping stone that allows for a gradual shift to the role of full-fledged health professional.

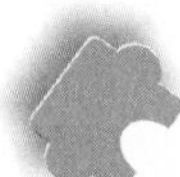

Networking

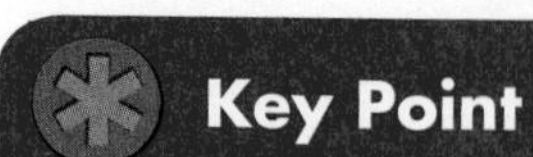

Key Point

Networking marshalling people, systems, agencies, or resources that a specific person needs at a specific time.

Networking means marshalling people, systems, agencies, or resources that a specific person needs at a specific time. A system here refers to a segment of society, for example, family or work. A network is a system of channels of actual or potential communication with different people or agencies.

In a business sense, networks often involve computer information or people, for example, business managers, politicians, or others who are good at networking. In a social sense, networks are people in a patient's life who interact with him or her, like family, friends, or business contacts.

An effective networker knows who has the key talents and empowers the user to use these talents. Rather than simply providing a list of resources, the good networker motivates the patient to utilize resources. The good networker also understands the power of networking. Many successful businessmen, entrepreneurs, managers, politicians and professionals are good networkers. In times past the Rolodex or "little black book" was the mark of a good networker. Today the e-mail list, cell contacts, or Facebook and LinkedIn contacts mark a good networker. E-mail has become a powerful networking tool with the ability to "cc" the same communication to multiple people.

Patients in a hospital usually have multiple health care providers caring for them. The physician is often the case manager or networker. Communication between disciplines is chiefly through the hospital chart, to which health professionals have open access (incidentally, confidentiality may be a problem here).

Outpatients often have a single professional caring for them, but networking or case management may still be required. Communication is by telephone, letter, e-mail, or FAX to other professionals. Confidentiality is generally easier to manage. Protocols are dictated by the Health Insurance Portability and Accountability Act of 1996 (HIPAA) regulations, which will be discussed in a later chapter.

For hospital health professionals the "corridor consultation" is a common means of communication. As the name implies, this is usually a brief chance meeting with another health professional during which clinical problems are discussed. Proximity certainly is valuable in this form of communication. As times change, the hospital corridor is less and less a means of networking. In addition, the hospital corridor is not a confidential place in which to discuss patient issues.

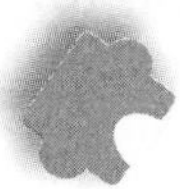

Modes of Interdisciplinary Communication

Interdisciplinary communication has always been a problem in the health care field.

CASE STUDY 10-3

Harry Goldblatt, a 78-year-old patient on a surgical floor, was referred by the floor nurse to the social worker Anita. Anita spoke to Harry and found out that his wife had just died from a heart attack and that an alcoholic son lived with him and disrupted his life. She discussed outpatient avenues for help for Harry and was a good empathetic listener for Harry's grieving.

However, after Anita completed the referral, the nurse called her back saying that Harry needed placement in a nursing facility because he was "still sundowning" and was agitated at nighttime. The nurse had not communicated the reason for the consultation or the necessary details.

Interdisciplinary communication needs to be specific and relevant to a case plan or problem. For instance, a nurse should not just call up a social worker and request a consultation. The social worker needs to know why the patient needs to be seen. Is it for social casework as the social worker assumed in this case? Is it to arrange a walker at home when the patient leaves the hospital? Or is it because the patient, despite the best efforts of the team, still seems to deny his heart attack and this denial could jeopardize his chance for a safe recovery?

All communication has legal ramifications. For example, when a phlebotomist takes blood, she might say, "The doctor has asked me to take some blood from you—OK?" It is true that, if she is silent, there is implied consent when the patient holds his or her arm still for the venipuncture, but the verbal communication makes it better. All written communication including e-mails creates a legal paper trail. Judgmental comments are not appropriate. Neutrally toned comments are more appropriate (e.g., "verbally abusive" rather than "foul-mouthed," "attentive family" rather than "demanding family," and "consultation lasted two hours" rather than "the patient was very time-consuming").

There are several ways that health practitioners communicate with one another: through case conferences; telephone calls; written communication like letters, forms, chart notes, and e-mails; and the medical record, either written or electronic.

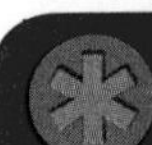

Key Point

Case conference ad hoc meeting of health care professionals focusing on a specific patient at a specific time.

Case Conferences

Multiple **case conferences** improve patient care and time efficiency. As noted earlier, in the ideal world, interdisciplinary communication is best conducted through a case conference. But to assemble six health practitioners for one hour to discuss one patient means that there must be a reasonable expectation that something significant will come out of the meeting that was unlikely to occur without the meeting. It is not uncommon for health professionals to go off on a tangent or to protect their turf rather than share pertinent information.

Generally, case conferences are held only when a patient cannot be adequately cared for without them. Case conferences may be held routinely with specific situations like the discharge of a geriatric patient from a skilled nursing facility. The conference would include the director of nursing, the patient's personal assigned day nurse, the patient's health aide, the physical therapist, the occupational therapist, the social worker, the patient, and the patient's significant other. Notice the physician and pharmacist are usually absent as they are not primarily employees of the nursing facility, and it is not efficient use of time for both of them to travel to the facility for such a conference. Everyone involved must be highly specific, and everyone must agree on a common focal point—in this case the ability of the patient to maintain independence at home.

Telephone Calls

Like other types of communication, telephone communication must be specific. If the message can reasonably be conveyed another way, for example, through a filled-out requisition form, then interruptions during patient care, telephone tag, etc., can be kept to a minimum.

Telephone technique is very important, not only in communicating with health practitioners but also in dealing with patients. If possible, answer

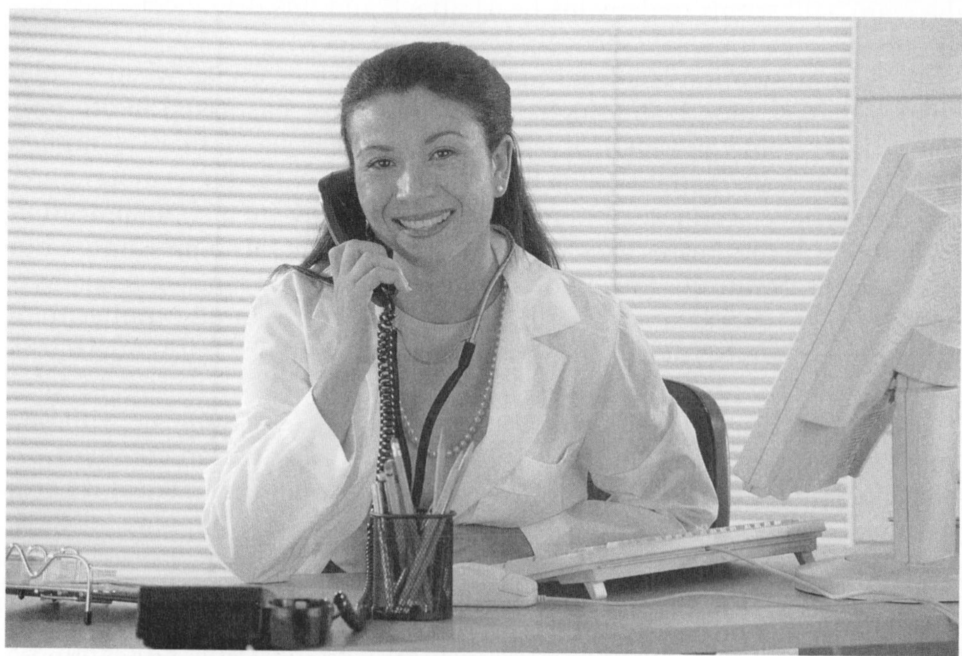

Telephone technique is very important for all levels of health professionals.

the telephone within three rings, and preferably after the first ring. Greet the caller and identify your department and yourself, for example, "Good morning. Pharmacy. John Reed speaking."

Because the telephone permits no nonverbal cues, it is especially important that you project your attitude (which will be friendly and professional) over the telephone. It is helpful if you smile while using the telephone. If you make the same facial expressions while listening on the phone as you would during face-to-face communication, your pauses and comments will come at the right time and will be more appropriate.

Being a good listener is even more important on the phone than in face-to-face communication. Because you cannot look the caller in the eye, it is important to use the caller's name.

If you cannot do what the caller asks, be sure to ask what should or can be done, for example, "I'm afraid I can't see your patient tomorrow, but would the next day be all right? Would you like me to call you after I've seen her or should I just write my comments on the chart?"

Written Communication: Letters, Forms, Notes, and E-mails

Written communication should be brief and specific. Because letters of referral document the communication in writing, it may actually be less time-consuming to write a letter than to try to reach someone on the telephone. Remember that it is unprofessional to make a referral without specific communication as to why the patient has been referred. Both the reason for referral and the answer to that reason should be communicated through accepted channels for every consultation, collaboration, or referral.

In all written communication, try to state things simply. Keep sentences short. Many years ago a label on a tube of glue read, "Optimal results from this product will be obtained by applying the minimal product to the maximal surface area." Someone noticed that the instructions would better read, "Apply thinly."

Avoid the passive voice (e.g., "John has been treated by Dr. Jones" should read: "Dr. Jones has treated John"). Take a course on writing. Proofread even if you have used spell check. Keep e-mails brief: use a brief subject line and a single short paragraph. Any more and it probably will not be read.

Medical Record

For hospitalized patients the medical record is the major form of interdisciplinary communication. Some notes are too short, and some are too long. Computer generation of progress notes in narrative form based on "macros" may look useful in court, but it is dangerous because it hinders communication. An ideal medical record is clear, concise, brief, legible, and accessible in one easily available chart. However, notes entered into an electronic record are easy to access by all who hold the correct password.

Medical records are frequently used in court litigation. What you write and whether it can be read may be pivotal in a malpractice case. Unfortunately, physicians tend to set the worst example by frequently writing illegible and sketchy notes.

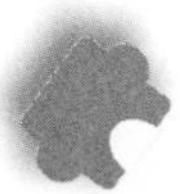

What Is a Team?

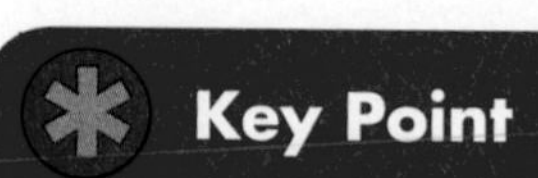

Task focus outcome toward which team is working.

A team is a group of individuals with a common purpose who communicate, collaborate, and consolidate knowledge. In most cases, there is some outcome beyond intellectual consolidation. A **task focus** is the outcome the team is working towards. Not all teams meet at set times around a table and deal with printed agendas. In the real world, most health practitioners are part of informal teams.

Each member of a team has his or her own position. That position entails the individual's personality as well as her or his perspective, team position, and expertise.

The personality of a team member may determine the person's ability to produce an effect. The person's power, team position, and flexibility are all reflections of his or her personality. Whether a person is an introvert or an extrovert, for instance, will affect how the person functions on the team. Personality may be expressed differently in team settings than in private settings. Examples of team personalities include catalyst, facilitator, devil's advocate, and boss.

Team position refers to a person's role. It may be a labeled position (team leader), an assumed position (physical therapist), or an unassumed position (devil's advocate). The generalist is the patient's mouthpiece to others within the team. Sometimes teams are leaderless. Sometimes the patient may be made team leader. The leader is ultimately responsible for how the team functions.

Some people naturally grab power; others are unassuming. Power in a team setting may be appointed or nonappointed. Power refers to the ability to exercise authority, in particular to punish or reward. Powerful people also tend to coerce team members to think as they do. This tendency can become stifling, inhibiting the free flow of ideas and resulting in a team in which all members tend to think alike.

Status refers to a person's position in the network pecking order. Power implies expression of control. Status implies rank, without necessarily being an expression of power. All team members have their own status, which affects how other members of the team react to them and their ideas.

Flexibility of personalities and roles in a team is important. If the team leader is absent, it is good if another can easily take the role of leader for that meeting. If there is disagreement, it is ideal if team members can accept the right to disagree without feeling angry or inadequate.

Team members often are appointed on the basis of expertise rather than personality. The hospice team, for example, contains a pharmacist, hospice nurse, physician, and so on. The area of expertise may be further defined, for example, by requiring the home care nurse and the hospital floor nurse to attend. The team member's labeled position is often simply the person's area of expertise; for example, pharmacist.

Team members all have their own unique perspective, which entails many factors beyond expertise and personality. For example, one X-ray technician may be a 60-year-old religious, widely traveled father who is new to the community whereas another X-ray technician may be a 27-year-old atheistic single mother. Such differences make each team member unique and special. Multiculturalism within the team is an advantage.

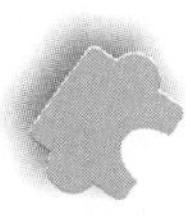

Some Requirements for Effective Teaming

A successful team requires much from its members: understanding, willingness, trust, and a focus on the patient as the center of the team's effort. Each team member must understand the roles of team members as well as the strengths and weaknesses of their personalities and their areas of expertise. Each team member must be willing to share some professional responsibilities when it is in the patient's best interest. Team members must trust that:

- Other team members will put the patient's needs over their own.
- The team will still function if one or two team members are absent, and team members will substitute for each other when necessary and safe.
- Other health professionals will take responsibility for their actions.
- Giving and receiving feedback is not an interpersonal battle, but it is necessary to optimal team function.

Finally, team members must focus on the patient as the center of the team's effort. It may be helpful to include the patient as a key member of the team. Doing so will enhance communication, increase control and responsibility for the patient, and decrease ethical dilemmas. If the patient is mentally fit, he or she may even be the ideal team leader.

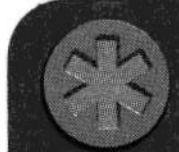

Key Point

Hospice support program for terminal patients emphasizing comfort and home care.

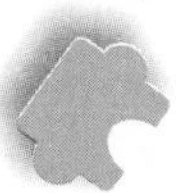

Examples of Health Care Teams

Examples of teams include discharge planning teams, social work teams, after care teams, cardiac rehabilitation teams, visiting nurse teams, and psychiatric casework teams. The list is almost endless. However, we will examine three in depth.

The Hospice Team

Hospice care was pioneered in the 1950s by Dame Cicely Saunders. It relies heavily on teamwork. The hospice approach emphasizes:

- Continuing care by a group of health practitioners.
- The acceptance of death as imminent (usually patients are accepted in such programs only if death is expected within six months). Quality of life rather than quantity of life is stressed. Hospice patients, therefore, always have Do Not Resuscitate (DNR) orders.
- A lot of time for talking, especially talking related to death and dying.
- The involvement of family and friends whenever possible.
- Maintaining the patient at home whenever possible. However the patient may be cared for also in a hospital, a skilled nursing facility, or a hospice center.

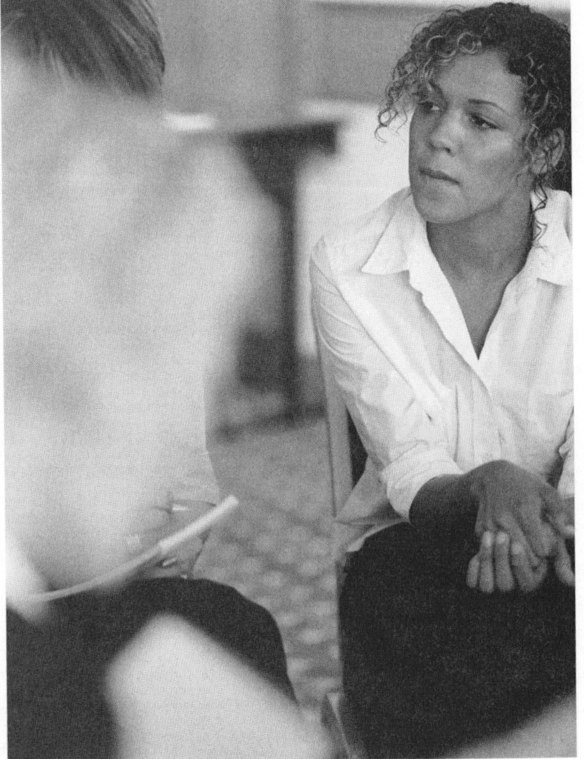

Hospice involves team work.

The hospice team is typically composed of a hospice coordinator (usually a nurse or social worker/psychologist), member of the clergy, pharmacist, physician, hospice director, patient's personal physician, hospital nurse, home nurse, social worker, trained volunteer, and psychologist or thanatologist. The patient typically interacts with the team, chiefly through the hospice nurse and often through trained volunteers, the patient's private physician, and the home visiting nurse. The pharmacist/home supplies specialist and physician program director may have little direct contact with the patient.

Regular, often weekly, meetings are held, and inpatients and outpatients in the program are monitored. The hospice coordinator may be in charge of the meetings, but the patient's personal primary care physician is in charge of the patient's overall care. Like any other team, the hospice team may have shy, overbearing, or sensitive members. Decisions are often made by consensus, however, and the decision-making process guides the primary care physician and establishes policy for the workers who have primary patient contact, especially the hospital nurse or home nurse. Relationships between team members are generally open and trusting. Communication after team meetings is usually good.

The Rehabilitation Ward Round

The ward round, which represents an informal team, is not necessarily scheduled. It may be "after lunch" or on "Friday mornings usually." The usual team members are the rehabilitation physician (may be an orthopedist, rheumatologist, physiatrist, or neurologist), physical therapists, occupational therapists, the rehabilitation coordination nurse, the floor nurse or charge nurse, the social worker or rehabilitation counselor, and involved patients. The purpose of the ward round is to monitor and give direction for coordinated patient rehabilitation. The patients typically are victims of strokes, auto accidents, or war and may have lost the use of limbs or have had amputations.

Anyone may be in charge; it may be the person with the dominant personality or it may vary from patient to patient. The meeting takes place at each patient's bedside. Even though various members of the team do not always show up, the team still functions, and in this respect roles may be shared. Although the rehabilitation nurse coordinator may be considered responsible, team members may regard the rounds more as a forum for exchanging information than as a management technique. Each member's role is especially important in complex cases in which family support, financial stability, occupation, housing, legal, or mental health issues come into play.

The Hospital Team

Of all the possible health care teams, perhaps the most important is the hospital team. It represents both a formal health network and an informal health network with people coming and going. There may be several teams within the hospital team. Communication is primarily through the patient's chart. Numerous health professionals may see the patient on a consultant, collaborative, or referral basis, or as members of various teams. The hospital is an instant network for the patient.

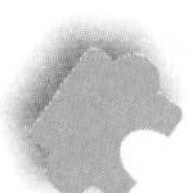

Who Is in Charge?

Logically, it might seem that the person with legal responsibility should be in charge, but responsibility can be transferred by appointing a team head. Alternatively, responsibility can lie with the case manager. A **team leader** heads a team that may be devoted to anything (for example, an infection control committee or care for 10 patients). A **case manager** handles a single patient only.

One way of selecting the team leader is to choose a professional who is good at networking. Managers in the business world are selected on the same principle. The best person to be case manager is usually the person who is also a good networker by training or aptitude. Such a person knows who has specific skills and where the resources are and can empower people to use them. This person can manage all aspects of the case for the patient.

Common case managers are physicians, social workers, nurses, physical therapists, occupational therapists, and psychologists. The case manager could be the patient as long as he or she is not depressed, psychologically disturbed, or psychologically immature and as long as the he or she retains insight. But most patients lack the health networking knowledge of professionals. Some patients are best managed by a particular health professional. For example, an indigent unwed pregnant teenager may be managed well by a social worker. A patient with multiple nursing needs, like ostomy, wounds, and home IV therapy, may be most aptly managed by a nurse. A patient with multiple medical problems and recurrent hospitalizations may be best managed by a physician. Although legally the physician is the patient's case manager in a hospital, this may not always be appropriate. The physician must be a real believer in the benefits of the team approach.

Outpatients may have anyone as a case manager. A good networker is the ideal person. In practice, it is often a social worker, nurse, psychologist, or physician when dealing with medical issues or a trained "case manager" for mental health or substance abuse issues.

The case manager is the person who is ultimately responsible for the patient's care and who must coordinate all aspects of the patient's health care. If we remember the definition of **health** as not simply the absence of disease but a state of complete physical, mental, and social well-being, it is clear that the patient's health encompasses a great deal. The primary emphasis must be on the patient's needs.

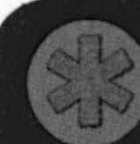

Key Points

Team leader person appointed to head a team.

Case manager person appointed to handle a specific patient.

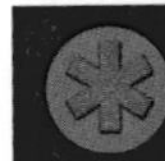

Key Point

Health not simply the absence of disease but a state of complete physical, mental, and social well-being.

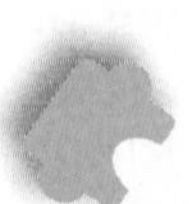

Health Information Technology

It seems that modern management and medicine is moving towards a series of **acronyms**. The acronym to beat all is TLA, which stands for three-letter acronym! So it is that **health information technology (HIT)** must be talked about as a catalogue of systems referred to by acronyms as follows.

1. Physician office–based
    - EHR or EMR
    - Practice management software

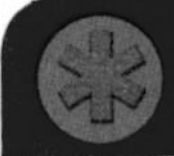

Key Points

Acronym series of capital letters standing for a phrase.

HIT acronym for health information technology, the use of computers in medicine.

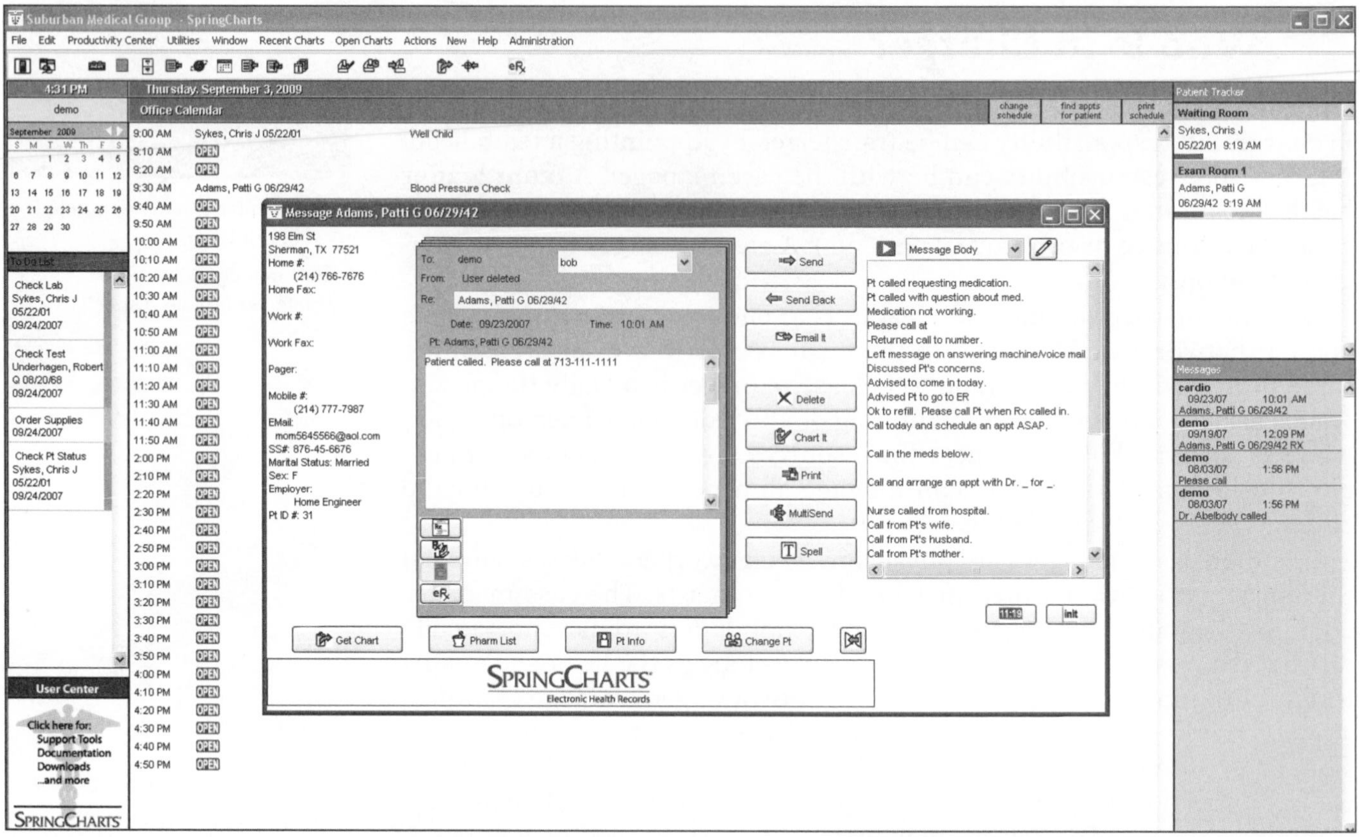

Typical computer screen for practice management software

- Drug-prescribing software
- Patient sign-in systems

2. Hospital-based (uniting architecture is HIS, or hospital information system)
    - EHR
    - CPOE
    - PACS
    - LAN or WAN
    - Internal systems like Pyxis

Physician Office–Based Health Information Technology

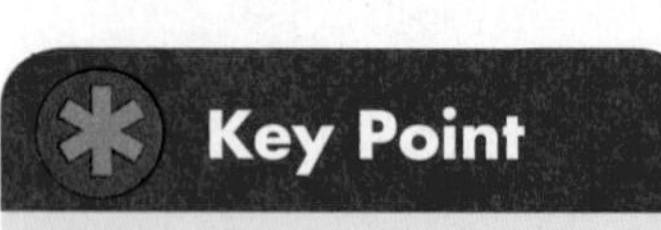

Key Point

EHR acronym for electronic health record, information technology replaces old paper physician or hospital chart.

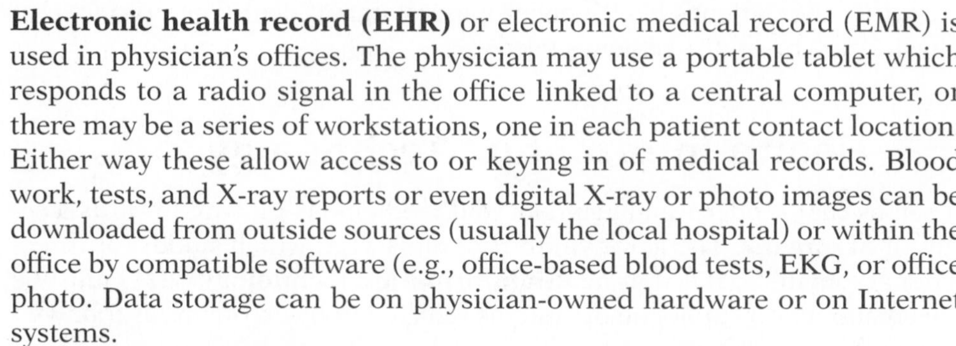

Electronic health record (EHR) or electronic medical record (EMR) is used in physician's offices. The physician may use a portable tablet which responds to a radio signal in the office linked to a central computer, or there may be a series of workstations, one in each patient contact location. Either way these allow access to or keying in of medical records. Blood work, tests, and X-ray reports or even digital X-ray or photo images can be downloaded from outside sources (usually the local hospital) or within the office by compatible software (e.g., office-based blood tests, EKG, or office photo. Data storage can be on physician-owned hardware or on Internet systems.

The EHR may include computerized decision support systems (which help physicians when they are unsure about a diagnosis) and links to patient e-mail that can be made part of the electronic record.

Practice management software includes billing software. This may be seamlessly linked to or "integrated" into an EHR system. This enables sharing of the patient database, patient demographics, and patient diagnoses required for billing. The billing software electronically bills third parties, prints monthly patient balance bills, and creates management reports. It is often linked to patient scheduling software.

Drug-prescribing software enables physicians to order drugs in the EHR or without an EHR. Information is then automatically transmitted by the Web or by fax as an authorized prescription to the pharmacy of the patient's choice. The software may include drug information and drug interactions.

Patient sign-in systems are not very common in the United States but are common in Europe. The patient registers that he or she has arrived at the office for an appointment, avoiding face-to-face receptionist time. The system may also allow the patient to key in other information (e.g., medication list, or change in insurance information).

Hospital-Based Hospital Information Systems

The uniting architecture of the hospital-based computer systems is called HIS, an acronym for hospital information systems. But this does not always mean the systems are united. Unfortunately they are often separate.

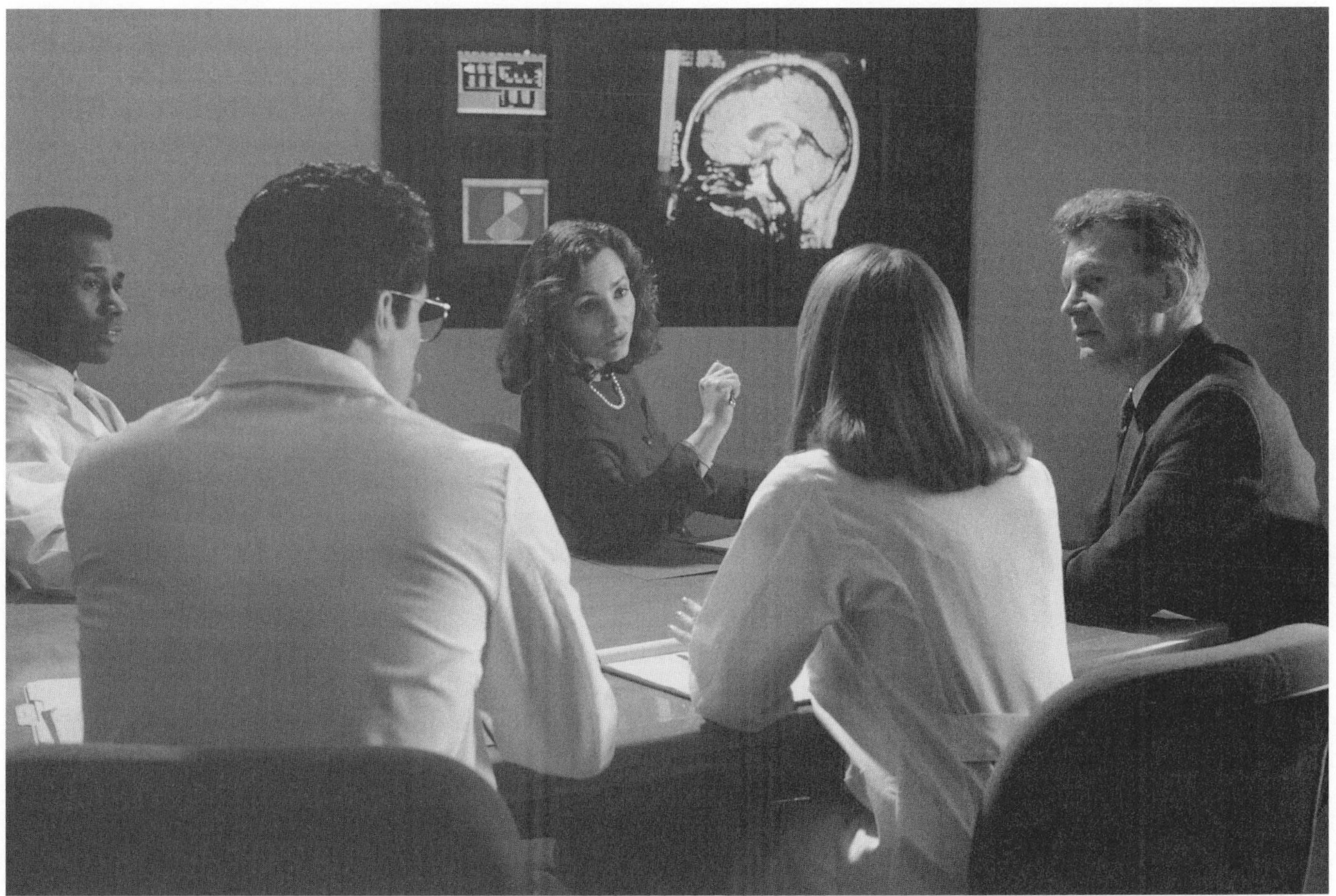

X-ray specialists using PACS. There is no hard copy, only computer files.

EHR may also be used for the hospital chart, or for one department only like the emergency room record.

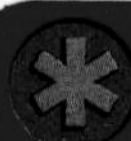

Key Points

CPOE acronym for computerized physician order entry, a system that replaces written orders for physician, nurses and allied health professionals.

PACS acronym for picture archiving and communication system, which stores and retrieves imaging studies on computer.

Computerized physician order entry (CPOE) is data entry for physician orders. As well as pharmacy orders, nurse, therapist, and other orders may be entered in the chart. This has the potential to reduce medical errors by approximately 80 percent so is currently being pushed, even if there is no EHR.

A **picture archiving and communication system (PACS)** stores X-rays, computed tomography (CT) scans, ultrasounds, and other imaging studies and replaces hard copy X-rays. There are no hard copy X-ray films archives, only hard disc storage with hard disc backup systems. The PACS may be linked with a LAN (local area network) or WAN (wide area network) to physicians offices. It may be Web-based (i.e., there is an Internet portal). Thus a CT scan could be done of your abdomen in Montana at 2 a.m. and read by a radiologist in New Zealand or India within minutes, with the report returned via the Internet minutes later to the local emergency room. The next day the CT scan and reports can be seen by the attending physician on his or her office computer screen.

Hospitals commonly use other internal systems, for example, pharmacy supply systems like Pyxis, a computer-based dispensing system, that try to reduce errors. Pyxis is a large cart with a computer on top. The nurse has to sign in, enter the drug or equipment required, and the drawer that contains it opens.

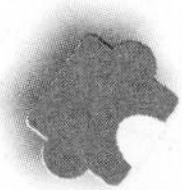

American Recovery and Reinvestment Act 2009

The American Recovery and Reinvestment Act (ARRA) of 2009 included a $17 billion plus taxpayer stimulus for health care information technology in physicians' offices and hospitals. The funds will be administered through Medicare and Medicaid over five years.

Physicians who are "meaningful EHR users" may receive up to $44,000 over five years. However the government has still not released the definition of "meaningful user requirements." Actual costs of EHR implementation per physician are estimated to be in the range of $40,000 to $70,000. Clearly, the government wants physicians to become used to using EHRs.

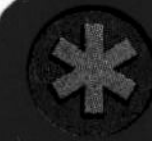

Key Point

e-prescribing electronic means to send prescriptions direct to pharmacy.

In addition, each physician who uses electronic prescribing (also called **e-prescribing**) will receive a 2 percent Medicare bonus starting in 2009, which will turn into a 2 percent penalty for not using e-prescribing by 2014. Hospitals will receive similar incentives to go over to EHR.

Hospitals have been slow to convert to HIS. Approximately 1.5 percent of U.S. hospitals have a fully integrated HIS. In England primary care physicians have widely adopted EHR systems, but the minority of hospitals have adopted EHR and very few hospitals have an integrated HIS. For hospitals (as opposed to primary care), this may be because of a more diverse range of uses, a larger number of programs with interoperability problems, a larger number of more diverse users, and greater problems with privacy protection. In addition, over the last 30 years English primary care physicians have worked with the government on incentives for EHR. But hospitals have not had the same incentives and have treated HIT as a cost center, not a benefit center.

This is not to say that hospitals do not use computers. They use computers for scheduling, for financials, for word processing and medical records, for administration, for lab results, and for billing. But hospitals are not synthesizing all this data—it exists on separate systems that do not communicate with one another, and that is what is meant by a not–fully-integrated HIS.

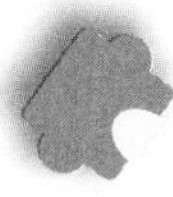

Advantages and Disadvantages of Health Information Technology

Advantages of Health Information Technology

- HIS networks all players together, giving instant access to all information. This may avoid a percentage of hospital admissions because previous test results are not accessible. It may also avoid duplication of tests, which are often repeated because a timely result is not available.
- HIT may be instrumental in malpractice prevention.
- HIT improves billing accuracy.
- Data are useful for follow-up tickler files for repeat examinations and follow-ups for questionable mammograms and imaging studies, chronic disease states, and cancer.
- Data are useful for health maintenance (e.g., routine vaccinations, colonoscopies, mammograms, PAP smears, and physical exams).
- Data are useful for statistical purposes (e.g., incidence of disease in various situations that could yield new information). Data are also useful for early detection of infectious disease outbreaks.
- Data are useful for clinical trials.
- HIT reduces medical errors (e.g., CPOE may reduce errors by up to 80 percent).
- HIT allows instant access to changing drug formularies of different insurance companies and drug interactions before prescribing.
- HIT may improve health care quality.
- HIT reduces paperwork and health care administrative costs.
- HIT allows better tracking of chronic disease states.
- HIT may change the nature of teams with more equal and less hierarchical structure.

Over the long haul, computers, software, and user training may be expensive, but we live in the computer age and old paper systems will be increasingly displaced by computerized systems.

Disadvantages of Health Information Technology

- The cost of implementation is high for the physician's office for EHR alone, with a steep learning curve, more time spent, and ongoing software and hardware updates that cost perhaps $5,000 a year per user. One survey showed that 50 percent of physicians who adopted EHR subsequently abandoned it because of problems. Only 17 percent of physicians in the United States use an EHR.

- HIPAA made EHR access stricter than paper record access, but still there are concerns about implementing these standards. Privacy is still a problem, especially in Web-based systems (e.g., a hacker can access information; office receptionists can access the hospital records of their neighbors).
- Insurance company access needs to be limited, but when a patient is applying for life insurance, too much information may be sent, which the insurance company may archive for life.
- It is difficult to incorporate the old paper records into EHR. The old records can be scanned, but this is time-consuming and occupies a lot of storage space and often is still not integrated into the record.
- **Interoperability** is still low. Interoperability is the ability of one computer system or network to interact with another. Interoperability is low between physicians—there are about 20–30 EHRs available and in use, and virtually none of them are interoperable or relational. There is no point in having 20 different EHR systems in the country that cannot communicate with each other. Likewise, systems are incompatible between hospitals or even within hospitals; for example, one may have to sign in once for PACS, a second time for access to the EHR of the emergency admission, and a third time for the hospital lab work on line. However, some large organizations like the Veterans Administration have good within-system interoperability. ARRA makes interoperability a requirement for qualifying EHRs, though the standards for interoperability have not yet been announced. EHRs will need to be integrated with government health information exchanges (HIE).

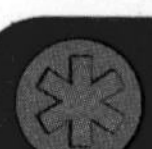

Key Point

Interoperability the ability of one computer system or network to interact with another.

- The health professional looks more at the computer screen than the patient. Recall Chapter 1—this promotes poor body language and poor nonverbal communication.
- **Legacy** is an important part of any EHR or HIT. This means that the system cannot be accessed in years to come. Recall floppy discs—they are now virtually impossible to use. Imagine an office with a $100,000 EHR system with four physicians plus staff of 12, who over the years have become skilled in its use, suddenly being told their system would no longer be supported because the company is being bought out or going bankrupt, despite assurances to the contrary over the years. What happens to the medical records? Changing formats make old EHRs difficult to access. How are records accessed after a physician retires?

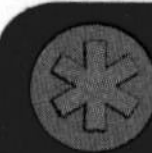

Key Point

Legacy a system whose design contains hardware and software elements that may be unsupportable in later years when more advanced systems replace it.

- Computer crashes and down time are inevitable. This means staff cannot work efficiently during that down time. Everyone is on hold and frustrated.
- GIGO still applies. GIGO is an acronym for garbage in, garbage out. It is true that a lab test will probably be accurate. However, many physician EHRs contain drop down boxes and check off boxes that prompt macros that generate information with no basis in reality. One physician described the process as "check box hell." A six-page report that a patient's ear wax was removed is unlikely to contain accurate or pertinent information beyond that the ear wax was removed.

Summary

Times change and this is reflected in changing roles of health care providers. Health care professionals are more involved in management, communication, and computers. Communication is vital for both intra- and interdisciplinary communication. Health professional roles are defined by the patient, the job description, professional specialty training, your own perception, or by liability concerns. As patients see different health professionals, the terms consultant, collaborator and referral source need to be defined.

This chapter focused on examples of the ideal team, rather than on informal teaming. Different methods of interdisciplinary communication were discussed, as well as who is in charge of the team (team leader) and of the patient (case manager). This chapter examined requirements for effective teaming and how each member's position in a team encompasses personality, perspective, team position, and expertise. The vital role of networking among different health professionals was presented.

The aspiring health professional needs to be skilled not only at communicating with patients but also with other health professionals and, increasingly, in handling information technology. Important acronyms for computerized systems were defined. How will these systems become implemented in America, which has been slower to implement them than Europe? ARRA is influencing implementation of computerization in both health professionals' offices and in hospitals.

Chapter Review

Key Term Review

Acronym: Series of capital letters standing for a phrase.

Case conference: Ad hoc meeting of health care professionals focusing on a specific patient at a specific time.

Case manager: Person appointed to handle a specific patient.

Collaborators: Two people working together toward a common end for material information or to transfer patient care.

Computerized physician order entry (CPOE): A system that replaces written orders for physician, nurses, and allied health professionals.

Consultant: Temporary adviser on current problems.

Crisis intervention: Brief therapy to resolve a major crisis in a patient's life.

Electronic health record (EHR): Information technology that replaces old paper physician or hospital charts.

e-prescribe: Electronic means to send prescriptions direct to pharmacy.

Formal network: Team that is apparent and obvious, assembled for exchange through defined relationships in an organized structure.

Health: Not simply the absence of disease but a state of complete physical, mental, and social well-being.

Health information technology (HIT): Use of computers in medicine.

Hospice: Support program for terminal patients emphasizing comfort and home care.

Informal network: Team that is hidden, with no set rules or procedures to follow and no permanent structure.

Interdisciplinary communication: Communication between members of different health specialties.

Interoperability: The ability of one computer system or network to interact with another.

Intradisciplinary communication: Communication between members of the same health specialty.

Legacy: A system whose design contains hardware and software elements that may be unsupportable in later years when more advanced systems replace it.

Networking: Marshalling people, systems, agencies, and/or resources that a specific person needs at a specific time.

Picture archiving and communication system (PACS): A system that stores and retrieves imaging studies on computer.

Referral source: Another person to supply information or care for the patient.

Role: All behaviors expected from a person who occupies a particular position and status.

Task focus: The outcome that a team is working towards.

Team leader: Person appointed to head a team.

Turf: Territorial rights within an area of expertise.

Chapter Review Questions

1. What is the significance of the difference between inter- and intradisciplinary communication?
2. Describe a network in your school. Is it formal or informal or hidden or revealed?
3. How would you answer a patient who complains that anyone can look in his chart in the hospital and that the information is not confidential?
4. Design a form for interdisciplinary communication to go in a patient's chart. What are the important ingredients of this form?
5. List the items of telephone technique that constitute good telephone manners.
6. Give an example of a team in which you have been involved. What was your role, who was in charge, and what was the purpose of the team? What were the major problems encountered in fulfilling that end?
7. What is a case manager?
8. What is a team leader?
9. List the different factors that characterize a team member's position on a team.

Case Study Critical Thinking Questions

1. In Case Study 10-1 could Jim's insomnia also be from low back pain? Could this indicate a more ominous problem? How would you analyze Jack's role and protect him from malpractice? Would you do the same thing yourself?
2. In Case Study 10-1 Jack finds that each follow-up visit is taken up more by Jim's grieving process than by physical therapy. Is it an appropriate role for Jack to devote time to this? If Jack refers Jim to another health professional, what are the chances of Jim attending, being satisfied, and feeling a connection with someone other than Jack?
3. In Case Study 10-1 is it appropriate for Jack as a physical therapist to help Jim through his grieving?
4. In Case Study 10-2 the surgeon absolutely insists on range of motion exercises for both legs. Should the physical therapist perform range of motion exercises only on the unaffected limb without telling anyone? Would it make a difference whether the patient did or did not have pain in the affected leg?
5. In Case Study 10-2 should the physical therapist ask the patient whether she wants to have range of motion exercises to the limb that will be amputated?
6. In Case Study 10-2 should the physical therapist discuss amputation with Esther to help her with anticipatory grief?
7. In Case Study 10-3 should Anita have asked the nurse first the reason for the consultation?
8. In Case Study 10-3 does Anita have any responsibility to go any further than arranging for placement in a skilled nursing facility?
9. In Case Study 10-3 Anita talks to Harry and discovers that not only his son but he, too, has an alcohol problem, which was denied in the patient's record. What should she do and to whom should she talk?

References

1. American Academy of Family Practice analysis of EHR implementation. www.aafp.org/online/en/home/publications/news/news-now/practice-management/20090513pricewater-rpt.html
2. Computer use by hospitals and physicians www.ahrq.gov/research/computer.htm
3. Health and Human Services www.hhs.gov/healthit/
4. Health Resources and Services Administration www.hrsa.gov/healthit/
5. Healthcare Information and Management Systems Society and the 2009 HIT stimulus www.himss.org/EconomicStimulus
6. Hospice care www.nlm.nih.gov/medlineplus/hospicecare.html
7. How to write well www.uweb.engr.washington.edu/education/engtoolchest/WrittenComm.pdf
8. Medscape article on EHR implementation. www.medscape.com/viewarticle/590460

Additional Readings

1. Baber, A., Waymon, L. *Make Your Contact Count: Networking Know-how for Business and Career Success.* New York: American Management Association, 2007.
2. Dattilio, F. M., Freeman, A. *Cognitive-Behavioral Strategies in Crisis Intervention.* New York: Guilford Press, 2007.
3. Davis, N., LaCour, M. *Health Information Technology, Second Edition.* Philadelphia: Saunders, 2007.
4. D'Ettorre, P., Hughes, D. P. *Sociobiology of Communication: An Interdisciplinary Perspective.* OUP, US. 2008.
5. Englebardt, S. P., Nelson, R. *Health Care Informatics: An Interdisciplinary Approach.* Mosby, 2002.
6. Lipnack, J, Stamps, J. *Virtual Teams: People Working Across Boundaries with Technology.* John Wiley and Sons, 2000.
7. www.ama-assn.org/ama/pub/health-system-reform/index.shtml American Medical Association's vision of health care reform.
8. www.cchit.org Certification Commission for Health Information Technology.
9. www.ahima.org American Health Information Management Association.
10. www.himss.org/ASP/index.asp Health Information and Management Systems Society.

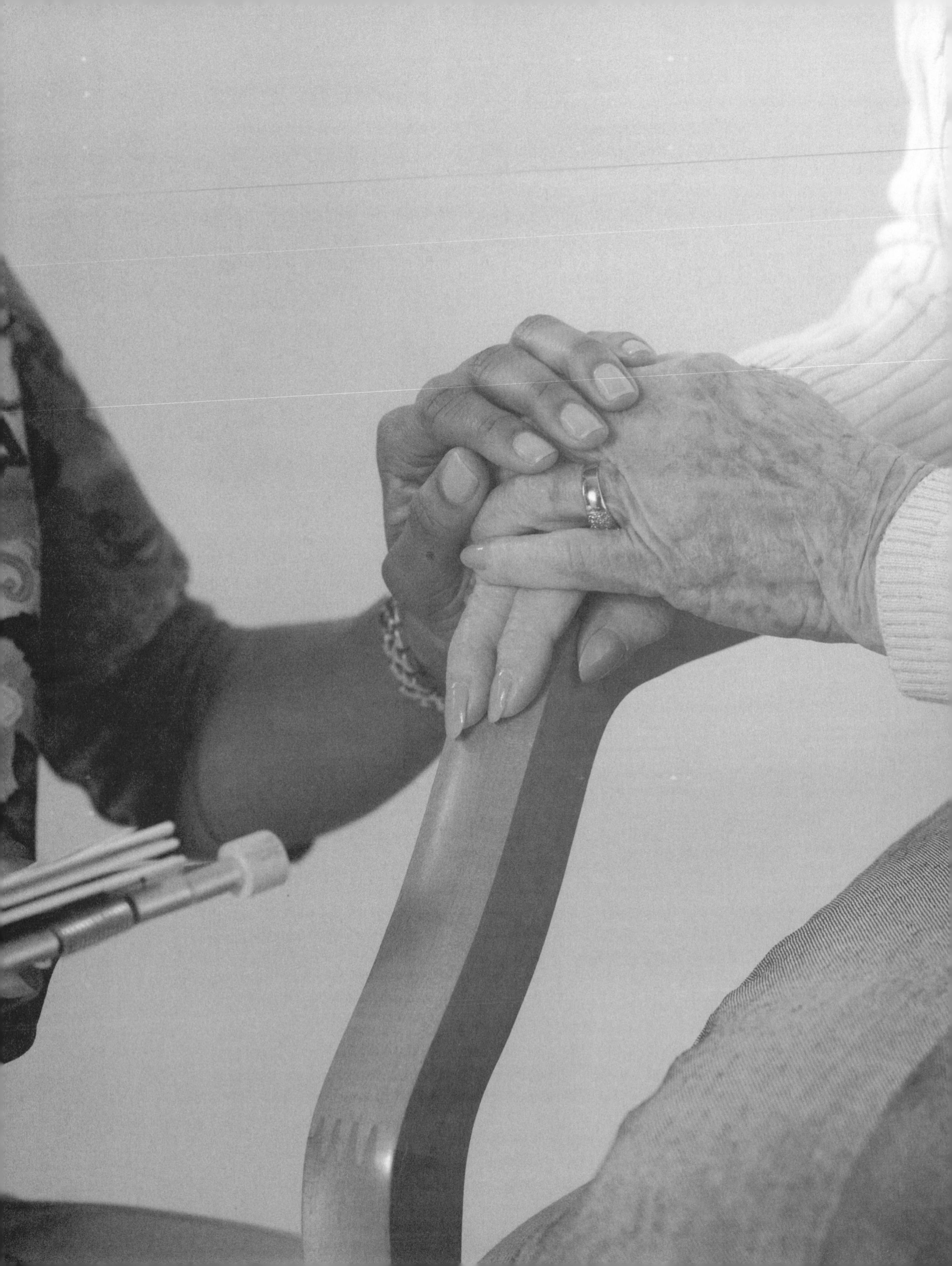

Professional Ethics

Learning Outcomes

After reading this chapter, you should be able to:

11.1 Define the term *ethics.*

11.2 Differentiate between an ethical code and a legal one.

11.3 Explain the concepts of beneficence, nonmalfeasance, autonomy, and justice.

11.4 Describe ethical principals for a health care provider and how they are applied.

11.5 List pitfalls in conducting research on humans.

11.6 Explain how ethical concepts are applied in practice.

11.7 Compare *evaluation, objectivity,* and *informing* within an ethical context.

11.8 List the components of informed consent.

11.9 Analyze a variety of ethical dilemmas.

11.10 Describe the Health Insurance Portability and Accountability Act and the role of the government and outside agencies in protecting patient rights.

Key Terms

Absolute
Autonomy
Beneficence
Competence
Confidentiality
Decorum
Degree
Ethics
Etiquette
Hippocratic Oath
Health Insurance Portability and Accountability Act (HIPPA)
Informed consent
Institutional review boards (IRBs)
Justice
Nonmalfeasance
Patient's Bill of Rights
Professional responsibility
Risk–benefit ratio
Sanctions
Torts

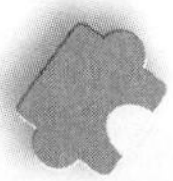

Defining Ethics

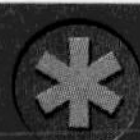

Key Points

Ethics a set of standards and codes held as essential by professionals for the welfare of their patients and their professional standing.

Etiquette 19th century medical code used to guide professional conduct without relying on the term *morality* but based on the presumption of "an upright man instructed in the art of healing."

Decorum term used for the medical etiquette of the Hippocratic Oath.

Hippocratic Oath oath sworn by new physicians declaring that they place the welfare of their patients first and will do no harm.

Ethics are codes of moral behaviors that enable the health care provider to distinguish right from wrong. But whose view of moral behavior should be used? Who should decide right from wrong and in which culture and at which time and place? Although ethical and moral standards are often linked, they are, of necessity, separate constructs.

During the 19th century, medical codes were frequently called **etiquettes**. The word *etiquette* is useful because it avoids the problems of defining morality. An etiquette presumes an "upright man instructed in the art of healing." **Decorum** is more literally the medical etiquette of the **Hippocratic Oath** (the oath new physicians take that sets a high standard of care and demands that doctors do no harm; all other health providers model their practice after this code). This etiquette chiefly governs the professional contacts of members and defines professional courtesy.

Well-intentioned, educated people disagree on many of the issues related to modern health care. Some moral questions evoke striking moral consensus (for example, western cultures would agree that child abuse is immoral). But issues of health care ethics seem always to evoke persistent disagreements (for example, abortion, right-to-die, confidentiality in relation to communicable diseases, drug testing).

The ethics of the American Psychological Association offer a pragmatic view. Here the term *ethics* refers to a set of guidelines for professionals primarily designed to ensure public or consumer safety. A professional claims the right to profess something, and ethical guidelines define the scope of that professing so the public can be reasonably certain of what the knowledge and practice of a given professional entails. It is important that the patient can trust the health professional. Knowing that a health professional is highly ethical helps the patient's trust to develop. Any violation of ethical principles represents a violation of public trust—a violation of all patients. Such violations also undermine and harm the status of all professionals.

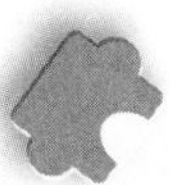

Ethical versus Legal Codes

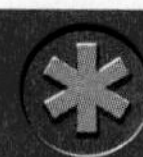

Key Points

Absolute total, all or nothing.

Degree a step in a series.

Torts laws that define what constitutes a legal injury and establish the circumstances under which one person may be held liable for another's injury. Torts cover intentional acts and accidents.

Sanctions penalties for noncompliance.

Ethics differ from the law in two major ways. First, an ethical principle tends to be **absolute**. That is, either the health professional did or did not behave in an ethical manner. By contrast, legal decisions usually involve a qualifying factor of **degree**. Both **torts** (civil actions involving harm or injury) and criminal law focus on a degree of negligence or intention to do harm. The more rigid view of professional ethics stems from a conviction that the public needs to believe in exemplary conduct from health professionals. This is a matter of public trust. The consumer must be able to believe that the health professional acts to protect and enhance the well-being of the consumer, not in any self-serving manner. The consequences of legal and ethical violations also differ. Legal convictions generally result in fines, probation and service, or incarceration. Ethical violations result in **sanctions**, including the possibilities of reprimand, censure or expulsion, and loss of membership for the most severe breaches of ethics. If a legal conviction is sufficiently serious (a felony, or serious crime, rather than a misdemeanor), professional organizations may also impose corresponding sanctions against the offending member.

There have been many instances in which acquittal from legal charges did not release the professional from sanctions for unethical behavior. A behavior or practice can, therefore, be legally acceptable but professionally unethical.

For behavior judged to be inappropriate but not clearly unethical, members can be sanctioned through a variety of methods. Consider the following example:

CASE STUDY 11-1

A physical therapist in private practice has been regularly treating a patient who cannot pay for services. This patient is also a carpenter. The physical therapist suggests that the patient work off some of his debt by putting an addition on the therapist's home. The carpenter agrees but makes some building errors that result in major roof leaks and additional expenses for the therapist. When the carpenter comes in for treatment, the physical therapist has difficulty remaining objective about the patient's care.

This relationship is not unethical (although it would be for many mental health workers and those in substance abuse treatment where no out of work contact is permitted), but the health professional is guilty of using poor judgment. In such a case, educative advisory sanctions (cease and desist orders) would constitute typical action from the professional organization. That is, the therapist would be educated about the error in judgment and told to either stop using the carpenter's services or to stop treating the carpenter as a patient.

To summarize, the definition of ethics focuses on two principles: concern for the protection of the public and concern for the knowledge and fitness of the health practitioner. It is little wonder that ethics are heavily emphasized on most licensure examinations. A breach of ethics is an embarrassment to all members of a profession and constitutes harm to the public the profession purports to serve.

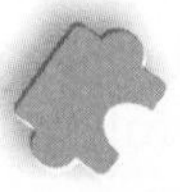

Relationship between Health Professional and Patient

There are a number of themes that are helpful in guiding thinking when dealing with ethical and legal issues with patients.

Beneficence. Licensed practitioners practice the profession of their choice for the benefit of the patient. Their primary duty is to use their professional expertise for the patient's well-being.

Nonmalfeasance. This means weighing the risks and benefits for all courses of action with patients. Most of the time this value judgment is automatic, but at times decisions require more thought. Then the doctrine of *primum non nocere* applies: *Above all else do no harm.*

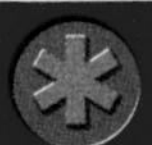

Key Points

Beneficence the use of a professional's expertise for patient well-being.

Nonmalfeasance doing no harm.

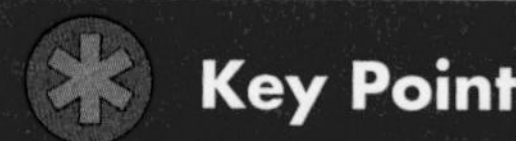

Key Point

Autonomy the individual right of a patient to exercise own judgment.

Autonomy. Autonomy of the patient means respecting the patient's right as an individual. An adult of sound mind has a right to make decisions about his or her own life unless there is danger to third parties. Examples of dangers to third parties include infectious disease, denying a spouse income, and homicide. Another issue of patient autonomy is quality of life. Patients have the right to refuse a treatment if it violates their standard of dignity. If, for example, a patient refuses a barium enema (and understands the risks) because it is undignified, this must be respected. The right of a cancer patient to die in peace without invasive or undignified procedures must also be respected.

Autonomy of the health professional means that each health professional is morally independent and cannot let others influence her or his decisions. The allied health professions are becoming increasingly independent from physicians. As this autonomy increases, exposure to malpractice also increases. Therefore, all health practitioners must become more aware of malpractice issues.

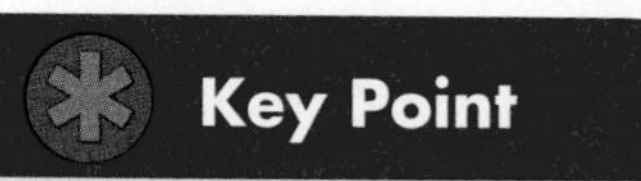

Key Point

Justice a sense of fairness.

Justice. A sense of fairness must exist in the relationship between the allied health professional and the patient. Malpractice exists, after all, as a legal recourse or redress for any breach in the relationship between the health professional and the patient. Justice must also exist in the relationship between society and the patient. For example, a psychologist cannot allow a homicidal patient complete autonomy despite the supposed sanctity of patient confidentiality. If a psychologist believes there is a reasonable risk of violence or death to a person, the psychologist also has a duty toward that victim.

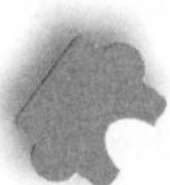

Overview of Ethical Principles

All health professionals share a common code of ethics. Although wording of various codes may differ slightly from profession to profession, the basic underlying intent does not. For example, the American Physical Therapy Association is just as concerned about the problem of a member sexually abusing a patient as the American Medical Association is—both consider such abuse a tremendous violation of ethics.

The following review of ethical principles was adapted from the *American Psychologist*. It offers a foundation of ethics that is common to all health professionals. This commonality of principles is easy to understand when we accept that all health professional organizations charge their members with basic responsibilities to the public in ten areas:

- Professional responsibility.
- Competence.
- Moral and legal standards.
- Public statements.
- Confidentiality.
- Welfare of the consumer.
- Professional relationships.
- Assessment techniques.
- Care and use of laboratory animals.
- Research with human subjects (this is a special case).

Professional Responsibility

The principle of **professional responsibility** means that health professionals must accept the consequences of their own actions. They must maintain the highest standard of their profession as practitioners, educators, and researchers.

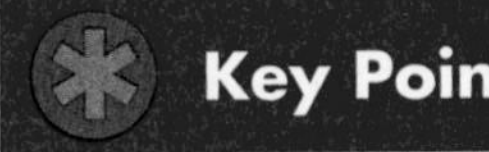

Professional responsibility acceptance of the consequences of their own actions by health professionals.

With respect to research, health professionals must never suppress, mislead, or distort their findings. They must choose the subjects they pursue for research carefully and must never accept a research project that could cloud their objectivity or create a conflict of interest. In all instances they must make full disclosure of the limitations of their findings.

As teachers, practitioners, or researchers and in a social context, health professionals must not misuse their influence. Consider the following example based on an article published in the *American Journal of Public Health* (1975).

CASE STUDY 11-2

A man named Theodore D. Sterling, Ph.D., reviewed the American Cancer Society studies linking smoking to lung cancer and published his findings in an article entitled "A Critical Reassessment of the Evidence Bearing on Smoking as a Cause of Lung Cancer." He concluded that the studies were poorly done, biased, and worthless. He further attempted to convince readers that smoking had no influence on lung cancer. Much of Sterling's work was seen as biased.

Without reading the document, what opinion do you formulate when we tell you that Sterling's research was funded by the American Tobacco Institute?

Competence

The principle of **competence** also requires that a high standard of skills be maintained. Health professionals must accurately represent their education, training, specialties, limitations, and boundaries. Duties must be performed in conjunction with careful preparation. If a health professional suffers a health or personal problem (for example, alcoholism or bereavement) that creates conflict with the person's professional effectiveness, she or he must refrain from practicing or must seek the help of other professionals to determine what actions he or she needs to take. For example, although some practitioners may be able to work effectively while partially impaired, an objective opinion should be sought to determine the degree of limitation. The following example relates to competence in terms of educational training and boundaries:

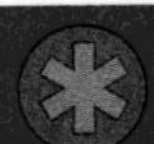

Key Point

Competence the ability to perform according to the standards of the profession.

CASE STUDY 11-3

An occupational therapist who works in a small general hospital is asked to help fill in for a few weeks while a physical therapist colleague has her baby. The occupational therapist has a strong general knowledge and has often seen physical therapists in action. Would it be ethical for her to teach walking with a prosthetic device?

Teaching walking with a prosthetic device is probably not ethical unless the physical therapy staff could prepare and supervise this activity.

Moral and Legal Standards

Health care providers must live up to the same standard of moral and legal behavior expected of any other citizen, except when such behavior might compromise their ability to fulfill their professional duties. Health practitioners must be aware of prevailing community standards and must not act in a way that would jeopardize their ability to perform their professional duties. They must always consider the possible impact their actions may have on the public. Further, health professionals must never act to violate or limit the legal or civil rights of others.

CASE STUDY 11-4

A health professional at a small private college (which had established itself with a value for premarital abstinence) is asked by a number of students he sees at the health center about contraception. In response, he wages an all-out campaign to teach human sexuality and contraception to the students. He places brochures in the infirmary, the dorms, and the hallways of classrooms. He hangs many posters that promote specific contraceptive devices and that feature explicit photos of the human anatomy. Many of the students, their parents, and the faculty are offended by this action.

Is this health professional guilty of ethical misconduct? Yes, the health professional's views are clearly unacceptable when the standard of this community is taken into consideration.

Public Statements

Health practitioners may make public statements or advertise their services only to the extent of assisting the public to make informed choices and only within the scope permitted by their professional association. Health professionals must accurately represent their own credentials. In no way should they use fear to solicit patients, but, of course, they should make no misleading or false claims about available services or outcomes of treatment. Health professionals should not induce any member of the media to promote them or their services. The name of an individual's professional association should never be used in such a way as to imply endorsement of a product by that association.

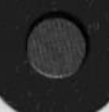

CASE STUDY 11-5

A dietitian advertises that services are available for help with weight loss. Credentials, hours, the address, professional affiliations, and fees are listed in a pamphlet. This statement appears at the end of the copy: "If every diet and gimmick has failed, this is the place for you."

This last statement represents a breach of ethics because it implies success without any scientific evaluation that back ups such a claim.

Confidentiality

The patient has the right to expect that the details of his or her health care will be shared only among those health practitioners who require the information in order to perform their duties. This is the essence of **confidentiality**. (See HIPAA discussion below.) Among professional groups, patient information can be shared outside of a practice only if the patient gives written consent. In no instance is information about a patient's health to be shared for any non–health-related purpose. Health care providers must always guard the patient's privacy and must not invade that privacy unless they are medically required to do so. Health care workers must also provide reasonable security for records and any written information about patients.

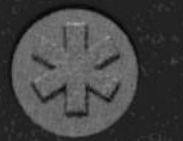

Key Point

Confidentiality the nondisclosure of information.

Health professionals who write or lecture about actual cases must have prior written consent or must adequately disguise the case to protect the patient's identity. When professionals work with those who are unable to give informed consent, the best interest of the patient takes precedence.

Health professionals might need to inquire about a patient's sexual contacts from a given point in time should a venereal disease be diagnosed. They do not, however, need to know what positions they have sex in. Such questions betray idle curiosity. Further, should the health professional's best friend live next door to this patient, no overt or covert disclosure of the patient's diagnosis could be made.

Welfare of the Consumer

Health practitioners must act to protect the welfare of their patients. Conflicts may arise between the needs of the patient and those of an institution offering service. Conflicts may also arise between the needs of the patient and the needs of the health professional. When such conflicts occur, the health professional is responsible for seeing that they are clarified and that all concerned parties are informed.

Health professionals must be aware of their own needs and not use their influence and position to further their needs at the expense of the consumer. Patients are not to be exploited sexually or otherwise. Health practitioners do not engage in sexual harassment of either patients or other professionals.

Before treatment, health care providers inform the consumer about all financial arrangements. Health professionals do not accept financial remuneration for referring patients. When a health care provider believes that a patient is not benefiting or progressing from the services, the provider terminates treatment and refers the patient for appropriate follow-up elsewhere.

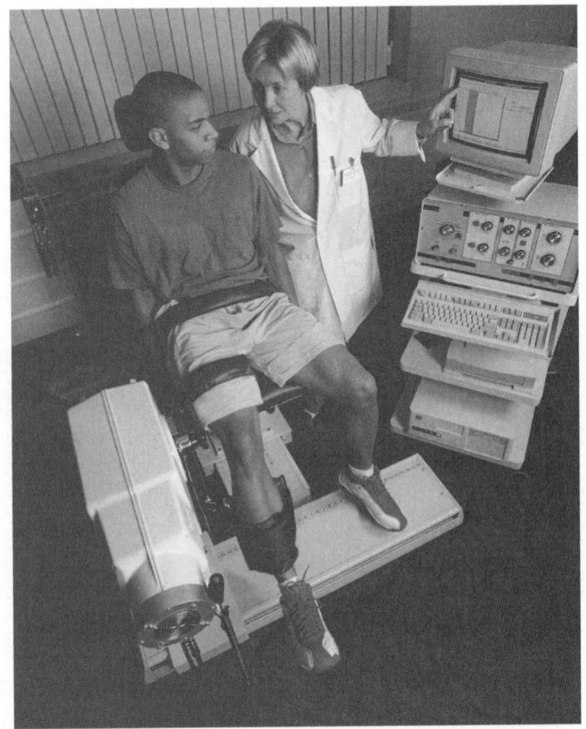

The physical therapist has the welfare of the patient primarily in mind.

CASE STUDY 11-6

The physical therapy department that John works in continues to accept patients for treatment even after their ultrasound machines have broken down. Therapists offer the patients alternative treatments but feel uneasy because they know they cannot provide the best care. Still, what can John do? The hospital administrator insists that the department not turn away patients who have insurance.

Clearly, John is bound by ethical standards to explain the treatment limitations to prospective patients. Further, he needs to make it clear to the administration that he will not compromise his treatment standards.

Professional Relationships

Health professionals know and understand the competencies of other health professionals. They use available resources to ensure the best possible patient outcomes. Health professionals conduct research within the ethical guidelines and standards of their profession and the institutions for which they work. In the case of publications, health professionals assign credit proportionately with the size of the contribution.

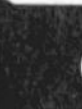

CASE STUDY 11-7

A patient keeps complaining of persistent morning diarrhea. The psychologist repeatedly tells the patient it is a reaction to stress. The patient is treated for stress for 18 months until a conversation between another health professional and the patient reveals the possibility of lactose intolerance.

The psychologist is bound ethically to know the limitations of treatment and the potentially valuable role of other health professionals. The practitioner failed to act ethically by not referring the patient to a physician.

When health professionals become aware of ethical violations by other health professionals, they attempt to resolve the problem first informally and then formally if necessary.

CASE STUDY 11-8

A student health professional reports to the clinical supervisor that a clinical professor has continued to ask her for dates, even though she has not encouraged him, and feels uncomfortable having to repeatedly turn down the advances of someone who must grade her.

The clinical supervisor speaks to the professor, who readily agrees to stop requesting dates. The matter has been handled informally. Should the professor continue to seek dates with this student, the supervisor would have to make a formal request. It is always preferable to resolve such matters simply and quietly.

Health professionals must also refrain from gratuitous comments about other health professionals. It is not possible to know all details of a relationship between a patient and another professional. It is therefore inappropriate to suggest to the patient that they go elsewhere or seek a second opinion or that the other professional is incompetent. If one health professional feels that another health professional has issues that might seriously impair patient care, then those issues must be addressed, but not through the patient.

Assessment Techniques

Health practitioners develop and use only those assessment techniques that meet a high standard. The welfare of the patient is uppermost in considerations related to assessment techniques. Health care providers explain the use, meaning, and validity of all assessments to the patient in understandable language. Further, health providers do not encourage the use of assessment techniques by untrained or unqualified people.

CASE STUDY 11-9

A firm that specializes in the sale of psychologic tests frequently makes large volume sales to a health school graduate program. The graduate students then test volunteers and publish the results on such measures as internal/external locus of control, depression, assertiveness, empathy, and self-efficacy.

The problem here is that the students are not really trained to administer or interpret these tests. The test company is not concerned because it is being well paid for the tests. But the volunteers and the public are being misled into assuming that the test results are valid and meaningful.

Care and Use of Animals

Animals should be used in experiments only for a true advancement in knowledge or for the development of human skills. No undue harm should ever be inflicted on an animal. Animals should be cared for humanely. Once it is appropriate to terminate an animal's life, it should be done rapidly and painlessly.

CASE STUDY 11-10

A researcher who uses rats does not provide food for them on the weekends because it is an inconvenience to the researcher and because the amount of food the rats eat is not essential to the experiment.

This researcher is guilty of inhumane treatment. Starving the rats two days each week causes them discomfort and might cause unnecessarily cruel death.

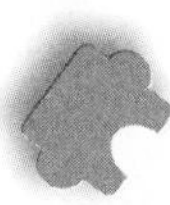

Research with Human Subjects

Following the horrors of the Tuskegee experiments, in which prisoners from Alabama were intentionally infected with syphilis and followed for 30 years without treatment, the then Department of Health, Education, and Welfare established guidelines for human research. These guidelines became law with the National Research Act of 1974.

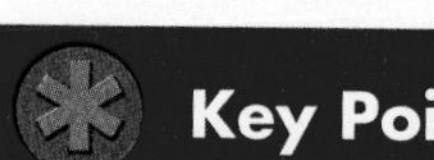

Key Point

Institutional review boards (IRBs) independent ethics committees that oversee medical research on humans.

Title 45 of the Code of Federal Regulations governs the role of **institutional review boards (IRBs)**. All research that receives any government funding must be overseen by IRBs regulated by the Department of Health and Human Services. The IRBs are independent ethics committees that oversee medical research on humans.

Since 1974 any researcher or institution wishing to receive federal funds has had to comply with these regulations. Because these guidelines also reflect sound ethical practices, health professional organizations have accepted them almost universally.

Health practitioners who wish to conduct research on human subjects must weigh the risks and benefits involved, make arrangements for the issues surrounding prior informed consent, determine whether the research could be conducted without the use of human subjects, and deal with the promises made to subjects.

Prior Informed Consent

Researchers cannot always adequately judge the benefit of a given experiment. Further, any risk is best judged by those who are going to take the risk in conjunction with the researcher. Before an experiment can be conducted, the researcher must gain the written informed consent of the subject or the subject's legal representative. Subjects must be informed of:

- The nature, purpose, and methodology of the research.
- The possible risks and benefits.
- What compensation will be made to them should anything go wrong as a result of the experiment.
- The fact that they can withdraw from the experiment at any time.

In cases in which advanced notice of experimental conditions might render the experiment meaningless, a researcher must consult with experts to change the design in a manner that will permit prior informed consent or, if this fails, must submit the research proposal for review to gain permission to perform a research deception. The review board of the institution that employs the health professional usually can best determine whether the risk–benefit ratio is worthy of approving a deception.

If a deception is approved, the health professional must:

- Agree to debrief each subject immediately after the experiment has been completed.
- Compensate any subject who has been injured by the deception.
- Withdraw the data of any subject who objects.

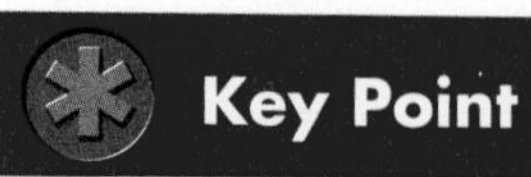

Key Point

Risk–benefit ratio assessment of the risk versus the benefit of treatment or a research experiment to make a decision.

Risk versus Benefit Ratio

The risk–benefit ratio must be favorable. If an experiment carries moderate risks with possible major benefits, the **risk–benefit ratio** is appropriately balanced. An example might be the experimental use of a drug that could cure colon cancer. A patient suffering from colon cancer would gladly risk a side effect, such as loss of hair, for the potential benefit of saving his or her life. But what if the experiment involved injecting volunteers with cancer cells to see how the body's immune system might fight off the cancer? Certainly, the ratio here would be heavy on the risk side, and the experiment would offer no obvious benefit. When health professionals are determining what type of research to conduct, a key part of decision making revolves around the risks–benefits ratio. Obviously, the ideal experiment would involve no risk to the human subject and a possible major gain.

Experimentation without Human Subjects

Could the experiment be done without human subjects? This question must be one of the first a researcher asks. If an experiment can be conducted validly without using human subjects, this is ideal. However, there are obvious benefits to conducting research on humans if humans are the population that the findings are designed to serve. One of the major criticisms of early cigarette/lung cancer research was that it dealt with the effects of a cigarette smoked by a mouse, not a human.

If an experiment with human subjects involves little or no risk, it may be labeled *expedited* and given institutional approval with little review. Examples include collection of nail clippings or excreta, tests dealing with normal educational practices, and benign inventories or questionnaires. Research that involves minors or pregnant women or that entails such activities as exercise or probing psychologic inquiry requires full and objective review.

Promises to Subjects

Only outcomes that are realistic should be mentioned to subjects as potential benefits. Subjects who are asked to volunteer for experiments should make their decisions freely, on the basis of an informed understanding of the experiment. They should not be harassed, induced, deceived, bribed, or coerced into volunteering. (For example, if a college professor tells students that they must participate in an experiment or flunk the course, the students have the right to protest this action as coercive.) If rewards, such as copies of the results, are promised to subjects, they should be delivered. If subjects are told that their answers are anonymous, this must be true. If subjects are told that their answers will be kept confidential, they must be kept confidential or they must be disguised beyond any possible recognition.

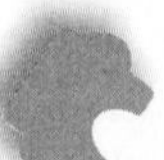

Applying Ethical Concepts in Practice

Although allied health students "become proficient in the technical aspects of their career field, they lack the skills in decision-making related to ethical and moral concerns." If this statement, which was made by a prominent allied health school dean in 1979, is still true, we must focus on building the skills to remedy the problem. The fact that studying the absolutes of the basic sciences is so different from studying the complex dilemmas of ethical and moral judgments may contribute to the difficulties students have. In any case, health professionals must learn to work within

Patient's Bill of Rights

1. The patient has the right to considerate and respectful care.
2. The patient has the right to know, by name, the physician responsible for coordinating his or her care at the Clinical Center.
3. The patient has the right to obtain from his or her physician complete current information about diagnosis, treatment, and prognosis in easily understandable terms. If it is medically inadvisable to give such information to the patients, it will be given to a legally authorized representative.
4. The patient has the right to receive from his or her physician information necessary to give informed consent prior to the start of any procedure or treatment. Except in emergencies this will include, but not necessarily be limited to, a description of the specific procedure or treatment, any risks involved, and the probable duration of any incapacitation. When there are alternatives to therapeutically designed research protocols, the patient has the right to know about them. The patient also has the right to know the name of the person responsible for directing the procedures or treatment.
5. The patient has the right to refuse to participate in research, to refuse treatment to the extent permitted by law, and has the right to be informed of the medical consequences of these actions including possible dismissal from the study and discharge from the institution. If discharge would jeopardize the patient's health, he or she has the right to remain under Clinical Center care until discharge or transfer is medically advisable.
6. The patient has the right to be transferred tvo another facility when his or her participation in the Clinical Center study is terminated, providing the transfer is medically permissible, the patient has been informed of the needs for and alternatives to such a transfer, and the facility has agreed to accept the patient.
7. The patient has the right to privacy concerning the medical care program. Case discussion, consultation, examination, and treatment are confidential and will be conducted discreetly. The patient has the right to expect that all communications and records pertaining to care will be treated as confidential to the extent permitted by law.
8. The patient has the right to routine services whenever hospitalized at the Clinical Center in connection with the active protocol for which he or she is eligible; these services will generally include diagnostic procedures and medical treatment deemed necessary and advisable by the professional staff. Complicating chronic conditions will be noted, reported to the patient, and treated as necessary without the assumption of long-term responsibility for their management. The patient may be returned for long-term or definitive care of these conditions to the referring physician or to other appropriate medical resources.
9. The patient has the right to expect that medical information about him or her discovered at the Clinical Center, as well as an account of his or her medical program here, will be communicated to the referring physician.
10. The patient has the right, at any time during the medical program, to designate additional physicians or organizations to receive medical updates. The patient should inform the Outpatient Department staff of these additions.
11. The patient has the right to know in advance what appointment times and physicians are available and where to go for continuity of care provided by the Clinical Center when such care is required under the study for which the patient was admitted.

the dynamic and complex health care system to form a meaningful working value system. They must borrow from philosophy, logic, and ethics to help develop their thinking.

Consider for a moment the **Patient's Bill of Rights**. The patient has the right to respectful care, complete medical information, information requisite for informed consent, refusal of treatment, privacy, confidentiality, response to requests for service, information on other institutions touching on her or his care, refusal of participation in research projects, continuity of care, examination and explanation of financial charges, and knowledge of current hospital regulations.

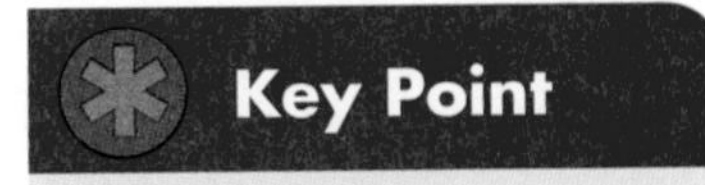

Patient's Bill of Rights list of a patient's rights.

There are similarities between these rights and the ethical principles just considered. The patient's right to know the diagnosis and the right to confidentiality and dignity in treatment correspond directly with the principles of assessment techniques, confidentiality, and welfare of the consumer. There apparently is a clear relationship between the professional's ethics and the patient's needs. Unfortunately, this relationship is often muddy. In the paragraphs that follow, we point out some of the most difficult ethical questions a health care provider must face.

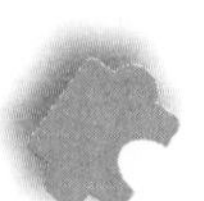

Evaluation, Objectivity, and Informing

What constitutes an "evaluation?" How far do health professionals go when evaluating a patient? When do they draw the line on testing? Is this decision based on probability tables, the patient's expressed concerns, cost effectiveness, time effectiveness, a presumed value for the patient's life, the patient's income, or the need to use or not to use some types of equipment? Would the same examinations be performed on two 76-year-old men if one were the president of the United States and the other a street person? As the government gets more involved in health care, what happens when it refuses to pay for expensive tests or treatments? Is that ethical?

What does "objective" mean? Health practitioners may think that they evaluate and treat patients objectively, but this may be only partly true. Just looking at the questions in the previous paragraph casts doubt on any human being's ability to be objective. The age, social status, disease prognosis, income, gender, family dynamics, and even personality of the patient may affect health professionals' objectivity. Provided there are some safeguards, being subjective may even be a necessary part of the service provided. Because we are human beings, our own histories also color our ability to be objective. Yet, strictly speaking, the ethical principles of health professionals are based on an assumption of objectivity.

How *informed* is informed? We believe that the patient has a right to know his or her diagnosis. Is this true in every case? Should one ever give out partial information either to protect the patient from a harsh truth or to persuade the patient that he or she must comply with our solution? Are deceptions, such as the use of placebos, ever justified if the end result is likely to be improved health?

Most of us would agree that there may be times when a "degree of informed" is sufficient and necessary. But a judgment that wavers from an absolute interpretation of informed is subjective, open to criticism, and potentially unethical.

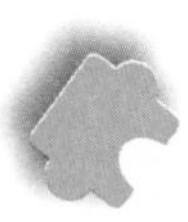

Paternalism, Consumerism, and Informed Consent

In generations past, the practice of medicine was paternalistic (i.e., health practitioners did what they felt was best for the patient without feeling the need to impart information and various pros and cons). Today the practice of medicine has moved to consumeristic (i.e., patients must be reasonably informed of the risks versus the benefits of tests and treatments and involved in decision making about their own health care).

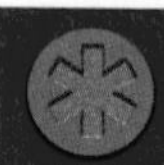

Key Point

Informed consent
Knowledgeable permission—patient reasonably informed about the pros and cons of a test or treatment.

Informed consent means that the patient is reasonably informed about the pros and cons of a test or treatment. Informed consent may be written, verbal, or implied. Written informed consent for a procedure like surgery requires that the patient understand:

1. What the procedure involves (e.g., general anesthesia, a surgical scar, going on the ventilator).
2. The risks of the procedure (e.g., hemorrhage, infection, death).
3. The benefits of the procedure (e.g., removing a cancer with chance of cure).
4. The alternatives to the procedure (e.g., radiotherapy, chemotherapy, or nothing).
5. The risks and benefits of the alternative procedure.
6. The risks and benefits of not doing the procedure.

A signed consent form is not the same thing as informed consent. The practitioner still needs to involve the patients in all the elements of decision making listed in the previous list.

Informed consent may be verbal and not written. For example, when a physical therapist performs cervical traction, there must be reasonable communication with the patient. She might say, "I would like to see if we can help your neck pain by using traction. This halter fits round your jaw and will be tight and this is expected. We'll start off for five minutes, and if at any time you feel you want to stop, for any reason, just push this button. Is that OK? Do you have any questions?" Although this is not written consent, it communicates with the patient and allows him or her to participate in decision making.

Implied consent means that the patient acknowledges what you are doing and does not object. For example such a lengthy introduction is unnecessary for a venipuncture if the patient extends his or her arm ready for the procedure. If not, the phlebotomist might say, "Good morning Mrs. Smith, I am going to take some blood from your arm. OK?"

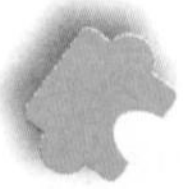

Examples of Some Ethical Dilemmas

There are thousands of ethical dilemmas that health professionals must face. The most dramatic of these conflicts, such as right-to-die issues, are commonly in the press. Recall the Karen Quinlan case, in which court orders were required to remove her from life support equipment.

Health care workers routinely must cope with difficult questions that are filled with both professional and personal conflict. Consider the following example of ethical conflicts, which deal with human immunodeficiency virus (HIV), genetic engineering, and transplants.

Human Immunodeficiency Virus

Years ago there was a dilemma of whether people with HIV should have all their blood specimens labeled as "suspect HIV." This has now been resolved by the Universal Precaution standards. To maintain patient confidentiality and to protect health care providers, all blood and body fluids are labeled and handled under the federally mandated Universal Precaution standards. This means all potentially infected materials are considered "high risk." All specimens are now considered contaminated (carrying any communicable disease) and are collected, handled, and processed by using specific required guidelines to minimize the risk of exposure. These guidelines also protect patients from the potential hazard of contamination by the health care professional. Although this does not eliminate the issue of specific warnings, it does increase safety and provide confidentiality, because a specimen need not be specifically labeled as "suspicious for HIV."

The latest information regarding Universal Precautions can be found on the Centers of Disease Control (CDC) site at www.cdc.gov.

Genetic engineering and artificial insemination

What scientists and researchers have seen as breakthroughs, many lay people have seen as proof of moral decay. "Tampering" with the unborn, promoting pregnancy where "God may not have willed one," determining gender before birth, and aborting an imperfect child are all seen as immoral and horrifying acts by some segments of society. Certainly, the potential of genetic engineering raises concerns for the species. For example, is it right to develop a baby specification kit whereby would-be parents could take a pill and predict the size, gender, IQ, appearance, and longevity of their child? What ultimate impact would that have on society? Would everyone look alike 30 years from now? Although this possibility may seem farfetched, scientists must deal with this view of the future.

Transplants

The scientific and medical advances related to the transplantation of human body parts have raised other ethical dilemmas. What constitutes death? Who gets the organs when there are not enough to meet the demand? What is the value or expense of saving a life? Which lives can society afford to save? Is it moral to ask a grieving relative for the organs of a lost loved one? Are artificial devices like the artificial heart worth transplanting? What constitutes undue risk or experimentation on a human subject with respect to transplant surgery?

CASE STUDY 11-11

Connie, a young woman with two small children, had suffered severe renal (kidney) failure and was on kidney dialysis three times a week. She felt unwell—tired, lethargic, and bloated—most of the time. She also had to follow a strict diet and severely limit the

(continued)

CASE STUDY 11-11 *(continued)*

fluids she drank. It became increasingly difficult for her to function and play a meaningful role in raising her sons. She finally decided to risk kidney transplant.

Because of her weakened health, the only realistic chance Connie had for survival was with an organ donated by a relative, which would minimize the chance of her body rejecting the kidney. Connie reported that she was an only child and that her father was her closest living relative other than her tiny sons, whose kidneys would be too small for her body. When her father was interviewed, however, he revealed that Connie had a severely retarded sister who had spent her entire life in an institution. The father was willing to authorize a transplant from his retarded daughter to Connie. There was no way that the retarded daughter could give her consent to the operation.

An organization that protects the rights of the incompetent took issue with this transplant arrangement. They went to court on the retarded daughter's behalf. Connie then went to the institution where her sister lived to help her decide what to do. Although she had been vaguely aware that this sister existed, she had not seen her in over 25 years. What she saw so shocked and saddened her that she refused to pursue taking her sister's kidney. She believed that her sister had suffered so much all through life that she had no right to inflict more suffering for her own gain. Three years later, Connie died of a heart attack following a dialysis treatment.

This case study raises many ethical considerations: How does one get informed consent from the mentally incompetent? Who has the right to speak for the incompetent? Does a severely ill patient have the right to refuse a lifesaving treatment? What role should the health professional play in this complex drama?

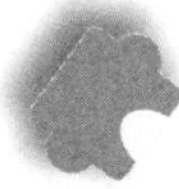

HIPAA and the Role of the Government

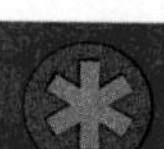

Key Point

Health Insurance Portability and Accountability Act (HIPAA) legal standard applied to protect privacy and security of patient information, especially when insurance reimbursements are made and information is exchanged

The **Health Insurance Portability and Accountability Act (HIPAA)** is also known as the Privacy Rule and applies to all communication of patient information whether electronically transmitted or in oral or written form.

The Security Rule of HIPAA regulations applies to the manner in which information is stored electronically.

The intentions of HIPAA are:

1. To protect the privacy and security of patient information, especially when information needs to be exchanged between agents such as medical offices to third-party payers.
2. To limit the information transmitted to only that which is essential.
3. To ensure that office personnel with no need to know details of patients' health cannot have access to those patients' records.
4. To inform patients about to whom, and under what circumstances, information is communicated.
5. To provide standards for information to be protected.

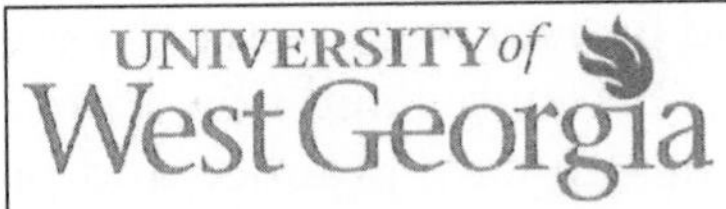

Department of Health Services
Carrollton, Georgia 30118-4700

UNIVERSITY OF WEST GEORGIA HEALTH SERVICES
AUTHORIZATION FOR DISCLOSURE OR USE OF PROTECTED HEALTH INFORMATION

Please complete this form in its entirety. Items not checked or blanks unfilled will be considered as non-applicable or specifically not authorized for release. This release is not valid if it does not contain the patient's orginal signature or if it has expired as described below.

I hereby authorize: University of West Georgia
Health Services
1601 Maple Street
Carrollton, GA 30118
678-839-6452

To disclose the following information from the health records of:

Name ____
Last First MI

Date of Birth: ________________ Social Security No.________________

This information is to be disclosed to: (Name of provider or entity authorized to disclose your information):

____
____
____

For the purpose of (Choose One) _____Continued Medical Care _____Personal _____Insurance
The following may be released (please check all that apply):

_____The entire medical record
_____Medical data related to:
( ) Specific condition(s):______________________________
( ) Specific dates of service: ______________________________
( ) Specific test(s):______________________________

I understand that this may include information relating to: Acquired immunodeficiency syndrome (AIDS)/human immunodeficiency virus (HIV); Behavioral health service/psychiatric care; treatment for alcohol and/or drug abuse; and sexually transmitted diseases.

Affirmation of Release:
By signing below I give my permission to the University of West Georgia, Health Services to release only the information I have selected on this form to the above named entry. I understand that this release is valid for up to one year from the date of signature and I may revoke this authorization at any time, except to the extent that action has been taken in reliance on this authorization or, if applicable, during a contestability period. Any revocation or refusal to sign this authorization will not effect treatment or payment. I understand that a revocation must be in writing and sent to University of West Georgia, Health Services, 1601 Maple Street, Carrollton, GA 30118. The revocation must include: patients desire to revoke this authorization; the patient's signature and date of letter. As a patient I also have the right to payment for copying cost. I further understand that if the person or entity that receives the above specified information is not a health care provider, health plan or healthcare clearinghouse covered by the federal privacy regulations or a business associate of these entities, the information described above may be redisclosed by the recipient and no longer protected by the regulations. I also understand that I have a right to receive a copy of this authorization if I request one.

______________________________________ ________________
Signature of Patient/Guardian/Legal Representative Date Signed

Tel 678-839-6452 • Fax 678-839-0656
The University System of Georgia • Affirmative Action/Equal Opportunity Institution

HIPAA compliant patient release form for medical records.

Confidentiality, informed consent, and patient welfare are the essence of ethical behavior. HIPAA regulations are reasonable and flow from an ethical perspective. They serve to help the health care practice and practitioners remain aware of the patients' right to privacy. And with the advent of electronic transmissions, HIPAA regulations set a standard for managing these newer elements of record keeping and record sharing.

How an office manages client records that are maintained electronically raises concerns if all members of the office have equal access to that information even though they are not treating that individual. Therefore, codes and passwords limit the ability of people within the same office to open confidential records. What can be transmitted by fax also has a distinct set of guidelines. HIPAA is somewhat more lenient regarding information that may be sent by faxes as they go to a limited locale. However, there are very strict prohibitions against sending details of patient records via e-mail when that patient is identifiable because it is so much more difficult to have a secure site guaranteeing private transmittal only.

Psychiatric and substance abuse records are treated differently. For example, 42 CFR refers to the Code of Federal Regulations, Title 42, last revised in 2003. It singles out records on alcohol and drug abuse, imposing stricter confidentiality requirements.

Today most busy health care offices have trained at least one person to serve as the HIPAA compliance expert so that questions may be answered with authority as they arise. Most offices also train all new employees to be certain they are HIPAA knowledgeable. Whereas this adds work and takes staff time, it is prudent to be certain we err on the side of protecting patient confidentiality to remain ethical, or "HIPAA compliant," in the health care workplace.

Summary

This chapter defined ethics as a set of guidelines for professionals that are designed to ensure public rights. The area of ethics encompasses both an understanding of professional responsibilities and an understanding of the professional's limitations. Consequences for a breach of ethics can be imposed by professional organizations. These consequences are different from the punishments typically handed down for legally defined misconduct. The relationship between the health professional and the patient was discussed in terms of beneficence, nonmalfeasance, autonomy, and justice.

All health professional organizations charge their members with basic responsibilities to the public in 10 areas: professional responsibility, competence, moral and legal standards, public statements, confidentiality, welfare of the consumer, professional relationships, assessment techniques, use of animals, and research with human subjects. Understanding these principles can increase the health professional's skill in making ethical judgments. Themes such as prior informed consent and the risk–benefit ratio are key concepts for future health professionals to understand.

A philosophical view of ethical concepts in health care requires that we, as health professionals, question the absolute definition of such constructs as evaluation, objectivity, and informing. Informed consent is an important example of the need to involve the patient in information sharing and decisions about their own health care. Informed consent can be written, verbal, or implied.

Health professionals currently face many ethical dilemmas. Public safety versus an individual right to confidentiality of a patient with acquired immune deficiency syndrome (AIDS), society's views, and the possible risks of genetic engineering, and the multiple conflicts of transplant surgery are examples critical to our time.

HIPAA guidelines and standards inform health professionals of how to manage information while simultaneously protecting patients' rights. A practice that is HIPAA compliant is one that practices a highly ethical standard.

Chapter Review

Key Term Review

Absolute: Total, all or nothing.

Autonomy: The individual right of a patient to exercise own judgment.

Beneficence: The use of a professional's expertise for patient well-being.

Competence: The ability to perform according to the standards of the profession.

Confidentiality: The nondisclosure of information.

Decorum: Term used for the medical etiquette of the Hippocratic Oath.

Degree: A step in a series.

Ethics: A set of standards and codes held as essential by professionals for the welfare of their patients and their professional standing.

Etiquette: 19th century medical code used to guide professional conduct without relying on the term *morality* but based on the presumption of "an upright man instructed in the art of healing."

Hippocratic Oath: Oath sworn to by new physicians declaring that they place the welfare of their patients first and will do no harm.

Health Insurance Portability and Accountability Act (HIPPA): Legal standard applied to protect the privacy and security of patient information, especially when insurance reimbursements are made and information is exchanged.

Informed consent: Knowledgeable permission—patient reasonably informed about the pros and cons of a test or treatment.

Institutional review boards (IRBs): Independent ethics committees that oversee medical research on humans.

Justice: A sense of fairness.

Nonmalfeasance: Doing no harm.

Patient's Bill of Rights: List of a patient's rights.

Professional responsibility: Acceptance of the consequences of their own actions by health professionals.

Risk–benefit ratio: Weighing relative gain over possible loss.

Sanctions: Penalties for noncompliance.

Torts: Laws that define what constitutes a legal injury and establish the circumstances under which one person may be held liable for another's injury. Torts cover intentional acts and accidents.

Chapter Review Questions

1. What ethical violations do you believe would be extreme enough to require loss of licensure or the right to practice?
2. Can you think of a health care example in which the health professional might be found guilty of a crime (legally responsible) but not in violation of an ethical principle?
3. Can you describe an experiment using human subjects in which a deception might be justified?
4. You visit a dietitian for advice on how to lose weight. She tells you that she can sell you a vitamin product that will help you lose weight. Is this ethical behavior? Should she be reported to any professional or licensing agencies?

5. Your mother has terminal cancer and is going to a skilled nursing facility. The nursing facility director tells you that they will not accept any patient with a "Do Not Resuscitate" order as that is against their religious beliefs. Should you report this to the State Department of Health? What if your physician says that it is perfectly acceptable behavior and that, if you have a problem with it, you should simply go elsewhere?
6. You smell alcohol on your therapist's breath during a therapy session. But she seems to be perfectly cogent. What would you say? Would you report her to any agency?

Case Study Critical Thinking Questions

1. In Case Study 11-1 was the physical therapist unethical or guilty of poor boundaries? Explain.
2. In Case Study 11-2 should there be a ban on research sponsored by commercial interests? What about the liquor industry? What about the tobacco industry? What about the pharmaceutical industry? What about universities? How do you keep research objective?
3. In Case Study 11-3 what harm is there in an occupational therapist filling in for a physical therapist?
4. Refer to Case Study 11-4. Assume you work with a physician group. A patient asks you about having a termination of pregnancy. You are a Roman Catholic. What would you do?
5. With reference to Case Study 11-5, what is the ethical issue involved in referring to the achievements of one's clinical practice?
6. Refer to Case Study 11-6. Your boss asks you to use more modalities for physical therapy in order to increase billings. You realize that it is common for physical therapists in private practice to use multiple modalities and that your job could be in jeopardy. How would you handle the issue?
7. Refer to Case Study 11-7. Any health professional who is giving advice outside of his or her scope of practice or not referring the patient when he or she is unable to help is guilty of what? Explain.
8. Using Case Study 11-8 as a reference, is it ever advisable to handle ethical matters informally?
9. Examine Case Study 11-9. What is the problem with the students conducting the tests?
10. Case Study 11-10 points out the necessity of humane treatment of experimental animals. Is such an ethical principle necessary?
11. Case Study 11-11 has many facets. Think about all of these and discuss with your class.

References

1. www.fda.gov/ScienceResearch/SpecialTopics/RunningClinicalTrials Institutional Review Boards
2. www.ama-assn.org/ama/no-index/physician-resources/2498.shtml American Medical Association's Code of Medical Ethics.
3. www.pbs.org/wgbh/nova/doctors/oath_classical.html Hippocratic Oath.
4. www.hhs.gov/ohrp/informconsfaq.html Informed Consent.
5. www.hhs.gov/ocr/privacy/hipaa/understanding/index.html HIPAA
6. www.cc.nih.gov/participate/patientinfo/legal/bill_of_rights.shtml Patient's Bill of Rights

Additional Reading

1. Bennett, B., et al. *Assessing and Managing Risk in Psychological Practice: An Individualized Approach*. Rockville, MD: The Trust, 2006.
2. Brahams, D. "The Hasty British Ban on Commercial Surrogacy." *Hastings Center Report* 17(1):16–19; 1987.
3. Daniel, E., ed. *Taking Sides*. Dushkin Publishing Co., 1998.
4. Krager, D., Krager, C. *HIPAA for Medical Office Personnel* Clifton Park, NY: Delmar Learning, 2005.
5. Nicholl, D. S. T. *An Introduction to Genetic Engineering,* New York: Cambridge University Press, 2008.
6. Pence, G., *Medical Ethics: Accounts of the Cases that Shaped and Define Medical Ethics*. New York: McGraw Hill, 2007.
7. Plomer, A. *The Law and Ethics of Medical Research: International Bioethics and Human Rights*. New York: Routledge-Cavendish, 2005.
8. Pozgar, G. D. *Legal Aspects of Health Care Administration*, 2nd ed. Aspen Law & Business, 1999.

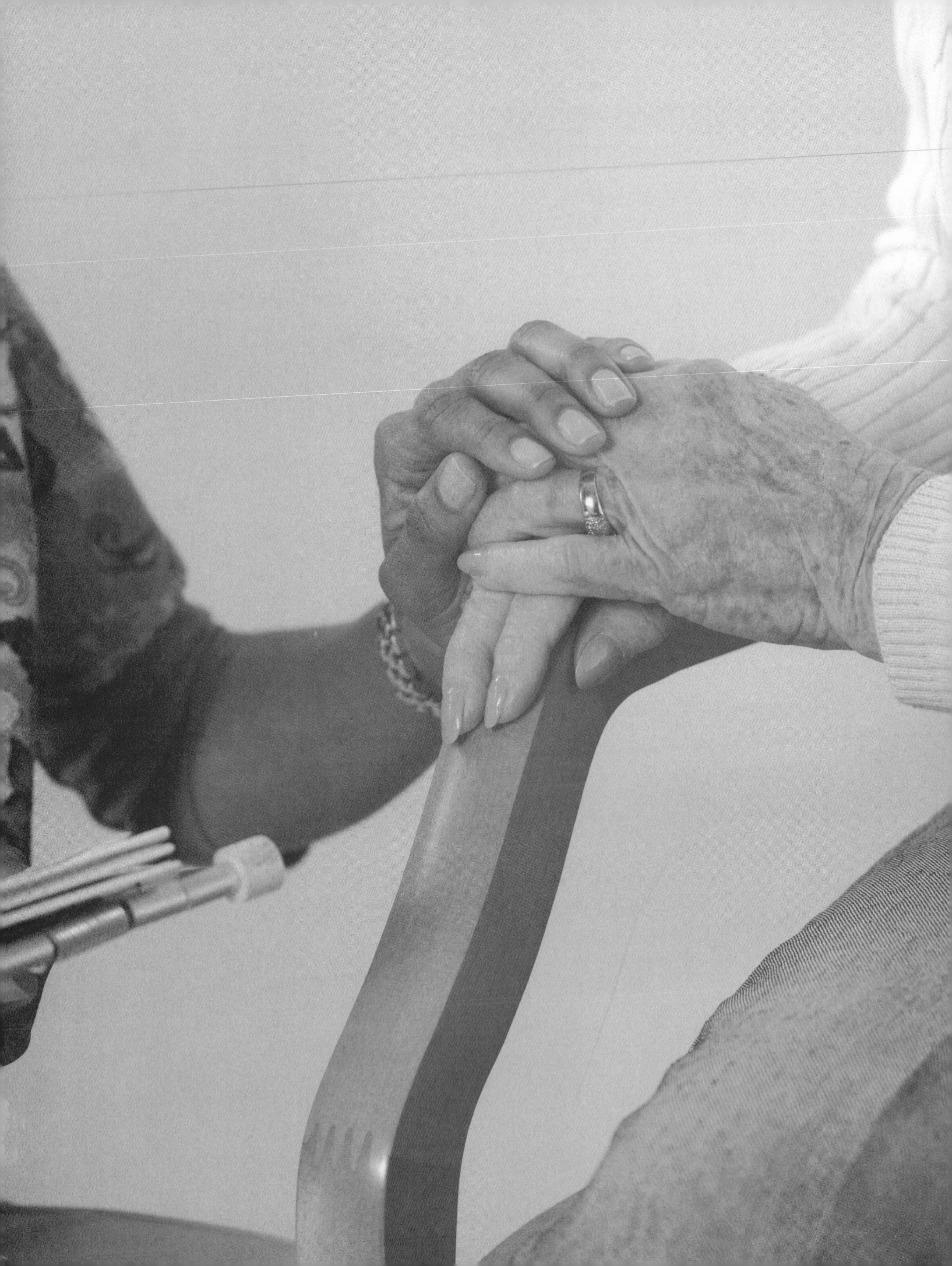

Abuse, Impairment, and Discrimination

chapter 12

Learning Outcomes

After reading this chapter, you should be able to:

12.1 Define physical and mental abuse, exploitation, and neglect and identify common threads that run through the different types of abuse.

12.2 Understand and manage elder abuse.

12.3 Describe spouse abuse and ways to manage it.

12.4 Recognize child abuse and ways to manage it.

12.5 Explain the term *liberated minor*.

12.6 List the signs of rape and be able to show empathy to a rape victim.

12.7 Recognize the different forms of mental incompetence.

12.8 Differentiate between mental incompetence and impairment.

12.9 Discuss rehabilitation, adaptation, and emotional and legal issues for the disabled.

Key Terms

Abuse
Americans with Disabilities Act (ADA)
Assault
Battery
Cognitive impairment
Conservator
Denial
Disability
Discreditable
Discredited
Discrimination
Exploitation
Liberated minor
Mental incompetence
Neglect
Power of attorney
Prejudice
Pro re nata (p.r.n.)
Rape
Restraint
Stigma

Abuse

Abuse, impairment, and discrimination are important topics for all health professionals. Five to 20 percent of all people have been abused during their life. Health professionals also frequently deal with patients with physical or mental impairments. Unless health professionals have sensitivity to these issues, they will not be able to communicate effectively with huge numbers of their patients.

It should be recalled that the definition of health is not simply the absence of disease but a state of total physical, mental, and social well-being.

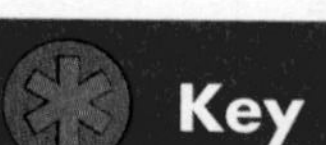

Key Point

Abuse willful infliction of physical or mental pain through acts of commission or omission.

Abuse is the willful infliction of physical or mental pain through acts of commission or omission. Abuse can include deprivation of services necessary to maintain health.

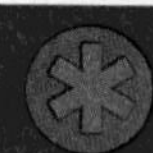

Key Point

Exploitation taking advantage of another person, usually financially.

Exploitation is the process of taking advantage of another. In the case of the elderly, exploitation is using the elder's resources for financial or personal gain. (Although the victim appears to have given consent, there is obvious misuse of their trust or incompetence. Exploitation reflects back to our definition of informed consent and raises the issue of knowing consent.)

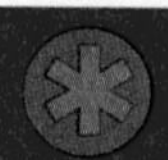

Key Point

Neglect willful infliction of physical or mental pain through acts of omission.

Neglect is the willful infliction of physical or mental pain through acts of omission. Neglect refers particularly to the deprivation of services necessary to maintain health.

Types of abuse are:

- Physical abuse: the willful infliction of physical pain (e.g., hitting, restraining, confining, drugging, sexual abuse).
- Mental abuse: the willful infliction of emotional pain (e.g., threatening, ridiculing, ignoring, isolating).
- Financial exploitation: using checks and credit cards, forging signatures, and stealing cash from a client for personal benefit. "Rackets" like fake charities and investment fraud are often operated by befriending a lonely elder. Obsession with limiting the cost of caring for an elderly person is another form of financial exploitation; for example if they need new dentures, they need to be provided.
- Neglect: the intentional or unintentional abandonment of an elder who needs care or leaving young infants belted in a car while going into a store.
- Health care abuse: charging for care not given, double-billing, fraudulent remedies.

There are some common themes that run through abuse:

- The abused child often becomes an abusing adult (12 percent in one study).
- The chronic fear suffered by the abused may create a state akin to posttraumatic stress disorder. Think of the recent horrific case of Jaycee Dugard, an 11-year-old, who was abducted by a child molester Phillip Garrido. Jaycee was held for 18 years and repeatedly raped by Garrido.
- The association with substance abuse.
- Social isolation of the abused and the abuser. The abuser does not want others to know what is going on for fear of getting found out, and the abused is not allowed by the abuser to have friends.
- Underreporting and underdiagnosis.

- Difficulty in treatment: The abuser will not come in for treatment. The abused will often deny abuse or not follow up with appointments.
- Denial by the abused and the abuser that there is any abuse going on.

Abuse of the Elderly

Abuse of the elderly is denounced in countries where the elderly are revered. In 2008 there were approximately 39 million people over 65 in the United States. In the National Center on Elder Abuse Study in 2004 there were 564,747 reports of elder abuse to adult protective services, of which 191,908 were substantiated. Thus about 1.2 percent of people over 65 were reported as abused. For those over 80 years old the percentage is much higher. It is also estimated that multiple cases go unreported—perhaps 7 percent more. As defined previously, abuse includes not only active abuse but also passive abuse or neglect as well as exploitation (usually financial in the elderly) and violation of rights.

It is important to distinguish between reported, suspected, and substantiated abuse. Many cases of abuse are never reported. It is estimated that only one in six cases of elder abuse is reported. By contrast, it is estimated that only one in three cases of child abuse is reported. If a case is reported, it is often investigated. But just because a case is unsubstantiated, it does not mean it did not occur and it may still be suspected. Elder abuse is difficult to prove because the abuser often denies it, and the abused may be confused or retract statement for fear of retribution or being put in a nursing home.

With the elderly, neglect, which is certainly the most common form of abuse, includes particularly isolation, inattention, and withholding physical or mental care that would undoubtedly be offered to a younger person.

Restraints

Although persons of any age may have to be restrained in a hospital, it is most common among the elderly. Is restraining a patient a form of abuse? To answer this question, consider the primary interests of the patient and take other patients into account. It is reasonable to restrain a patient when there is a risk that the patient may injure himself, herself, or others. If, for example, a patient might pull out intravenous lines, try to commit suicide, or try to hit others, restraint may be reasonable.

Reasonable medical **restraint** usually consists of a material vest with tapes tied to the bed or the back of a chair, and padded side rails on the bed. For a very violent patient—for example, an acutely manic or intoxicated patient—a four-point restraint might be used. Such a restraint consists of leather cuffs for the ankles and wrists that anchor the patient to a bed or stretcher. In cases in which a patient simply has to be watched carefully, putting the patient in a chair with a Velcro fastening lap restraint easily undoable by the patient and positioning the chair opposite the nursing station in a hospital or nursing home might suffice. Although the patient would not be tied down and, traditionally, no physician's order would be needed, this arrangement nevertheless would still be a form of restraint. In grey areas such as this, health care providers must weigh the risk to the patient of being unrestrained against the psychologic trauma of being restrained. Formerly, cross chair tables were used as a form of restraint. These were trays that attached to each arm of an arm chair that prevented the patient getting

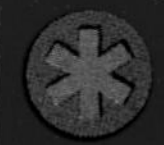

Key Point

Restraint limitation of physical or verbal activity by chemical restraint (sedating drugs) or physical restraints (tying patient down).

out of the chair. However, use of these has stopped because some patients slipped down the chair and strangled themselves.

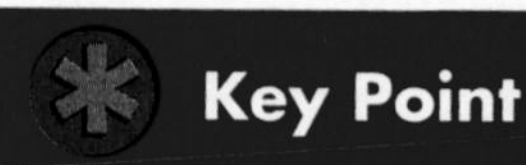

pro re nata (p.r.n.)—Latin for *if necessary.*

Restraint may be physical, chemical, or emotional. Chemical restraint, which is using drugs, accomplishes the same end as physical restraint. Straitjackets became virtually extinct with the advent of major tranquilizers in the 1950s. Giving a patient tranquilizing drugs calls for the same consideration as deciding whether to use physical restraint. If, for example, a patient shouts all night long, keeping others awake, and the physician orders that tranquilizers be used on an "as necessary" basis, also called **pro re nata (p.r.n.)**, the nurse has a duty not simply to give p.r.n. sedatives but to ask what the benefit of the sedation is to the patient and to what extent she or he may be violating the individual patient's rights by administering medication. Also, the nurse must balance these two considerations against what is fair to the other patients. The nurse's role is not simply to administer the restraint but to use judgment in deciding whether to administer it. Unfortunately, there seems to be a direct relationship between poverty and long-term chemical restraint. In the past, indigent mental patients have spent decades sedated.

Emotional restraint consists of withholding normal social responsiveness. Walking out on a patient halfway through a sentence, avoiding eye contact with a patient, and shutting a door to quiet a patient's shouting are all forms of emotional restraint. Emotional restraint tends to represent the ordinary subconscious behavior of both family members and health practitioners. It usually is not weighed and considered as physical and chemical restraints are. If emotional restraint is to be used, it should be decided upon in advance and discussed with other professionals. Emotional restraint should not be allowed to be an outlet for the health professional's frustrations.

Recognizing Elder Abuse

CASE STUDY 12-1

Judith is taken by her son, Ken, to the dentist. Judith, who has dementia, has had three front teeth fall out. Cindy, the dental assistant, sees Judith in the waiting room and notes a swollen lip with some bruising. Ken gets up to walk into the dental suite with his mother Judith. However, Cindy knows about elder abuse and cleverly tells Ken that the dentist has to treat her alone.

When Judith comes into the dental suite, Cindy asks her what happened. Judith starts, "Well, it was all my fault." Cindy, rather than waiting for a lie asks, "What was your fault?" Judith says, "I shouldn't have done it." Cindy asks, "Shouldn't have done what?" Judith replies, "I was bad." Cindy, sensing Judith's reluctance to come to the point, asks, "How were you bad?" Judith realizes that if she were to say anything against Ken, she might have to live the rest of her life in a nursing home because Ken would not look after her any more. So Judith says, "I fell." Cindy replies, "Did anyone push you?" Judith says, "No." Cindy says, "Does anyone do things to you that aren't right?" Judith pauses and then starts crying, "Yes, he hit me." The dentist reports the case to the state, and an ombudsman investigates and finds that Judith's son, Ken, has a gambling problem and is constantly trying to get money from his mother. Ultimately, Ken attends counseling and Gamblers Anonymous. He is heartbroken that he hit his mother and vows he will continue caring for her. The ombudsman arranges for social work follow-up to ensure that further physical abuse does not occur.

The elderly recipient of abuse commonly is female, white, and over 75 years old. Elderly victims commonly suffer from one or more physical or mental impairments and are economically, physically, or mentally dependent. Excessive dependence makes people especially vulnerable to abuse.

The abuser is commonly a female relative, usually a daughter, of the abused who has served as caretaker for the victim for many years (averaging about 10 years). The abuser is over 50 years old in 75 percent of the cases and is commonly the least socially integrated of the siblings, often being unmarried or unemployed. It is common for abusers of the elderly to have been abused themselves as children. Steinmetz found that one in two adults who were abused as children abused their parents in later years whereas only 1 in 400 adults who were not abused as children abused their parents later. Ninety percent of those who abuse the elderly are clinically depressed. It is common for the abuser to be intoxicated with drugs or alcohol or to be under mental stress during abusive acts.

The home where the victim and the abuser live may have locks on the doors of the bedroom, kitchen, and other rooms and locks on the phone or kitchen cabinets (to restrict communication or food). Although a vulnerable elder may recall how to operate a hardwired phone, a cell phone requires more skill. The home may lack appropriate aids for daily living.

An abused elderly person commonly reacts to his or her situation by:

- Becoming depressed.
- Presenting multiple medical problems.
- Being hypercritical of caregivers or professional attendants.
- Regressing to childlike behavior.
- Denying any abuse.

The abuser commonly reacts to the health care provider by:

- Being hostile toward the victim or the attendant.
- Showing excessive concern over the elderly person.
- Being obsessed with control or the burdens of caregiving.
- Denying any abuse.

The following is a typical example of how abuse of an elderly person develops.

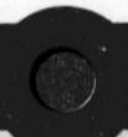

CASE STUDY 12-2

Marian is the youngest of four daughters. Aged 42, she is still unmarried, although she became engaged about a year ago. Marian's mother has suffered from dementia for the last six years. After a bout with pneumonia and a stay in the hospital, it became obvious that she could not return to her home alone. All Marian's sisters have their own families and naturally turned to Marian to care for their mother. Marian felt guilty. It had only been five years ago that she got her own apartment, and she wondered whether her departure contributed to her mother's downhill course.

So her mother came to live in Marian's apartment. Initially things went well, but after several months Marian's fiancé, who had begun to see himself as married to two women, broke off the engagement. Marian was heartbroken and angry. She resented having to be a caretaker for her mother and having to eke out a meager income as a

(continued)

CASE STUDY 12-2 *(continued)*

psychiatric aide. Soon after her fiancé broke their engagement, Marian discovered that a bottle of wine after dinner eased her sorrow. Her mother was beginning to become disturbed at night, waking up several times each night and sometimes wandering out of the house. Marian had to get up from a sound sleep to put her mother back to bed and had difficulty functioning at work the next day. Her mother behaved better during the day, but at times she was incontinent of both stool and urine. She was also falling down from time to time. Sometimes she would switch on the gas stove and forget to light it. Marian disconnected the gas and bought a microwave.

A month ago, much to the outrage of her sisters and their families, Marian, at the end of her tether, applied to a nursing home to accept her mother. But her mother put on a good show when they visited the social worker at the nursing home. She denied all problems and refused to go to the nursing home. Marian's relatives all sided with her mother and said she should stay at home and have Marian look after her.

The following week Marian lost her job for shouting at a patient. She began to drink more. One afternoon, when Marian went out shopping, her mother called up her neighbor and claimed she had been abandoned. When the neighbor questioned Marian, Marian got angry and reprimanded her mother. The same thing happened a few days later. When it happened a third time, Marian lost her temper and slapped her mother across the face. Now when Marian goes out shopping, she locks her mother in her room, and, because she does not want her to fall while she is away, she also ties her to a chair with a vest restraint she stole from the nursing home.

Increasingly, Marian is resorting to hitting her mother when she is incontinent or disturbs her sleep and restraining her during the day when she wants to watch television undisturbed. Marian frequently cries, especially when she has to clean the feces and urine from her treasured furniture and the floor. Marian feels she has been abandoned by her family and sentenced to a life of hell.

Management and Legal Issues in Elder Abuse

The Elder Abuse Prevention Identification and Treatment Act was passed by Congress in 1985; it was modeled after the Child Abuse Act of 1974. This act defines abuse, exploitation, and neglect.

Usually a case of abuse is identified by a health professional—nurse, physical therapist, occupational therapist, social worker, or physician—especially with home visits or hospital admissions. Each state has different laws, but many states make it mandatory for a number of health care providers, including orderlies and aides, to report abuse. In addition, the law specifically declares any such reporter be immune from civil or criminal liability.

A report of abuse is generally made to the regional ombudsman for the elderly. (An ombudsman is an official appointed to investigate complaints on behalf of the public.) Usually a form for protective services is filled out at the same time. The ombudsman then becomes responsible for ensuring that the person in question receives adequate protection. If the elder is mentally competent, he or she can refuse services. Typically, however, a visiting nurse follows the patient at home. The nurse provides general support to the caregiver, involves other family members, may arrange a companion to allow the caregiver a rest, and monitors progress. The abuser may need the services of a social worker or psychologist, particularly if she has a history of being abused or if substance abuse, major depression, or poor social integration is involved. There is often a tendency to adopt a hidden prejudice against the abuser, which hinders providing satisfactory care for the elder. Recall the case study. How would you feel in Marian's place?

If the situation does not improve, the elder has to be removed from his or her home and from the caregiver. Removal usually involves placement in a skilled nursing facility or intermediate care facility.

If an elderly person refuses care but appears to lack insight, conservatorship proceedings (discussed in the Issues of Impairment section of this chapter) may be initiated.

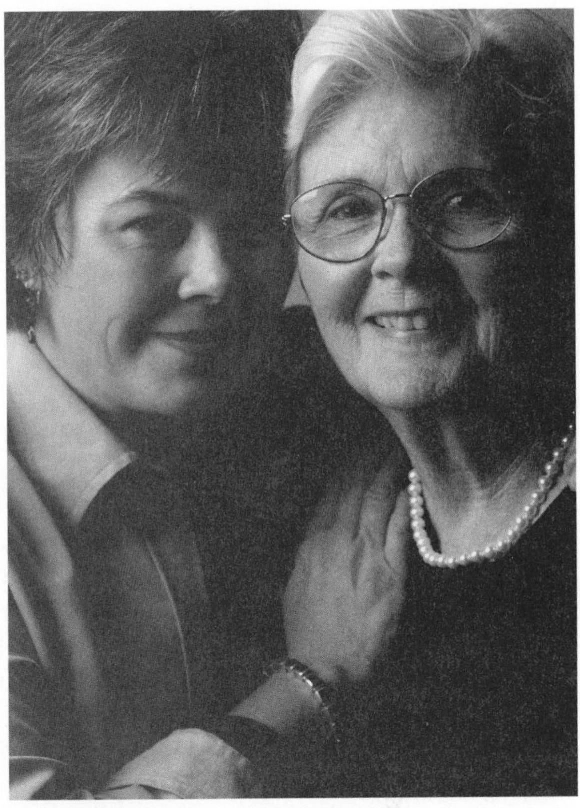

This could be Marion and her mom.

Spouse Abuse

Trainor and Mihorean (2001) in "Statistics Canada" reported 12-month wife abuse rates of 3 percent. The WHO in 2002 reported 20–50 percent of women in various populations around the world have experienced spouse abuse at some point in their lives. A common thread running through all types of abuse is a history of abuse. Eighty percent of male spouse abusers have a history of witnessing or experiencing abuse as a child.

There are two chief theories explaining abuse. The *dynamic theory* states that abuse represents repressed rage from receiving abuse, which is now being expressed through more abuse. In medieval times, some kings used a

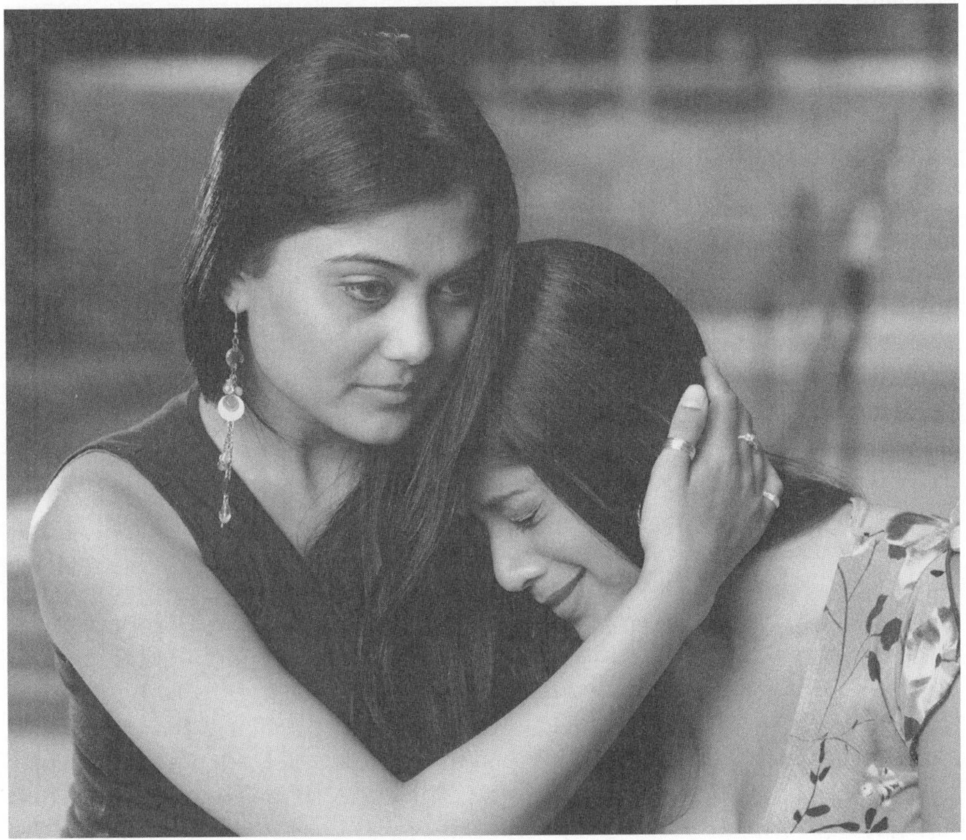

Abuse can happen at any age and in many forms. What can you in your role as a health care provider do to help the abused? And the abuser?

beating boy rather than punish their own children for wrongdoing. Each time the prince did something wrong, the beating boy got the birch. In modern society, the beating boy would be called an abused child. The abused child grows up wanting to "take it out on others" when anything upsets him. The anger he repressed at being abused he now expresses by abusing others.

The *learning theory* of abuse states that people are socialized to use abuse in their important relationships. In particular, as children they see that assertiveness by the abused is usually punished and they witness that violence by the abuser is the appropriate way to exert authority. As adults, abused children abuse their spouses or their own children and later may abuse their own parents if the right situation arises.

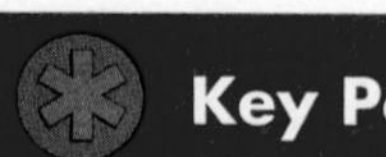

Key Point

Denial psychologic mechanism in which conflict in mind is resolved by disavowal of that conflict.

As discussed in Chapters 3 and 4, **denial** is one of many psychologic mechanisms for dealing with events or conflicts that our minds cannot handle. Denial is extremely common in all forms of abuse.

Denial also has a psychologic effect on the health care provider: it tends to prejudice her or him. If you, as a health practitioner, were to ask a man whether he hit his wife and he broke into tears and confessed, you could at least feel some empathy. But if the man denied what you knew to be true, you would feel deceived and probably less empathic.

Typically, the spouse, usually female, appears with a significant injury, for instance a fractured jaw from being punched in the face. She eventually admits that her husband did it. When her husband is confronted, however, he says they were only playing around or it was the first time it's ever happened. If pressured, he says there is no problem or his wife needs to change or she hit him. Commonly the man is intoxicated during the physical abuse.

Willful infliction of mental pain is also a form of abuse. Verbal and emotional abuse can be just as devastating as physical abuse, and to describe a man as "henpecked" can trivialize a potentially powerful and very common form of abuse.

Characteristics of Spouse Abusers and Their Relationships

As mentioned earlier, spouse abusers frequently have been abused themselves. Men who abuse their wives usually are socially isolated. They have few or no friends to talk to. They feel shame and low self-esteem. They are frequently alcoholic. Ceasing to abuse their spouse is only one of many adjustments they need to make.

Because the abuser is socially isolated, his relationship with his wife is usually very intense. She may be the only person he relates to, and he has a tragic problem in expressing that relationship: he finds it difficult to differentiate between himself and his wife. He becomes disappointed, for example, when she does not anticipate his every need, and he may become jealous and paranoid if she relates to other people. With his low self-esteem, social isolation, and inadequate coping mechanisms, violence represents a moment of reward in exerting his power. Following a violent expression of power, he not only feels very guilty but also fears losing his only relationship. The wife also fears loss of the relationship. This fear leads to a period of intensification of the relationship, a honeymoon period, while he atones for his violence because he fears she will leave him. These cycles often repeat themselves. Sometimes increasing violence is necessary to gain the same effect. Sometimes the wife is forced to have unwilling sex—sexual abuse—which may also be regarded as marital rape in many situations and it is illegal.

Management and Legal Issues in Spouse Abuse

As with the elderly, excessive dependency fosters abuse. Because the abuser needs to control his wife, he tries to foster dependency. He will not allow her to work. He may control all the money. He may not allow her to leave the house unless he knows the reason and he sets time limits: "Make sure you're back in an hour with those groceries; no dilly-dallying." He may move the family to a distant town to intensify his relationship with his wife and remove her from her social contacts.

Her dependency makes separation difficult. Where could she go if she left? He might come after her and injure her seriously. What would happen to the kids? She cannot leave them alone with him. She cannot provide for them. She has no money, no job, no housing, no social contacts, no coping mechanism, and no willpower left.

CASE STUDY 12-3

Carla goes to the dietitian, David, because she wants to lose weight. David notes that Carla has bruises on the inner forearms and asks how she got them. Carla replies that she fell.

David wonders how putting her arms out to break a fall would cause multiple bruises on the inside of both arms. He says "Carla, do people sometimes do things to you that you don't want them to do?" Carla looks down and says, "No." David says, "Carla, if you fell, those bruises would be in a different place." Carla says nothing. David says, "Is there anything else I can help you with? Is there anything else you would like to tell me?" Carla still looks down, then, after a pause says that she just wants advice on how to lose weight. At the end of the appointment, David gives Carla a card with a toll free number for the nearest spousal abuse hotline. This is an example of denial.

It is not surprising therefore, that both wife and husband deny that abuse has occurred. To break through the denial, the threat of exposure must be stepped up. If necessary, this may have to be accomplished by having the husband arrested for spouse abuse. Ideal treatment is for the husband to go to group therapy sessions with other spouse abusers. Such sessions are both educational and ego-strengthening. The abuser will be accepted into a group of abusers. The therapy will address the issues of shame, jealousy, low self-esteem, and relating only to one person. Violence and power cannot be used in group therapy. For the first time, the abuser may learn about normal relationships and how to behave in a normal relationship.

Meanwhile, the wife may live with her children in a shelter for abused women. Through group work she will be given a chance to develop esteem, willpower, independence, and new coping mechanisms. A goal for her will be to learn to tell her husband what her limits are: "You may never hit me again. If you do, I will file for divorce. No more second chances!" Often the location of the center is secret to avoid the risk of the husband finding her. He may punish his wife (and possibly his children) for bringing shame on him by exposing their intimate secret.

After both spouses have spent some time apart in counseling, they may go through joint counseling if the wife will accept it. Alternatively, they may separate or divorce. If there is significant substance abuse, that must be dealt with before the other issues.

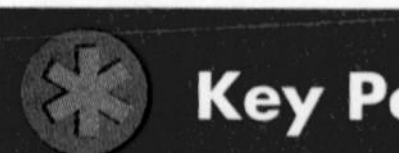

Key Points

Assault verbal abuse or threats of physical abuse.

Battery actual physical violence, involving physical contact with other person.

Few laws address spouse abuse specifically. Physical violence may result in arrest for assault and battery. Legally speaking, **assault** means verbal abuse or threats whereas **battery** means physical abuse. The most common advocate for the abused spouse is the social worker, counselor, or psychologist, who commonly is called to the emergency room to see a patient with significant injuries.

If an abused patient asks what she should do, the only safe response a health practitioner can make is to tell her to get to a place of safety. Once a wife has been hit, she is going to be hit again. As health care providers, it is our responsibility to ensure the victim's physical safety before we initiate any other services.

In cases of domestic violence, the police are frequently called in by the abused spouse, by neighbors, or by the children. If violence is obvious or if the wife is willing to bring action against her husband, the police can arrest him. Unfortunately, because she fears later punishment, the wife often denies the abuse or retracts the charge. This further alienates the police, who may have been called to the same household many times.

Unfortunately reporting of spouse abuse (i.e., abuse of a mate under the age of 65), unlike elder abuse or child abuse, is not mandated in most states. The abused spouse may also apply for a protective order, which is a civil court order that restricts the contact the abuser may have with the abused. The judge may specify the form of contact and conditions and exceptions. The order is then issued by a court. It protects the abused from harm or harassment and is cost free to any domestic violence, stalking, or sex abuse victim. The problem is that many abusers will violate a protective order.

A temporary restraining order to prevent domestic violence is also called a protective order. Once a protective order is in effect, the police can arrest the abuser for contravening a court order (e.g., telling the abused at work that he will kill her). The order may prohibit violence, the threat of violence, harassment, or even proximity to the abused. None of these are arrestable offenses without the protective order.

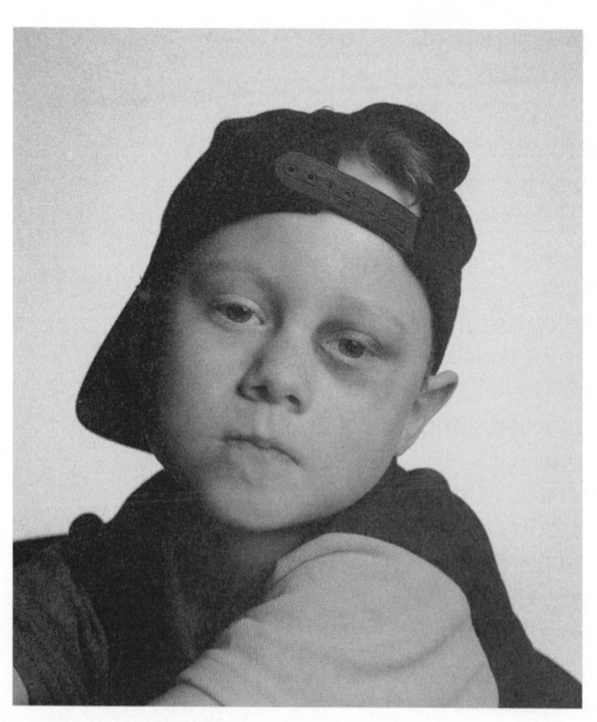

What caused those bruises?

Child Abuse

Psychologic abuse in children has also been called psychologic maltreatment, mental cruelty, and emotional abuse. Such abuse includes rejection, terrorizing, isolation, exploitation, and mis-socializing. Abuse may begin when the child is an infant and may be presented as failure to thrive (when a newborn baby does not put on weight). Sexual abuse of children is also common.

The National Abuse and Neglect Data System (NCANDS) collects statistics on child abuse (see Table 12-1.)

Table 12-1 Child Abuse Statistics USA2007 (NCANDS)

48.5 million children total
2.1 million reports of abuse
1 million reports of abuse after screening
450,000 substantiated abuse cases after investigation
1,760 estimated deaths from abuse

Seventy percent of reports by professionals were substantiated, but only 22 percent of reports by nonprofessionals were substantiated. Of the substantiated cases 62 percent involved neglect, 13 percent multiple maltreatments, 10 percent physical abuse, 7 percent sexual abuse, 4 percent psychologic abuse, and 5 percent "other."

Physical acts of commission include multiple fractures, cigarette burns, rope burns, dunking scalds (the child's buttocks and genitalia have been lowered into too-hot water), subdural hematomas (bleeding between the membranes surrounding the brain that is almost always a sign of child abuse rather than trauma), torn lips, and multiple bruises. If these injuries are repeated or multiple, if there has been an obvious delay in calling for medical advice, or if there are recurrent complaints about the child's bad behavior, then physical injuries should be suspected as signs of abuse.

Physical acts of omission include starvation of an infant, leaving open fires or open bottles of pills unattended, and similar acts that threaten the child's life or safety.

Mental acts of commission include locking a child in his or her room or in the attic or recurrent shouting at a child with verbal abuse. This does not mean that children must never be shouted at or punished. For instance, if, despite being told not to, a young child continues to stick objects into electric sockets or play with matches, it may be appropriate to smack the child's hand or shout at her. However, a more appropriate behavior would be to buy outlet covers and substitute lighters for matches (always keeping them out of reach). But locking a three-year-old in a dark attic for three hours because he spilled some milk is abuse.

A recent case that received national attention was when an aunt had custody of a child who repeatedly wet the bed. To teach him a lesson she withheld liquids and the child died from dehydration.

Mental acts of omission include failing to provide adequate love or mental stimulation for the child, although such omission alone seldom is the basis of investigation for abuse.

Sexual abuse may present as any form of trauma to the child's genitalia, venereal disease in the child, or urinary symptoms. A child is most unlikely to complain of sexual abuse, usually because the abuser makes threats to prevent the child from telling anyone about "their secret" or uses his or her relationship to ensure that the abuse remains a secret. Recently, it was reported that only one mother in seven believes her child when the child reports incestuous relations with her father or stepfather.

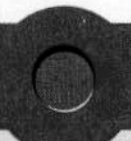

CASE STUDY 12-4

Tommy, aged six, is brought to the physical therapist, Angela, with a fractured foot for rehabilitation. Angela looks back over past records and notes that Tommy has had four other fractures before, involving his skull, his hand, bilateral rib fractures, and his right forearm. When Angela questions the mother, the mother is vague about details and just says they are all from "falls." Suspicious, Angela reports the case to the DCF, who find that two siblings have also been investigated as subjects of abuse.

Management and Legal Issues in Child Abuse

Child abuse was first labeled *the battered child syndrome* in 1962. This led to state child abuse and neglect reporting laws and subsequently to the Federal Child Abuse Prevention and Treatment Act of 1974, which was amended in 1986. Unless individual states comply with this act, they are denied federal funds.

It is illegal not to report a case of suspected child abuse. Not having proof of abuse is not reason enough to remain silent. The report is made to the Department of Child and Family Services, which assigns a caseworker to investigate. It is the responsibility of the social worker, not the person who reports the abuse, to decide whether the child has been abused. The reporter's only responsibility is to report anything suspicious. The agency will take action if it is actually or reasonably foreseeable that the injury is likely to result in protracted difficulties if the child is left untreated or in the home.

As with spouse and elder abuse, the abuser denies abuse, and often the abused denies it, too. The child may fear further acts of abuse if he or she tells.

The abuser, as well as the abused, needs help. There is a universal tendency to empathize with the abused and treat the abuser simply as a criminal. This chapter begins with elder abuse rather than child abuse because elders elicit less sympathy. Indeed, most can easily empathize with Marian in Case Study 12.2. In the section on spouse abuse, reasons were presented why some people become abusers. It is very difficult, however, for most people to empathize with child abusers. Remember that the person who abuses a child has problems, too. As noted, he or she probably was abused as a child. Substance abuse is often a problem. Child abusers have psychodynamic problems that are similar to those of other abusers. Child and family service agencies work with the entire family. The option of removing the child from the parents is seen as a last resort.

Sometimes people are wrongly accused of abuse. It is estimated that up to half the reported cases of child abuse are deemed to be unfounded. Such accusations take a toll on the approximately one million families who are reported, possibly falsely, for child abuse. Victims of Child Abuse Laws (VOCAL) is a support group that has sprung up to help such families. There has been much criticism of the handling of child abuse cases by social workers both in the United States and in Europe, mainly about children who died but also about false accusations.

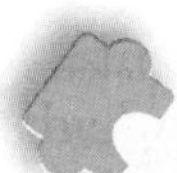

The Liberated or Emancipated Minor

Children, like adults, have certain rights. For instance, children of any age may own property, whether they acquired it through a gift or legacy or any other means. Children also have a right to be supported by their parents.

Generally speaking, parents exercise almost total authority over their children until they reach the age of majority, which in most states is 18. Beyond the age of majority the child becomes an adult; legally speaking, the young adult is his or her own free agent.

The **liberated minor** is a child who, because of circumstances, becomes his or her own agent before reaching the age of majority. In some states, the liberated minor is called an emancipated minor. For example, a boy who gets married in another state at age 16 and returns with a spouse and obtains gainful employment is a liberated minor. This boy's parent cannot direct his treatment or be considered by any health professional as his representative. All medical, social, psychologic, and legal decisions can be made by the liberated minor in this situation. Parents may also declare a child to be a liberated minor if they can no longer control the child and wish to absolve themselves of legal responsibility.

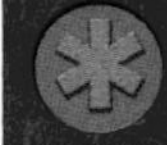

Key Point

Liberated minor child under 18 who is emancipated (i.e., a child who is free of parental control or power and may assume most of legal responsibilities of an adult).

The minor who at the age of 13 goes to a physician for treatment of venereal disease or goes to a social worker requesting help with an abortion is legally a liberated minor. Although generally the health professional would be wise to encourage such a child to communicate with her parents, the health professional is not obligated to tell the parent. And from a legal standpoint, the parent is not entitled to know.

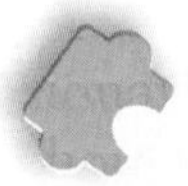

Rape

Rape is one form of sexual abuse. Other examples of sexual abuse include sexual harassment, sexual assault and battery, and sexual molestation of children. There are also several different types of rape, including date rape and statutory rape.

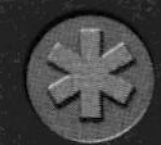

Key Point

Rape sexual penetration or its reasonable intent, without the subject's consent.

Sixteen percent of women and 3 percent of men report a sexual assault during their lifetime. Seventy-three percent of those raped know their assailant. In 2006 there were 272,350 reported victims of sexual assault (RAINN, 2008).

Rape is defined legally as penetration, or its reasonable intent, without the subject's consent. Penetration usually means penile penetration beyond the vaginal introitus, or in the case of anal intercourse, beyond the anal sphincter. The tying up of a woman and holding her at knifepoint while the perpetrator uses a candlestick rather than his penis to penetrate her also meets the definition of rape. To be able to consent, the subject must be of sound mind (not drugged, mentally retarded, or under age).

Sexual intercourse with a girl under the age of 16 is automatically defined as statutory rape because all state statutes say that people under the age of 16 cannot give consent. Sexual intercourse with a girl between the ages of 16 and 18 (the usual age of majority) is not automatically considered rape. At this age a girl is considered a liberated minor and can give consent.

Date rape, or being forced to have sex with someone simply because you have agreed to a date, is said to be extremely common. Unfortunately, this

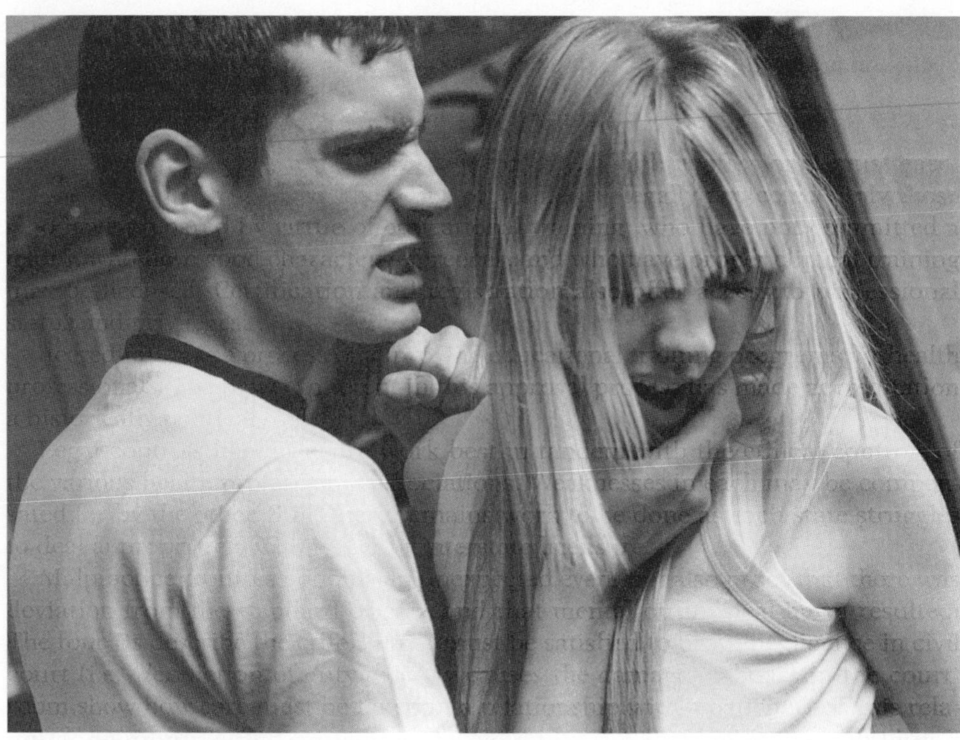

Date rape often goes unreported.

form of rape is rarely reported because the victim may blame herself, feel ashamed, or fear reprisals from a social network that she has in common with the rapist.

State and federal laws about rape change frequently. Some states say that the rapist can only be male; others say both males and females can be rapists. Rape can take place between a man and his wife.

Rape is an act of violence, and a demonstration of power. It is really an act of violence rather than lust. Most rapists actually despise or cannot relate to women.

The Psychologic Effects of Rape

Rape is an act of violence by the rapist and an act of abuse to the victim. Although rape usually entails a single incident, its effects can be as lasting as the effects of child, spouse, or elder abuse. Rape produces both acute trauma and psychologically long-lasting effects. It frequently causes a state akin to bereavement and acute trauma that takes time to get over. Some patients suffer from posttraumatic stress disorder related to the incident. The effect of being raped may vary depending on:

- The victim's previous sexual history.
- The victim's support systems.
- How much violence, pain, or mutilation was involved.
- The victim's age.
- The victim's religious beliefs.
- Whether the victim knew the rapist.
- The victim's marital status.
- Whether the victim has ever been raped before.

It is not surprising that rape victims frequently have subsequent sexual difficulties. The victim may react differently to her sexual partner. Simply associating sex with the violence of rape may create a feeling of panic with each subsequent sexual act. The victim's sexual partner, who can no longer relate in the same way as before, may not know how to behave. The victim feels drawn into her own world of sorrow; her partner feels bewildered by the loss of intimacy. Together they have been thrown into a different world. Victim assistance programs that include both individual and group therapy may be very valuable in this regard.

Management of Rape

Each state has a central regional office for sexual assault that oversees a number of local sexual assault centers.

If a patient reports a rape that occurred several weeks ago, there is unlikely to be documentable physical evidence of injury. Such a patient should be referred to a rape crisis center. If the rape is recent, the patient should be referred to the emergency room, where an established protocol is followed.

The protocol stresses that all services be on site; that all the history, examination, and tests meet legal standards for court challenges; and that the victim be treated with dignity and sensitivity and not be left alone at any time during the protocol. She must give written consent but can also refuse any question, exam, or test at any time.

The history includes past medical history, date and details of the assault, types of violation, mechanisms of injury, and activities after the assault. It also includes whether the rapist had the victim use drugs to facilitate sexual assault.

The examination includes a head-to-toe review for injuries, especially those proving force (e.g., bite marks, anal and vaginal injuries, and bruises on breasts and thighs). The patient is then photographed to preserve visual evidence of violence in case the patient wants to charge the rapist later. For the patient, this is often the most emotionally traumatic part of the proceedings.

A standard evidence collection kit uses specimens from the mouth, clothing, and bedding and bite marks, fingernail scrapings, pubic hair combings, and anal or vaginal smears to gain evidence of the rapist's DNA, as well as mouth swab for the patient's own DNA.

Urine or blood specimens for drug analysis with "chain of custody" forms (a legal term for the movement, location, and succession of the people responsible for evidence) are drawn. Specimens are also obtained for sexually transmitted diseases—syphilis, gonorrhea, chlamydia, trichomonas, hepatitis B and C, and human immunodeficiency virus (HIV)—and for pregnancy.

Emergency contraception; psychologic counseling; postexposure prophylaxis for HIV; follow-up HIV tests at one, three, and six months; antibiotic prophylaxis for sexually transmitted diseases; and hepatitis B vaccine are offered and the pros and cons discussed.

After discharge, the victim is given medical, mental health, and domestic violence follow-up as necessary and is referred to a crisis worker from the local sexual assault center. If she is willing, the patient makes a statement to the police. She is then asked whether she wishes to charge the rapist.

Ninety-four percent of rapists never spend a day in jail. Faced with the ordeal that follows a rape, it is not surprising that victims frequently refuse to be examined, to be photographed, to be interviewed by the police, or to make a charge. The courts, however, demand physical evidence.

Federal and state laws dealing with all forms of abuse (including abuse of the handicapped, which is discussed later in this chapter) are often quite similar in content. On the state level, these laws are administered through local branches and advocates, as shown in the accompanying box.

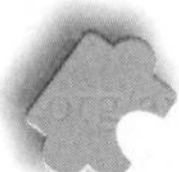

Issues of Impairment

This section deals with impairment and discrimination, a subtle form of abuse that is often sanctioned by large segments of society and may even be regarded as normal by some members of society. Listed in Table 12-2 are the state organizations and local advocates for various forms of abuse.

Mental Impairment and Mental Incompetence

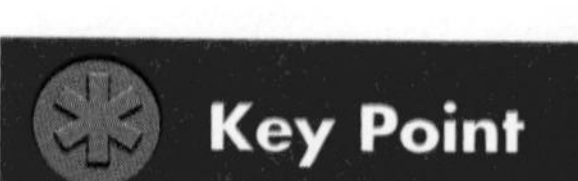

Key Point

Mental incompetence person's inability to make decisions in his or her own best interest.

Mental impairment is an actual physiological defect that can lead to mental incompetence. Mental incompetence tends to lead to appropriate societal responses. Mental impairment tends to lead to discrimination. **Mental incompetence** is the inability of a patient to make decisions that are in his or her own best interest. A toddler who walks into a fire is incompetent. A demented person who wanders down the middle of the road without

Table 12-2 State Organizations and Local Advocates for Various Forms of Abuse

Form of Abuse	State Organization	Local Advocate
Elder	Department of Aging	Regional ombudsman for the elderly
Spouse	State-subsidized regional community mental health service	Battered women's shelter designee
Child	State Department of Child and Family Services	Local-branch assigned case worker
Handicapped	Office for protection and advocacy for the handicapped (mental and physical)	None; each centralized state agency sends a specific person to investigate each case; homes for the mentally retarded may have resident social workers answerable to the state office
Sexual	State sexual assault center	Counselor at local rape crisis center or designee from victim assistance program

regard to traffic is incompetent. An elderly isolated woman who writes checks for life insurance, leaving herself insufficient money to eat, may be incompetent. It is impossible to know the workings of every mind. It is possible, for instance, that the visits this woman has from the insurance salesman to collect her insurance checks are the only form of social contact she has. Reflecting back to Maslow's hierarchy of needs in Chapter 3, it would not be surprising if she craves social contact more than food. Perhaps, therefore, she is not incompetent unless she does other things such as piling old newspapers next to an open fire or refusing medical care despite severe symptoms.

Although eccentricity must be respected in a free society, a patient who is living dangerously or is being abused, exploited, or neglected may not be able to recognize what is happening. The probate court appoints two types of **conservators** (or guardians): one who appropriates and takes charge of an elder's finances and one who takes charge of making decisions about the elder's mental, physical, and social health. The latter type of conservator may also decide whether the elderly person should be institutionalized. Typically, a bank trustee is appointed financial guardian whereas a relative or representative of the state is made responsible for the other areas of guardianship. Conservatorship proceedings also require a statement by a physician that the mental capacities of the elder are substantially and permanently impaired.

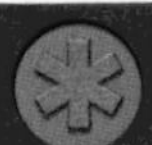

Key Point

Conservator person appointed by probate court to take care of financial and /or personal decision-making for an incompetent person.

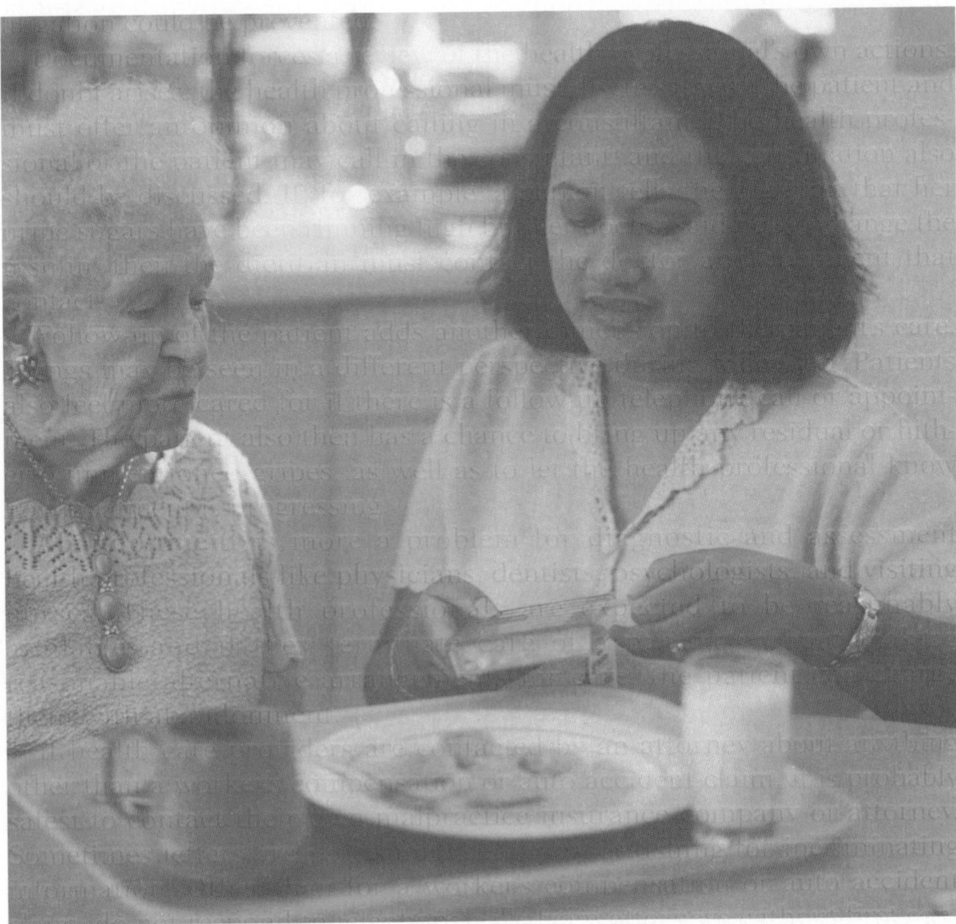

Is she competent?

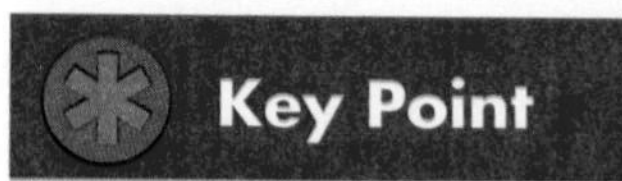

Power of attorney the granting of power by a competent person to another person to make specified decisions.

A competent person may grant to another the power to take charge of any specified decision (**power of attorney**). By contrast, conservatorship is usually made by a court to transfer authority for decision-making from the incompetent person to a competent one.

Such societal intervention is potentially dangerous. Supreme Court Justice Brandeis once warned that "experience should teach us to be most on our guard to protect liberty when the government's purposes are beneficent." Care must be taken when infringing on any person's rights, especially when the motive is to help them.

Social and emotional impairment sometimes results from mental impairment.

Lack of Insight

Mental competence describes the ability of a patient to make decisions in his or her best interest; insight describes the ability of a patient to understand his or her own problems. A certain degree of intellect is a prerequisite for insight as illustrated in the following:

Intellect ⟶ Insight ⟶ Competence

A patient may therefore be incompetent because of mental retardation or because of a lack of insight. Intelligent people may lack insight because of emotional, language, cultural, or other reasons. When lack of insight interferes with making decisions of self-interest, the patient may still be defined as incompetent.

Mental retardation and dementia both affect intellect. Examples of patients who typically lack insight are those who suffer from drug-related impairment, obsessive-compulsive disorders, and schizophrenia. Loss of insight can be difficult to judge in people who are reclusive, those who are excessively religious, and those who cannot speak the prevailing language.

Providing informed consent for surgery is only possible in a patient who has enough insight to see his or her problems in perspective. A patient may be legally competent enough to manage her own finances and everyday life but unable to understand the pros and cons of surgery when presented with complex facts in an anxiety-provoking situation. A mastectomy for possible cancer of the breast is an example of such a situation.

Cognitive Impairment

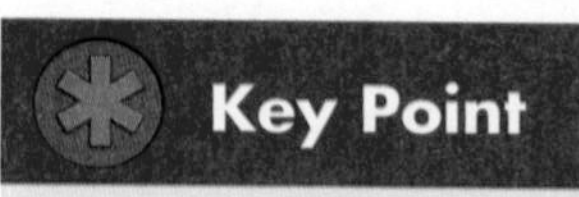

Cognitive impairment loss or absence of intellectual capacity.

Cognitive impairment used to be called mental retardation or dementia. The term cognitive impairment includes both, so one may have to specify whether the cognitive impairment is developmental or acquired.

Almost identical laws at the federal and state level protect the disabled from abuse. Mental and physical handicaps are both handled by the state office for protection and advocacy for handicapped and developmentally disabled persons. It is mandatory to report abuse of the mentally retarded. This is true for physicians, nurses, dentists, dental hygienists, physical therapists, osteopaths, optometrists, podiatrists, psychologists, social workers, teachers, speech pathologists, police officers, and any person paid for caring for persons in any facility serving mentally retarded people, as well as for private citizens. Any person who reports a suspected case of abuse in good faith is immune from civil or criminal liability. Failure to report a case can lead to a fine.

Emotional Impairment

Emotional illness carries a certain stigma. In some ways, certain of those stigmas have been removed by labeling certain illnesses as medical disease. Addiction, for instance, is now largely accepted as an illness rather than an immoral life.

Although emotionally impaired people have the same rights as all citizens, some people ignore the rights of the emotionally impaired. A man who sexually abuses his two-year-old daughter is undoubtedly emotionally or mentally ill. But he also has rights. He has a right to treatment, due process of law, and lack of discrimination. In actual practice, he will be heavily discriminated against, most of all by fellow prisoners, who pervasively condemn sexual abuse of children. Part of the problem is also the primitive moral or religious view that has impressed on society the idea that sexual abuse is a sin rather than an illness.

The religious rather than scientific view spills over into the whole of emotional illness. This causes deep-rooted feelings in people who then unconsciously discriminate against people who are emotionally ill.

Social Impairment

Social impairment refers to the inability of someone to integrate properly into the society in which they live. Although the impairment may be due to a relatively normal phenomenon like shyness, it may become a matter for discrimination. Social impairment associated with discrimination is **stigma**, which was discussed briefly in Chapter 3. Most people know or have met people who stutter or who are deaf, blind, physically unattractive, obese, alcoholic, illiterate, epileptic, or mentally ill. Indeed, the reader may acknowledge that they too have imperfections and have experienced times of feeling different, particularly as teenagers or in foreign countries. Stigma refers more to the social disgrace connected with a particular attribute than to the attribute itself.

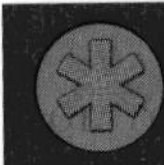

Key Points

Stigma feeling of social disgrace connected with a social impairment

Discredited description of a person with obvious social stigma

Discreditable description of a person with hidden social stigma.

A stigma typically causes psychologic mechanisms to come into play, particularly overcompensation, denial, rationalization, and inversion. Please review the discussion of defense mechanisms in Chapter 3. Stigma may also lead to depression or low self-esteem. A patient with polio who tries to become an Olympic athlete is overcompensating. An African-American patient who blames all his failures on skin color is rationalizing. A patient with an amputated arm who, rather than playing it down, goes to great lengths to flaunt her disability is displaying inversion. However the person who successfully challenges his or her disability, as in Lance Armstrong winning the Tour de France over and over again in spite of his history of cancer, is admired.

A stigma may be socially obvious (for example, stuttering or facial deformity), and the person may be labeled **discredited**. Or a stigma may be socially hidden (for example, when a person has had a colostomy or has epilepsy), and then the person may be labeled **discreditable**.

The discredited are uncertain how others will respond and may become self-conscious. They may compensate through defensiveness or aggression.

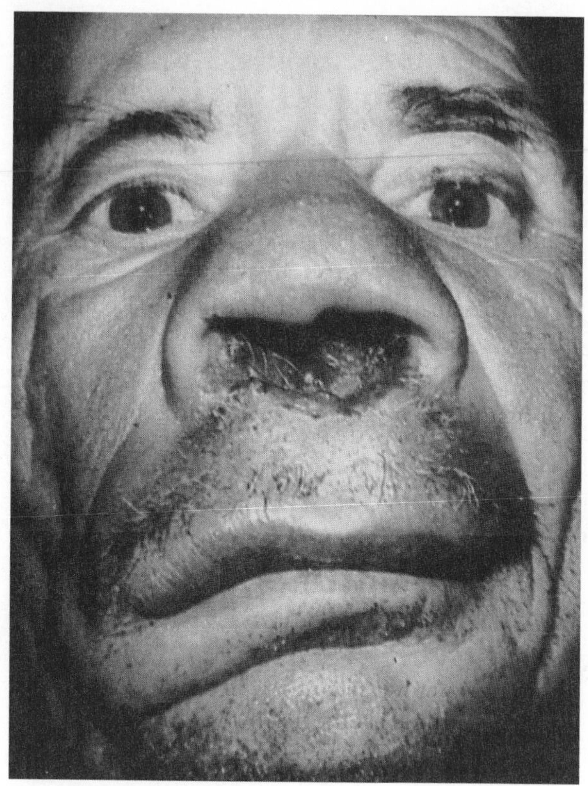
A discredited stigma

The average person may become confused about whether to ignore the stigma, talk about it, or make allowances for it. These problems can lead to strained and uncomfortable relationships. Some discredited persons become very adept at fielding comments, questions, and situations pertaining to the disability. "My Left Foot" is a great movie about a man with cerebral palsy who becomes a respected artist.

Although the discreditable person can hide the disability, he or she may be forced to reveal the disability at some later date, and this may cause conflicts. For example, the person may have to decide when in a relationship to tell the other person that she or he has had a colostomy. Some discreditable people cannot cope with such questions and choose to handle them by becoming socially or geographically mobile. Others may expose their stigma very early in a relationship in order to assume the role of the discredited. Recurrent genital herpes is another important example of this.

The stigmatized person may feel most comfortable with intimate contacts such as a parent, spouse, or health professional or with others who share the same stigma. Sharing the stigma with others is a support mechanism that may even be formalized into a support group. In this group the person learns from others how best to handle the outside world, and feels comfortable with fellow sufferers. (Kübler-Ross found that anger in the terminally ill against nonsufferers was eased by fellowship in a group.) On the other hand, the group exposes and emphasizes the stigma, and the patient may be ashamed of the stigma and the ghetto-like quality of the group. More and more amputees and those with spinal cord injuries from the gulf wars are achieving "normal lives" with the help of technology and good counseling although depression and posttraumatic stress disorder remain a major concern for all returning military.

Cultural Impairment

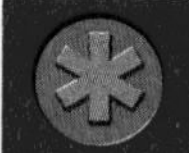
Key Point

Discrimination unfair treatment of person on the basis of group, class, or category to which that person belongs rather than on individual merit.

Prejudice prejudgment about a person

Cultural impairment is the inability of a patient to function optimally in society because of cultural attributes. Patients with a culture impairment face **discrimination**. Discrimination is derived from the Latin *discriminare,* which implies drawing lines of distinction between things. Discrimination typically involves color, sex, creed, age, and class. Examples include racism, sexism, ageism, class distinction, and religious creedism. Discrimination is in direct opposition to the concepts of civil rights and liberties. This is discussed further in Chapter 14.

Discrimination is different from prejudice. **Prejudice** is a prejudgment about an individual. *Prejudice is a belief. Discrimination is an action.* Discrimination means treating a person on the basis of their their belonging to a group rather than as an individual. By contrast, the person who is prejudiced thinks he or she knows all about an individual because of the person's sex, or age, or race, etc. An individual may be prejudiced but unwilling to discriminate because of the penalties involved or for reasons of conscience. An individual may discriminate even though it violates his or her own beliefs, for example for peer approval.

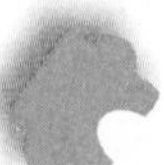

Disability

Disability is a physical or mental impairment that interferes with normal life. Disabled persons suffer from physical or mental handicap. Without legislation, protection, and advocacy, life for the disabled can be very difficult.

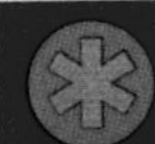

Key Point

Disability physical or mental impairment that interferes with normal life.

Rehabilitation for any handicap involves four major areas: medical, social, educational, and vocational. Medical rehabilitation involves particularly physical therapists, occupational therapists, and speech therapists. Social and educational rehabilitation often involves counselors, psychologists, and social workers. All of these health professionals must be familiar with the issues facing the disabled person. These issues include stigma; prejudice; discrimination; lack of insight; and the financial, physical, emotional, medical, sexual, and vocational aspects of disability.

The Bureau of Disability Determination is a federally funded state-run organization that determines whether disabled people will be paid a disability pension. The bureau also can refer a patient to the Department of Vocational Rehabilitation, a branch of the U.S. Department of Health and Human Services, where vocational specialists can enable the patient to become employable again.

In 1990 Congress passed the **Americans with Disabilities Act (ADA)**, to address discrimination of the disabled in the workplace. It was estimated at that time that there were 43 million Americans with physical or mental disabilities. The act is administered by the Equal Employment Opportunity Commission (EEOC), which also administers the provisions of the Civil Rights, Equal Pay, Pregnancy Discrimination, and Age Discrimination in Employment Acts.

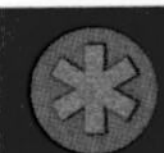

Key Point

Americans with Disabilities Act (ADA) administered by EEOC (Equal Employment Opportunity Commission)

The ADA requires all employers of 15 or more people to make reasonable accommodation, especially job restructuring or architectural changes, as long as this would not create undue hardship (i.e., being beyond the financial or operating resources of the company).

The ADA prohibits discrimination in applications; hiring, promotion; discharge; compensation; job training; or terms, conditions, and privileges of employment. However, the employer may disqualify the person if he or she still cannot perform the job required despite reasonable accommodation.

Summary

Abuse is the willful infliction of physical or mental pain by acts of omission or commission. This chapter presented several examples of elder, spouse, and sexual abuse. All forms of abuse are subjects of various federal and state laws with similar content. Examples were given of elder, spouse, and child abuse.

The concept of the liberated or emancipated minor was discussed. Also the many forms of sexual abuse were presented, including protocols for dealing with the rape victim.

A central theme in abuse is that abused people themselves often become abusers later in life. Abusers as well as the abused therefore need professional help. Most abused people are in dependent roles. When the abuse is of sufficient severity to threaten the immediate or future mental or physical health of a person, then the abused patient must be protected.

Mental impairment may involve incompetence, lack of insight, or mental retardation. Mental incompetence is commonly thought of as retardation or dementia. However, there are other dimensions in describing mental impairment, which is broken down into intellect, insight, and competence. Conservatorship, either financial, or making decisions on health care, was discussed, as well as power of attorney.

Mental impairment is divided into emotional, social, and cultural issues, including the concepts of discredited and discreditable stigma. Prejudice is contrasted with discrimination. Disability involving four major areas—medical, social, educational, and vocational—is a major area for specialization of a number of allied health professionals. The provisions of the Americans with Disabilities Act were also presented.

Chapter Review

Key Term Review

Abuse: Willful infliction of physical or mental pain through acts of commission or omission.

Americans with Disabilities Act (ADA): Act that addresses discrimination of the disabled in the workplace, administered by EEOC (Equal Employment Opportunity Commission).

Assault: Verbal abuse or threats of physical abuse.

Battery: Actual physical violence, involving physical contact with other person.

Cognitive impairment: Loss or absence of intellectual capacity.

Conservator: Person appointed by probate court to take care of financial and /or personal decision-making for an incompetent person.

Denial: Psychologic mechanism in which conflict in mind is resolved by denial of that conflict.

Disability: Physical or mental impairment that interferes with normal life.

Discreditable: Description of a person with hidden social stigma.

Discredited: Description of a person with obvious social stigma.

Discrimination: Unfair treatment of person based on group, class, or category to whom that person belongs rather than on individual merit.

Exploitation: Taking advantage of another person, usually financially.

Liberated minor: Child under 18 who is emancipated (i.e., a child who is free of parental control or power and may assume most of legal responsibilities of an adult).

Mental incompetence: Person's inability to make decisions in his or her own best interest.

Neglect: Willful infliction of physical or mental pain through acts of omission.

Power of attorney: The granting of power by a competent person to another to make specified decisions.

Prejudice: Prejudgment about a person.

Pro re nata (p.r.n.): Latin for *if necessary*.

Rape: Penetration or its reasonable intent, without the subject's consent.

Restraint: Limitation of physical or verbal activity by chemical restraint (sedating drugs) or physical restraints (tying patient down).

Stigma: Feeling of social disgrace connected with a social impairment.

Chapter Review Questions

1. Define abuse, neglect, and exploitation.
2. What does "physical, chemical, or emotional restraint" mean?
3. List types of abuse.
4. What are the two theories explaining abuse?
5. List three situations in which denial is commonly used.
6. What is the difference between assault and battery?
7. How should a health professional behave when a 13-year-old girl asks for treatment of venereal disease or help with an abortion? Should the case be discussed with the parent first?
8. List the five main recipients of abuse.
9. To which agency should each of these instances of abuse be reported?
10. What is mental incompetence?
11. How is social impairment different from stigma?

Case Study Critical Thinking Questions

1. Refer to Case Study 12-1. If you were the dential assistant, how would you have acted. What if Judith just said she "fell"? Would you explore the issue any further?
2. Refer to Case Study 12-2. How do you feel about Maria? Are you sympathetic? Do you feel guilty for feeling sympathetic?
3. In reference to Case Study 12-3 in which Carla denies spouse abuse to the dietician, what do you think happened to Carla? Lay out a likely scenario of what happened and where she ended up. Why do you think she came for dietary counseling?
4. Refer to Case Study 12-4. Did Angela do the right thing to report the case to DCF? What if there were no previous records and the family sued for wrongful accusation? Should Angela have sought more evidence before referring Tommy to DCF?

References

1. American Medical Association. www.ama-assn.org
2. National Center on Elder Abuse. www.ncea.aoa.gov
3. National Library of Medicine search site. www.nlm.nih.gov/medlineplus
4. Rape Abuse Incest National Network, 2008. www.rainn.org
5. Child abuse statistics, 2007. www.childwelfare.gov/pubs/factsheets/fatality.pdf
6. Child abuse statistics, 2007. www.acf.hhs.gov/programs/cb/pubs/cm07/cm07.pdf
7. 12% abused children become abusers. www.health24.com/child/Abuse/833-859,20875.asp
8. Rape protocol in New York State, 2005. www.albany.edu/sph/coned/healinghandouts.pdf
9. Elder abuse. www.preventelderabuse.org/elderabuse/physical.html
10. Child abuse. www.unh.edu/ccrc/physical-abuse
11. Domestic abuse hotline. http://dahmw.org
12. Child abuse government site. www.ojp.usdoj.gov/ovc/help/ca.htm
13. Trainor, C. and Mihorean, K. "Family Violence in Canada A Statistical Profile 2001." *Statistics Canada No 85 - 224 XIE*. Ottawa, Canada: Minister of Industry, 2001.

Additional Reading

1. Brewster, S. *Why Does He Do That? Inside the Minds of Angry and Controlling Men*. Emeryville, CA: Seal Press, 2006.
2. Cook, P. W. *Abused Men*. Westport, CT: Praeger Publishers, 2009.
3. Davis, L. *The Disability Studies Reader*, 2nd ed. Routledge, New York: BY, 2006.
4. Gil, E. *Helping Abused and Traumatized Children: Integrating Directive and Nondirective Approaches*. New York: Guilford Press, 2006.
5. Hellman, D. *When Is Discrimination Wrong?* Boston: Harvard, 2008.
6. Hinshaw., S. P. *The Mark of Shame: Stigma of Mental Illness and an Agenda for Change*. New York: Oxford University Press, 2007.
7. Holloway, M. *Driving with Dead People A Memoir.* New York: Simon Spotlight Entertainment, 2007.
8. Matsakis, A. *The Rape Recovery Handbook: Step-By-Step Help for Survivors of Sexual Assault*. Oakland, CA: Raincoast Books, 2003.
9. Silverstein, H. *Girls on the Stand: How Courts Fail Pregnant Minors*. New York: New York University Press, 2007.
10. Texas, N. Partnerships: Family Education about Mental Illness. www.namietexas.org. 2008.
11. Walls, J. *The Glass Castle A Memoir*. New York: Scribner, 2005.

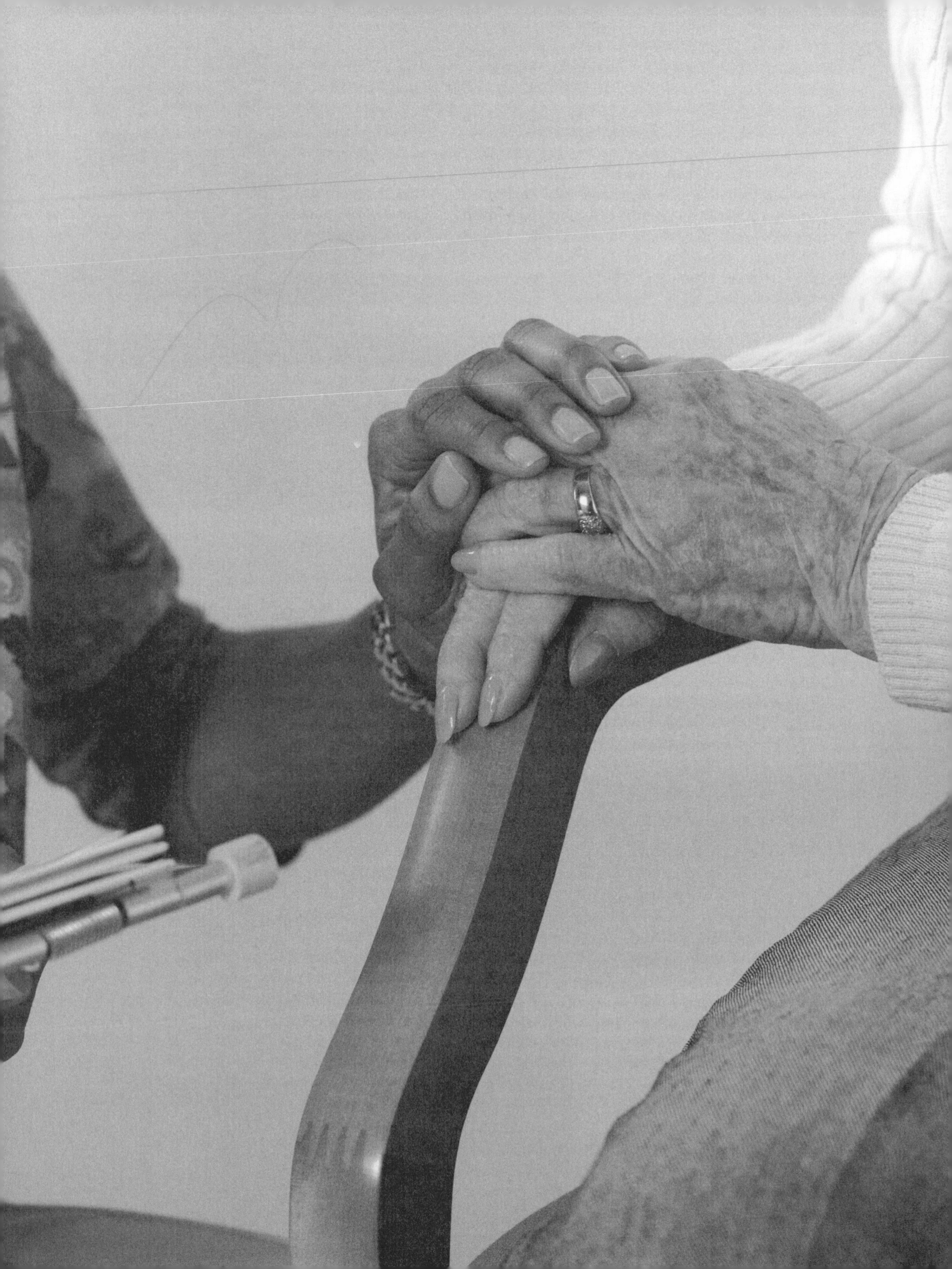

Legal Concerns

Learning Outcomes

After reading this chapter, you should be able:

13.1 Identify factors leading to the right to practice.
13.2 Discuss accreditation for the health professional.
13.3 Explain licensure for the health professional.
13.4 Describe how the public is protected from health practitioners.
13.5 Explain how negligence is determined.
13.6 List the chronological steps of a malpractice suit.
13.7 Critique the current malpractice system.
13.8 Understand how to prevent being sued.

Key Terms

Abandonment
Accreditation
Certification
Civil court
Criminal court
Deep pocket
Defendant
Expert witness
Flexner report
Four Ds of malpractice
Jury system
Licensure
Litigant
Maloccurrence
Malpractice
Negligence
Persistent vegetative state
Plaintiff
Rapport
Registration
SOAP
Standard of care
Statute of limitation
Tort

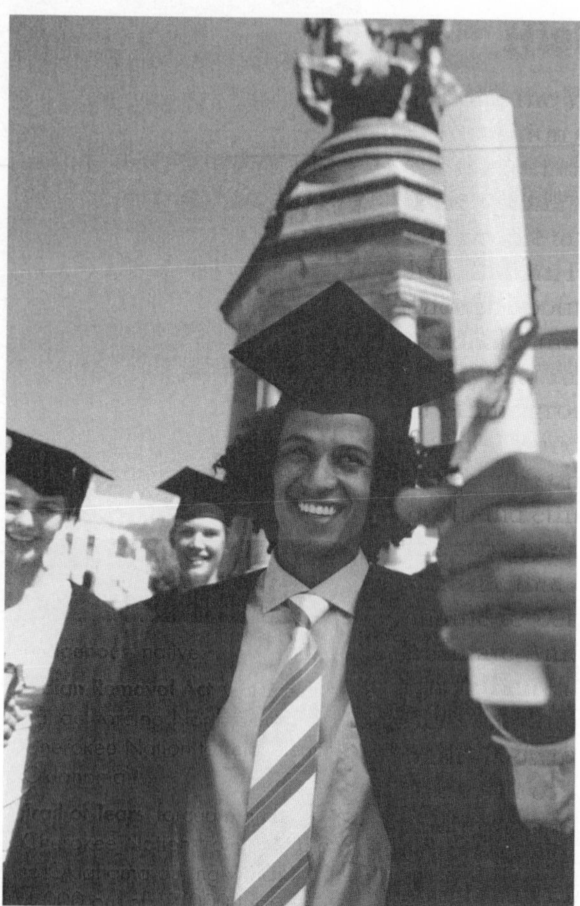

Graduation is a time of great joy, but also a time of new responsibilities.

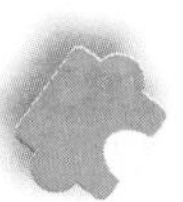

Occupational Regulation—The Right to Practice

In this country, the practice of health care is viewed, to a great extent, as a privilege. Health care providers must *earn* the right to practice. Depending on the health care specialty, earning this privilege may be fairly straightforward or quite complex, as reflected in our earlier discussion of health ethics. Ethical standards for health care professionals are guidelines intended to hold health professionals to exemplary standards. Because of these standards, the public can feel safe in placing its trust in the health care professional.

The right to practice is also based on an assumption of the value of the *rights of the patient.* Along with the privilege of being a health provider comes the *duty* of caring for the patient. When it comes to providing patient care, the health care provider is expected to accept extraordinary responsibility. Health professionals often work continuous shifts 24 hours per day; weekends and holidays must be covered by many health care workers. The needs of the patient must always be accommodated.

Earning the right to practice differs from specialty to specialty and, in some cases, differs from state to state. The first phase of this process is universally a learning stage. For some, this learning involves on-the-job, usually clinic-based, training; for others it is a combination of instructional and clinical training with heavy supervision. This latter type of program may span a few months or many years of both academic learning and supervised patient practice. In any case, the goal of the learning stage is to produce a competent health professional.

The learning stage is, however, only the beginning of access to the health professions. Most health professionals must also deal with certification or licensure exams. Further, individual educational programs must usually be accredited by professional organizations related to the type of training the school, college, or hospital claims to provide.

CASE STUDY 13-1

Ricardo, a physical therapist, got his license 30 years ago after physical therapy training in the Philippines. He is adored by all his patients, who refer many of their friends to him in independent solo practice. Each year he just signs his license application together with a check on the box that he has not been convicted of any crimes. However, he never interacts with other physical therapists in the area, never does any continuing education, and is basically just a "feel good" guy who uses modalities like hot packs, massage, range of motion, and ultrasound—the same modalities he has been using for the last 30 years. Should he continue to be licensed?

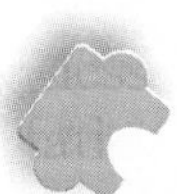

Occupational Regulation—Accreditation

Accreditation is the term used for the formal approval of an institution or educational program. If a program is judged to be of at least minimal acceptable standard, then accreditation is granted. Standards for accreditation are well-defined. Specific descriptions of these standards are published by the accrediting agencies and updated as necessary. The standards address such issues as the credentials of the teaching faculty, the number of hours a specific training program should involve, the curriculum, and the physical needs of a good teaching program. By the time these aspects of education have been delineated, the educational training program has some precise criteria to satisfy that help ensure standardization.

Key Point

Accreditation formal approval of an institution or educational program given by an outside agency.

Accreditation is said to be a voluntary process. That is, no hospital or school is forced to subject itself to review by an outside body. But, without accreditation, a nonprofit hospital or a teaching program might as well not exist. Insurance coverage, government subsidies, and grants are denied to nonaccredited programs. Graduates of nonaccredited teaching programs usually are denied access to the field for which they have trained. As discussed later in this chapter, being allowed to sit for a licensure exam usually is contingent upon holding a degree or certificate from an accredited educational program. So, although accreditation is a voluntary process, the sanctions against the nonaccredited are in many instances prohibitive.

Who Are the Accrediting Agencies?

The question of who the accrediting agencies should be has provoked political controversy within the health field for decades. In 1910, Abraham Flexner published a survey entitled “Medical Education in the United States and Canada” under a commission by the Carnegie Foundation. The **Flexner report** criticized many of the medical schools of the day. The American Medical Association (AMA) then took on the responsibility of accrediting these schools. Until recently, the Council on Medical Education of the AMA served as the accrediting agency for nearly all health care programs. On page 282 is a list of some Allied Health professionals together with their salary ranges.

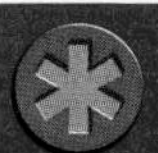

Key Point

Flexner Report Abraham Flexner’s report on the quality of medical education (1910) which, led to accreditation.

Although there are good reasons for AMA control of health care education, there are problems as well. As programs like nursing and physical therapy developed and matured, nurses and therapists began to understand their profession and its needs in a distinct manner. Eventually programs like nursing, pharmacy, physical therapy, and dietetics won the right to accredit their own educational programs. For many other health professional groups, accreditation is shared between the group’s professional association and the AMA. Many of these groups continue to lobby for total self-management of accreditation.

Another form of accreditation, this time of organizations, not individuals, is the Joint Commission, or JC (short for the Joint Commission on Accreditation of Healthcare Organizations). This is a private nonprofit organization that seeks to continuously improve the safety and quality of care provided by health care organizations. It is a monopoly. JC makes unannounced visits yearly to those organizations seeking accreditation,

Anesthesiologist Assistant $95,000
Physicians Assistant $71,000
Nuclear Medicine Technologist $67,429
Radiation Therapist $65,381
Perfusionist $60,000
Pathologist's Assistant $55,000
Physical Therapist $54,000
Speech Language Pathologist $52,694
Cytotech Supervisor $48,000
Cytotechnologist $46,000
Occupational Therapist $46,000
Orientation and Mobility Specialist $46,000
Specialist in Blood Bank Technology $45,000
Magnetic Resonance Technologist $44,410
Respiratory Therapist $41,537
Medical Librarian $41,000
Health Information Administrator $40,000
Ophthalmic Technician $39,000
Clinical Lab Technician / Medical Lab Technician $37,100
Radiographer $36,918
Dietician/Nutrionist $35,300
Electroneurodiagnostic Technologist $34,726
Occupational Therapy Assistant $33,000
Kinesiotherapist $32,500
Dental Lab Technician $31,780
Dental Assistant $32,198
Physical Therapist Assistant $30,000
Health Information Technician $30,000
Ophthalmic Dispensing Optician $27,000
Phlebotomist $24,315
Medical Assistant $22,650
Orthotist and Prosthetist $22,000
Pharmacy Technician $19,000
Ophthalmic Laboratory Technician $15,100

Some Allied Health career annual salaries in $ (Taken from Health Degrees.com as compiled from Bureau of Labor Statistics 2009) like hospitals, nursing homes, and visiting nursing agencies. Any facility that wants to receive Medicare funds must be JC-accredited.

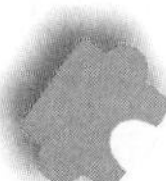

Occupational Regulation—Licensure

Licensure is a mechanism designed to assure patients that the care they receive from a professional meets a reasonable standard. Licensure is a function of state governments, so requirements for gaining access to licensure exams can vary somewhat from state to state. Many states will not recognize a license issued by another state if the requirements for licensure are not regarded as equivalent. On the whole, however, most states use a standardized examination process for a given profession. That means that the licensure exam taken by a would-be psychologist in Connecticut is the same as the one a candidate in California takes. Some states even have reciprocal agreements; if you are licensed by one state, certain other states will automatically honor that license (reciprocity). Although most states allow a grace period of practice with an out-of-state license, health professionals must rapidly take and pass the new state's exam.

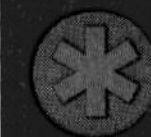

Key Point

Licensure mechanism designed to assure patients that the care they receive from a professional meets a reasonable standard.

Generally, the candidate health professional who seeks licensure must have graduated in good standing from an accredited educational program and can have no record of conviction of a felony (a serious crime). Also, letters of recommendation from practitioners who already are licensed in that field, sometimes called references, may be required. Such letters are expected to emphasize the character and ethical behavior of the candidate. In addition, many health professions demand that candidates complete a certain amount of supervised on-the-job training after graduation before they are permitted to take a licensure exam. To summarize, access to licensure involves:

- Graduation from an accredited educational program
- Lack of a serious criminal history
- Character references
- Proof of postgraduate training (for specified fields)

Weaknesses in Licensure

Relicensure, which means continuing to hold a license once it has been attained, has been criticized as too static. Generally, the health professional who wishes to keep his or her license simply pays a fee. This procedure raises major concerns in the area of professional competency.

Another weakness is that licensing mechanisms are usually general. That is, a license offers no legal control for specialty skills. For example, a physical therapist could, by virtue of the license, claim to be an expert in neurology when his or her primary emphasis actually is orthopedics. This discrepancy occurs because both neurology and orthopedics are within the scope of physical therapy practice. Later this chapter deals with how ethical standards work to control against general misrepresentation.

Certification as a Form of Licensure

Certain health professionals receive their credentials through **certification** rather than licensure. Certification attests that an individual has attained qualifications for a specified occupation. It differs from licensure in that it

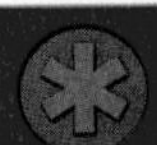

Key Point

Certification a testament that an individual has attained qualifications for a specified part of his or her occupation.

does not exclude others from outside professional groups from performing the same tasks. For example, a cytotechnologist is certified as able to perform specified tests. Although this certification is an important credential for the cytotechnologist, other clinical laboratory personnel can perform the same tests because there are no laws prohibiting them from so doing.

Another assurance mechanism for the training of a professional is the voluntary use of certification. Health professionals may use formal certification procedures beyond licensure to demonstrate their competency in a specialty area. Specialty boards may require candidates to complete educational and clinical training as well as to pass an examination. Such boards generally are linked to professional organizations, not to state licensure bodies. A licensed health professional may then declare that she or he also is certified to do whatever the specialization is and name the certifying body.

Registration

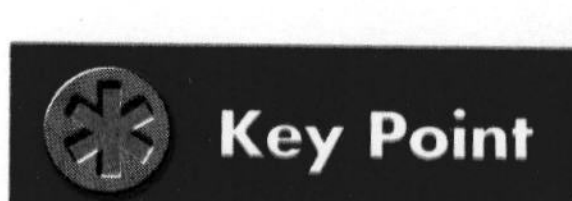

Registration a term often used interchangeably with both licensure and certification.

Registration is often used interchangeably with both licensure and certification. For example, registered nurses and registered dietitians are most appropriately thought of as licensed (nurses in all states are, in fact, licensed). State statutes recognize and protect their scope of practice. In some states only the titles are protected by the term *registered*; the regulation of practice is not. In these states the term *registered* takes on the same meaning as certification. Although certification has the same general intent as licensure, that is, to protect the public from incompetent practitioners, certification and some forms of registration do not have the force of the law behind them as licensing does.

A psychologist might get a degree in psychology, and then become *accredited* or *credentialed* as a clinical psychologist by the American Psychologist Association. She may then be *licensed* by the state that she practices in, and may have special expertise in a particular area in which she might obtain special *certification*.

She may also apply to a local hospital to be a practicing psychologist, where they would examine her qualifications, continuing education, and letters of reference. This process is also called *credentialing*.

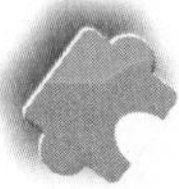

Protecting the Public

Chapter 11 points out that the goals of both ethical principles and legislation overlap considerably. That is, the ethics of today's health care professional must focus on ensuring public safety and protecting the public's trust. The legislation of the health professional's credentials is also aimed at protecting the public. Both legislation and ethical values assume the prominence of the patient's rights. Credentialed health practitioners accept a duty of serving and caring that puts the needs of the patient before all other considerations. What might once have been understood by virtue of etiquette is now spelled out in ethical principles and legislated statutes.

As mentioned in Chapter 11, the consequences of violating an ethical principle differ from the consequences of violating a law. Whereas violation of an ethical principle may result in sanctions such as reprimands, re-education, censure, or even expulsion from the profession, violation of the law may result in fines, imprisonment, or loss of licensure.

Although membership in a professional organization offers many benefits, it is not a necessary adjunct to practice. In states where one's profession is protected by licensure, however, loss of license equals loss of livelihood. The legal system carries the potential for more power via punishments than do the sanctions of the professional associations.

Legal and Ethical Controls Working Together

As mentioned earlier in this chapter, one of the weaknesses of licensure is the static nature of the license. That is, once a person has earned the privilege of a license, little effort is required to maintain that license. If sending in a renewal fee is all that is needed for relicensure, how does this really protect the public? What happens to the alcoholic, drug-dependent, or otherwise impaired health practitioner? And, what is even more often a risk, what guarantee does the public have of the continued education of its health care provider?

Say, for example, that a health professional entered the field some 20 years ago. Although she may have been bursting with knowledge and skill at that time, there is no way of knowing whether her knowledge and competency have continued to grow. Even with the best intentions of staying current, professionals with hectic and demanding practices can fall behind. It does not take many years of not having time to keep up with the journals to become out-of-date. Medical research and health care technology are advancing too rapidly for any practitioner to be judged fully competent if he or she does not make an effort to learn about new advancements in the field.

What can be done to protect the public from the technically stale professional? One possibility involves legislative directives that would tie relicensure to continuing education coursework. That is, no one would have their license renewed X number of years past examination unless they showed a transcript of relevant or approved courses they had completed during that time. Or, after X number of years, health professionals would be required to retake the state licensure exam. Many states already require that proof of continuing education be demonstrated for relicensure. Physicians and dietitians are two groups that require such updating. The requirement increases public respect for such professionals.

Another avenue of protection for the public exists in the area of ethical principles. Health professionals who are ethical and who are invested in membership within a professional organization must face the issues of responsibility and competency. Inherent in these principles is the tenet that health professionals must take responsibility for maintaining their own professional competency. To do less would be a violation of the public trust. Knowing that the health professional assumes this ethical responsibility helps us to believe that she or he would have great difficulty in ignoring the need for continuing education. Further, the ethical principle of competency helps to guard against the continued practice of an "unhealthy" professional. The alcoholic practitioner and his or her colleagues are duty bound to limit the practice of the impaired.

A second weakness of licensure laws is that they are too general in defining scope of practice. This generally leads to too little definition of precisely which specialties a given health professional is credentialed to perform. For example, a nurse primarily skilled in obstetrics and gynecology could, by virtue of licensure laws alone, claim to be a psychiatric nurse. Such a claim would be misleading to the public and therefore a violation of trust. One suggestion for controlling this problem has been the notion of a limited license. Such a license would attempt to restrict practice to those with educational training in a specific area related to their general health profession. Although limited licensure has some obvious benefits, it has not become a common practice, undoubtedly because of the complexity of screening and managing such a system and because of fear of the loss of flexibility that general licensure now affords.

Because limited licensure is not currently a reality, the burden of control falls on an assumption of ethical conduct. Once again, the principle of competence mandates that the ethical health professional *accurately* represent her or his education, training specialties, limitations, and boundaries and that she or he perform duties in conjunction with careful preparation. These behaviors serve as clear guidelines for those who wish to behave in an ethical and upright manner. The professional association is a watchdog in protecting the public from those who might exaggerate their capabilities.

CASE STUDY 13-2

Jake, a licensed social worker, was a woman's man. He had divorced four times and at the age of forty-two preferred to have a series of affairs and not marry again. He had worked in a small town in Minnesota for two years when affairs with three of his patients surfaced in the local newspaper. Complaints were made to the state health department, which only issued a warning. Six months later another complaint was made to the state health department after Jake had another brief sexual encounter with a patient, and Jake's license was suspended.

As he had registered and maintained licenses in three other states, South Dakota, Iowa and Illinois, he decided to move to South Dakota. There he lasted four years until his license was again suspended for multiple sexual improprieties. He then moved to Iowa.

When Controls Fail

The reader, cognizant of the weaknesses in licensure laws, no doubt will be aware of the possibilities for misuse. Misuse might occur through ignorance of a law's intent, although that is no defense. Misuse might also occur if health professionals have not fine-tuned their understanding of ethical principles. This is most likely to occur among those who are not active members of a professional association. Finally, misuse may occur among a small segment of health professionals whose intention it is to act fraudulently or with blatant disregard for public welfare. Recently a woman in Connecticut represented herself as a licensed registered nurse. She embellished this by stating she was named "Nurse of the Year" by the state nursing association, an award that did not even exist.

Sexually seductive behavior by male health professionals with female patients is one of the common examples of disregard for the public good.

Although female health professionals may be guilty of similar misconduct and patients may falsely accuse health professionals, this behavior by male health professionals bears further description.

Sexual impropriety with a patient is an obvious breach of ethical principles. A professional association typically expels a member from its ranks for life for such behavior. Legally, the offending health professional could be sued. Guilt in this matter could result in paying heavy damage fees to the patient and in loss of licensure. Although being expelled from a professional association may be damaging, the health professional is really injured financially through the legal system.

Can the public be protected from a health professional who seeks sex with his patients? Probably not. He need only cross the state border to set up a new practice, ostensibly with a clean slate. If he has not been found guilty of a felony, the new state may have no control over granting him a license. He may be licensed and receive the privilege of practicing by taking the new state's licensure exam, or he may receive it automatically if the new state has a reciprocal agreement with the old state. Another possibility is that he may hold multiple licenses. Many health professionals do this either as a safeguard against being restrained from practice should they lose one license or simply because they have lived in a number of different states. In any case, the problem is the same. States do not have reciprocity of licensure loss unless a felony has been committed. The culprit simply moves to another state. This lack of interfacing between state licensing bodies is a major frustration to those who have been mistreated by health professionals and is also a source of shame for ethical professionals. It remains a problem that needs resolving, although efforts are being made to track and list such persons.

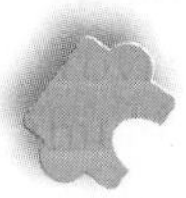

The American Legal System and Malpractice

All competent adults are responsible for their own actions. Allied health professionals are also responsible for their actions and are held to a reasonable **standard of care**—the degree of care and competence expected of a particular professional.

In America there are two court systems, the **civil court** and the **criminal court**. In a civil court the lawsuit is an action by private **litigants**—the parties to a suit are the **plaintiff** and the **defendant**. In a criminal court the government, represented by a prosecutor, brings an action against the defendant for a crime.

A **tort** is a civil wrong (excluding breach of contract) committed against a person or property. When a patient sues a health professional, the patient is the plaintiff, bringing an action in a civil court against the health professional (the defendant) for a tort.

Negligence is an unintentional tort, a wrong that a reasonable person would not have omitted or committed, and is the failure to exercise the proper standard of care. To prove negligence, first there must be a professional relationship established between the health professional and patient, and secondly the **four Ds of malpractice** or elements of negligence must be satisfied. The four Ds are:

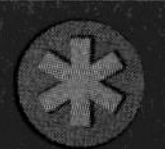

Key Points

Standard of care degree of care and competence expected of a particular professional.

Civil Court court that handles actions by private litigants.

Criminal Court court in which government prosecutor prosecutes defendant for crime.

Litigant person engaged in lawsuit against another person.

Plaintiff person who brings a suit.

Defendant person being sued.

Tort civil wrong (excluding breach of contract) against person or property that causes injury.

Negligence: unintentional tort that reasonable person would not have committed or omitted.

Four Ds of malpractice *Dereliction* of *duty* directly causes *damage*.

1. Duty of care that exists once a professional relationship has been established.
2. Dereliction of duty (i.e., deviation from the standard of care).
3. Damage to the patient, which must occur.
4. Direct cause (i.e., the deviation from the standard of care was the direct cause of the patient's injury).

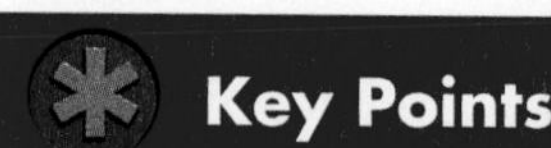

Malpractice maloccurrence that is actionable.

Maloccurrence untoward event (not necessarily actionable).

If a radiologic technologist takes an X-ray of the lumbar spine when an X-ray of the cervical spine was ordered, is this **malpractice**? No, it is not, because the patient has not suffered actual damage. Rather, it is a **maloccurrence**, a mistake that resulted in no damage. The two prerequisites for malpractice are mental or physical harm and deviation from the standard of care.

Mental or physical harm must obviously be significant. A medical malpractice case may cost $100,000 to take to court. If a mistake is made but no harm results, there is no malpractice. If, for example, the wrong hand is X-rayed, the mental or physical harm is insufficient to qualify as malpractice. If, however, the wrong hand is X-rayed, a malignant bone tumor is missed, and subsequently the patient needs an amputation, then harm has resulted.

Standard of care means what a usual health practitioner would have done in the same situation. Until a few years ago, location was included as part of the standards. Until then a country doctor was not expected to perform to the same standard as the university specialist. But now location is no longer a defense.

A physical therapist who manipulates a patient's neck when the patient has numb legs and recent urinary incontinence is not performing under the usual standard of care. If the patient becomes paraplegic, malpractice has occurred. If a physical therapist performs ultrasound and applies hot pack treatments to a patient with back pain, the usual standards of care have been applied. If this patient were to sue the physical therapist for erroneous treatment of cancer of the spine, the patient's attorney would have a difficult time. A physical therapist will treat a symptom, but a physician is the one who should have made the diagnosis. The usual standard of care does not include a physical therapist diagnosing cancer.

Other standards may be involved in malpractice. The most common malpractice suits involve surgical errors of commission. For example, the operating room technician gets the swab count wrong and leaves a swab in the patient. The patient subsequently develops an intraabdominal abscess that requires reoperation.

Errors of omission most commonly involve failure to diagnose, especially failure to diagnose cancer. For example, a physician's assistant is told by a patient about rectal bleeding and chooses to withhold the information from the chart or the physician. When the patient is later diagnosed with inoperable bowel cancer, there may be a basis for a suit.

Another error of omission in the United States is lack of informed consent. In an English case in the 1980s, a patient became paralyzed after disc surgery to the spine. Although the patient suffered damage, she still needed to show deviation from the usual standard of care. The patient said she was not informed of the risk of paralysis. U.S. courts would label this malpractice, but the English courts did not, instead saying that the physician had a duty to do what any similar physician would have done in the patient's best interest. Lack of information was not part of malpractice in England at that time. In the United States there is a *duty to inform.* Failure to do so, despite intent, is a form of malpractice.

How the Court Works

If a patient suffers damage and wants redress, he or she will see an attorney. The attorney must feel the case has merit because bringing a suit is very expensive and, if lost, the attorney may be out of pocket. Next the attorney requests copies of the patient's medical records.

The first phase of the suit is called pleading. The plaintiff's attorney files a complaint with the civil court. Summons are issued by the court and delivered by the sheriff to the defendant. The defendant then seeks an attorney who answers the summons.

The second phase is called pretrial discovery. A trial date is set by the court. Pretrial motions are made (e.g., modifying the initial complaint). The defendant is subpoenaed by the court for a deposition (sworn testimony given before both litigants' attorneys in the presence of a court stenographer). Sometimes there is an interrogatory, which is a written set of questions that require written answers.

At the end of this phase there may be a pretrial conference with the judge during which the attorneys discuss the case. Ninety percent of the time the case is settled out of court (i.e., never going to trial).

If the case does go to trial, the trial starts with jury selection, then the opening statements by each attorney, then the cross-examination of the witnesses, then the closing statements by each attorney. Following this, the jury deliberates, then comes up with a verdict that is handed to the judge, who makes the final judgment.

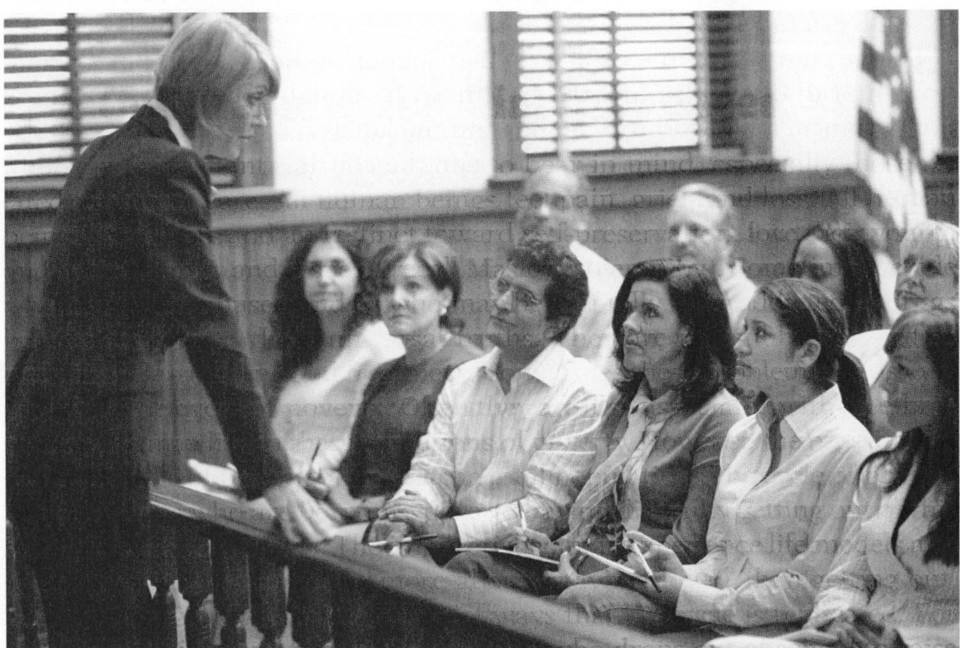

The jury system

Following the final judgment, there may either be an appeal to a higher court or the filing of posttrial motions.

Malpractice does occur. Not every health care provider has the patient's best interest at heart, and not every health practitioner is or will remain competent. Consumers must have the right to protection through the courts. If a maloccurrence (mistake) takes place and it was caused by an unreasonable action of a health professional, the patient must have recourse.

A court battle is usually an unpleasant experience for both the plaintiff and the defendant. It is common to wait three to five years for a case to come to court. This can take a heavy toll on the litigants. If, for example, a plaintiff cannot work because the wrong limb was amputated, a three-to-five-year wait is abusive. From the defendant's point of view, a three-to-five-year wait can also take a heavy emotional toll.

There are many other barriers to the patient's being able to obtain satisfaction from health care professionals: the imposing idea of a court battle, legal technicalities, the difficulty of proving malpractice, and worry over whether the patient will be shunned by health professionals in the community in which he or she lives.

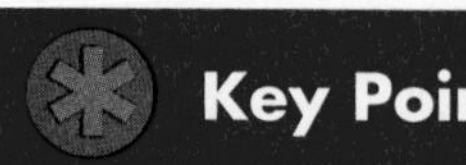

Key Point

Jury system A system in which a jury of public rather than judge decides on outcome of case.

The **jury system** is like a double-edged sword. On the one hand, it puts justice at the level of the common person. On the other hand, the complexity of many cases can make it difficult for an ordinary person to understand. If a social worker appears to have misjudged an abused patient's risk of death, is it fair to have untrained people judging the social worker? Explaining the wide perspective of a social worker to a jury during a court case is impossible. Jury members do not have the training to understand every complex issue; they gain much of their perspective from the prosecuting and defending attorneys. Given this situation, appeals to the emotions rather than the intellect are common.

Although both the prosecuting and defending attorneys have to be satisfied with the composition of the jury, who sits on the jury can be controlled to some extent.

Do the courts have the right to satisfy justice in the society–patient relationship rather than in just the health professional–patient relationship? For instance, if a laboratory technician mislabels a specimen and thereby delays a patient's diagnosis of AIDS, can the courts set an example with a $5 million award? They may, and the case may be appealed, and the appeal may be successful or unsuccessful. It is tempting to say that society will decide, but in practice the courts will decide.

Expert Witnesses

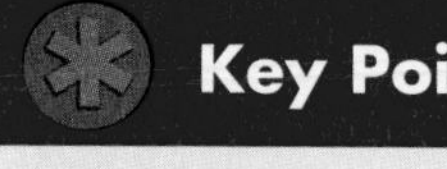

Key Point

Expert witness professional with education, training, skill, or experience in specific field beyond that of normal people.

The jury's lack of perspective is answered in part through the use of **expert witnesses**. Increasingly, however, expert witnesses are seen as "hired guns" who lack impartiality because they are paid by one side rather than by the court.

Expert witnesses not only testify as reference models but also set the standard of care. Health professionals have a duty to use reasonable professional care and to perform within the standards of practice. Standards of practice have traditionally differed between specialists and between communities. For example, the psychologist who specializes in eating disorders might be held more culpable for not recommending hospitalization of an anorectic than would a psychologist who specializes in sexual dysfunction.

Until recently, a laboratory technician who ran a small department in a country hospital was not expected to perform to the same standards as the person at a university teaching hospital. These ideas are now changing. The new thesis is that wherever you may practice, you were trained as others were trained and are expected to perform to the same standards. The small country hospital is expected to hire the same staff and perform to the same standard as the hospital in the city.

Statute of Limitation

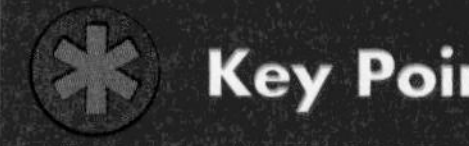
Key Point

Statute of limitation time beyond which a malpractice action cannot be brought.

Each state has a **statute of limitation** beyond which a malpractice action cannot be brought. Limitations change from time to time as state legislatures adjust their laws. In Connecticut, for example, the statute of limitations is two years from the time of malpractice. But, if a patient did not discover the malpractice within that time because he or she was not told or it went unnoticed, the patient has three years from the time of discovery. A common occurrence is a swab left inside that leads to an infection several years later. If the patient is told what happened at the time it occurs, he has two years to sue. If, however, the patient discovers the swab four years later when symptoms appear, he has three years from that time of discovery to sue.

What if a person who has had a withered arm since birth learns as an adult that it was caused by obstetric malpractice 20 years previously? Can the obstetrician be sued 20 years later? In Connecticut, a child's guardian is responsible for suing within two years of occurrence or three years of discovery. In some other states the child can sue later as an adult. In most cases the obstetrician's insurance company would be responsible for paying. But if the obstetrician has no malpractice insurance, he or she can be sued. If the obstetrician is dead, the estate can be sued. Although a situation like this example is feasible, it is a highly unlikely example.

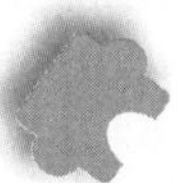

Costs of Malpractice

Deep Pocket versus Responsibility

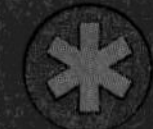
Key Point

Deep pocket slang for person with a lot of money.

It is common practice to name multiple respondents in a medical malpractice suit. One reason is that it is not always easy for attorneys to know in advance exactly who might be involved. Another reason is that awards may be higher where a **deep pocket** is found. A deep pocket refers to a person or institution with lots of money or high malpractice insurance. Commonly, several doctors and a hospital are named when it may be obvious from the start that only one doctor is to blame. Also, the allied health professional commonly is not named because the physician is considered to be "captain of the ship" for hospitalized patients. At present, litigants have no desire to prove a physical therapist or lab technician personally responsible for malpractice because, if a hospital or physician is involved, the captain-of-the-ship principle can be used and the captain is presumed to have deeper pockets.

Historically, allied health professionals seldom carried malpractice insurance because they were employed by others, especially hospitals or physicians. But allied health professionals become more autonomous by performing their profession independently. This autonomy applies, for example, to dietitians, social workers, physical and occupational therapists, speech therapists, and audiologists. Obviously, it would be difficult for health professionals such as radiologic technologists to practice independently.

Although the increased autonomy of many allied health professionals increases their exposure to malpractice, the majority of malpractice suits involve hospital inpatients. In hospitals, allied health professionals have exposure to malpractice only if they are practicing as independent outside contractors. Among hospital-employed health professionals, responsibility, however it is shared, is seen by the courts as the hospital's responsibility. This situation is reflected in the high malpractice insurance that hospitals carry and in the fact that most hospital-employed health practitioners carry low or no malpractice insurance. All other things being equal, the deep pocket is always the pocket that is pursued.

Fair Compensation

It is not always easy to decide what constitutes fair compensation. In a country where millionaires are still revered, a $1 million award may seem like a bonanza, yet a $5- or $10-million award may be difficult to understand. In 2007 a New York jury awarded a brain-injured man $109 million, a staggering award for a medical malpractice case. In determining what is fair compensation, courts consider such issues as economic loss, lump sum versus periodic payments, contingency fees, pain and suffering awards, and punitive damages.

Let us illustrate with the case of a 25-year-old male janitor earning $25,000 a year who has lost a limb because of a surgical mistake. He is unable to continue working. The economic loss of 40 years of lost wages at $25,000 per year is $1,000,000. This amount may be awarded as a lump sum or as payments of $25,000 per year. The patient may, however, receive disability income from the state. If he has private disability insurance, this could be taken into account, although it is often considered inadmissible evidence. Currently, many states allow lump sum payments, which would give him $1,000,000. Invested at five percent, this award would double his income.

But the patient's attorney may take up to one-third of this amount as a fee for handling the case. Under a contingency fee arrangement, the patient owes the attorney nothing if the case is lost. If the case is won, however, the patient owes the attorney a percentage of the total award. Some states are trying to limit contingency fees.

On top of the $1,000,000 for the loss of his limb, the patient may also be given a pain and suffering award and a punitive damages award. If he has phantom limb pain (pain where the limb was before the amputation) he may receive an additional award for pain and suffering. There have been attempts in some states to limit pain and suffering awards to, say, less than $500,000.

If the court wants to teach the surgeon a lesson, a punitive damages award may be added. What started as a fair replacement for income lost may end up as a $3 million award, with $1 million going to the attorney. Obviously, no amount of money can replace a lost limb, but the issue of determining fair compensation is a difficult one.

Cost to Society

The other factor in the equation of fair compensation is not how much the defendant gets but how much society pays. An obstetrician who pays a malpractice premium of $100,000 per year passes a substantial fee increase on to patients. If it costs $3,000 instead of $1,000 for total obstetric care, who pays the extra? All of society does, either out of pocket or through our medical insurance premiums or taxes.

Courts also make decisions about patients who are in a **persistent vegetative state** (prolonged coma). When Karen Quinlan lay in a coma on a ventilator at $600 a day, society was paying that cost, which amounted to almost $250,000 a year at that time.

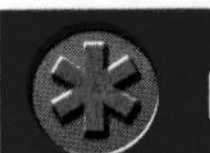

Key Point

Persistent vegetative state unresponsiveness of a patient to mental or verbal stimuli without signs of higher brain function; the patient is kept alive artificially.

The cost of malpractice to society also includes the cost of defensive medicine—the extra tests ordered and the extra days in the hospital. For example X-rays for back pain in a young healthy person, an MRI for migraine, or routine EKGs in young people going for surgery are usually unnecessary. The cesarean section rate in the United States is about 20–30 percent; 5–10 percent is considered optimal. Caregivers often feel that a cesarean reduces their risk of being sued or of losing a lawsuit. A conservative estimate of the cost of defensive medicine is 10 percent of the total cost of medical care. The total cost of medical care in the United States in 2009 is expected to reach $2.5 trillion. Thus at 10 percent defensive medicine could be costing us around $250 billion a year.

Malpractice insurance premiums rise and fall or stabilize for many reasons. Decreasing investment returns for insurance companies along with falling interest rates may have caused part of the rise in premiums. A number of state medical societies have started their own malpractice insurance companies (captive insurance companies), which puts malpractice defense more in the hands of physicians. As a result, there may be fewer tendencies to settle out of court rather than go to court. It is doubtful, however, that captive insurance companies will have that great an effect on costs to society.

Out-of-Court Settlements

As we have discussed, a medical malpractice case may involve multiple health professionals as well as an institution. Defense costs for an average medical malpractice case are about $100,000, and if the case goes to trial another $100,000 can be added to that. There is great pressure, therefore, to settle out of court. The average out-of-court settlement is estimated to be about one-third of what a malpractice award would have been. It is little wonder then that insurance companies are anxious to settle out of court. The problem is that cases of dubious merit frequently are settled rather than taken to court. A bird in the hand is worth two in the bush.

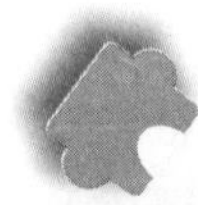

Preventing Suits

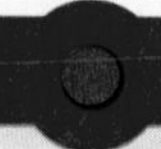

CASE STUDY 13-3

Sharon, a medical assistant, draws blood from Julia, a middle-aged lady with anorexia nervosa. During the procedure Julia suddenly shouts "Stop! You're hitting a nerve." Sharon, the medical assistant, tells Julia to be calm and continues to probe with her needle. Julia suddenly withdraws her arm and says, "I told you to stop, and you didn't." Sharon says she was only doing her job and that anyway Julia was always a difficult draw.

Following the procedure Julia seeks help from a neurologist because she has a numb area on her forearm that won't go away. The neurologist agrees that as it dated from the venipuncture it was likely that a nerve to the skin had been lacerated. Julia is angry, and she decides to sue Sharon rather than the physician she worked for and seeks legal advice.

The attorney says that the loss of skin sensation is a relatively minor injury and that she might get a settlement from the physician but a court case would not be worth the money. Julia tells the attorney she will pay the attorney his hourly rate because she just wants to teach Sharon a lesson. Why?

Good Communication

The old idea that the cause of suits is malpractice must be cast aside. Maloccurrence is needed for a successful suit, but as long as health care exists there will always be maloccurrences. Death, for example, is a maloccurrence and must come to everyone. *The most common reason that maloccurrence is taken to court is the lack of a relationship or the breakdown of the relationship between patient and health professional.* Patients seldom sue their counselors because, of all people, the counselor probably has listened most carefully to the patient's problems and has communicated with the patient.

Treating friends and relatives is a tricky area. If health practitioners decide to treat their friends and relatives as patients, they must do so with the same professionalism as they treat their regular patients. It is simply not true that friends and relatives do not sue. Actually, it is often inadvisable to treat close family members because they frequently end up being overtreated or undertreated, which in itself is poor health care. If health care providers treat their friends and relatives, it is important to keep records and to treat these patients in a professional setting.

An Informed Patient

Communication is the cornerstone of preventing malpractice suits. A maloccurrence not discussed with the patient may result in a successful suit. A maloccurrence that is discussed is not likely to result in a successful suit. Many physician malpractice insurance companies are now saying that a sincere apology for a mistake is a good, not a bad, thing and will make it less likely that the family will sue in the future.

Although the model of informed consent generally is for an invasive surgical procedure, informed consent also should be obtained for procedures such as podiatric surgery, bone marrow examinations by laboratory tech-

You have been given information about your condition and the recommended surgical, medical or diagnostic procedure(s) to be used. This consent form is designed to provide a written confirmation of such discussions by recording some of the more significant medical information given to you. It is intended to make you better informed so that you may give or withhold your consent to the proposed procedure(s).

1. **Condition:** Dr. ____________________ has explained to me that the following condition(s) exist in my case: ____________________
____
____

2. **Proposed Procedure(s):** I understand that the procedure(s) proposed for evaluating and treating my condition is/are: ____________
____
____

3. Right eye ____________ Left eye ____________

4. **Risks/Benefits of Proposed Procedure(s):**

   A. Just as there may be benefits to the procedure(s) proposed, I also understand that medical and surgical procedures involve risks. These risks include allergic reaction, bleeding, blood clots, infections, adverse side effects of drugs, blindness, and even loss of bodily function or life, as well as risks of transfusion reactions and the transmission of infectious disease, including Hepatitis and Acquired Immune Deficiency Syndrome, from the administration of blood and/or blood components.

   B. I also realize that there are particular risks associated with the procedure(s) proposed for me and that these risks include, but are not limited to, those enumerated in the addendum.

5. **Complications; Unforeseen Conditions; Results:** I am aware that in the practice of medicine, other unexpected risks or complications not discussed may occur. I also understand that during the course of the proposed procedure(s) unforeseen conditions may be revealed requiring the performance of additional procedures, and I authorize such procedures to be performed. I further acknowledge that no guarantees or promises have been made to me concerning the results of any procedure or treatment.

6. **Acknowledgments:** The available alternatives, some of which include ______________, the potential benefits and risks of the proposed procedure(s), and the likely result without such treatment, ______________, have been explained to me. I understand what has been discussed with me as well as the contents of this consent form, and have been given the opportunity to ask questions and have received satisfactory answers.

7. **Consent to Procedure(s) and Treatment:** Having read this form and talked with the physicians, my signature below acknowledges that: I voluntarily give my authorization and consent to the performance of the procedure(s) described above (including the administration of blood and disposal of tissue) by my physician and/or his/her associates assisted by hospital personnel and other trained persons as well as the presence of observers.

____ ____________________

Patient (or person authorized to sign for patient) Date

____ ____________________

Witness Date

Example of informed consent

nicians, and neck manipulation by chiropractors. Please also review the section in Chapter 11 on informed consent.

Documentation

A common stance taken by the courts is that if it was not written down, it did not happen. Unfortunately, this stance has led to a deplorable proliferation of hospital charts that make it difficult to find the forest for the trees. The advent of EHR has exacerbated the problem. But if, for example, a physical therapist writes that the left arm was treated and the patient later sues for right arm pain, the physical therapist's case is probably sound.

Good records are the cornerstone of defense in a malpractice suit. Records should be legible, signed, and dated, and they should document the reasoning that led to significant decisions and to the treatment provided. The ideal way to keep good records is to follow the **SOAP** (subjective, objective, assessment, plan) format, which is as follows:

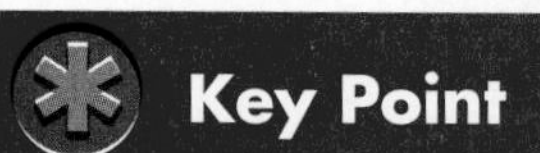

Key Point

SOAP method of record-keeping; acronym stands for *s*ubjective, *o*bjective, *a*ssessment, *p*lan.

S Subjective is what the patient says: "I take insulin for diabetes."

O Objective is what is observed: The patient has two packs of Oreo cookies and a Burger King wrapper on her bedside stand.

A Assessment is an evaluation of the situation: Diabetic noncompliant with diet.

P Plan is what the health professional will or did do: Discussed 1,400 calorie ADA diet and gave patient informational brochures.

Rapport

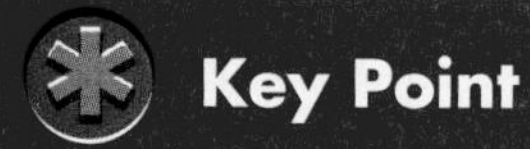

Key Point

Rapport sympathetic connection to patient established by genuine interest and correct body language.

Rapport with the patient may sound like a vague thing, but it is a crucial aspect of treatment, as the reader will recall by reviewing Chapter 2.

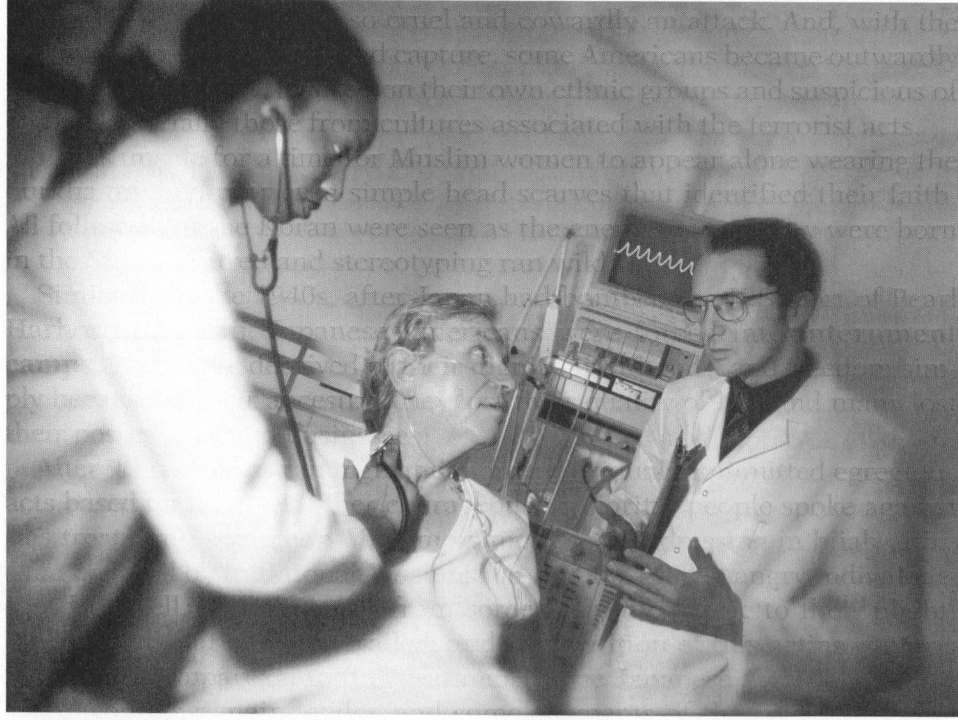

Explaining a procedure to a patient

Listening and smiling and using body language that communicates that the health professional is available may seem like a flimsy way to prevent malpractice, but it is really at the root of the matter. *Maloccurrence usually results in a lawsuit because the patient feels wronged by the health professional.* The best defense is to maintain a highly professional stance, be available, be a good listener, smile, communicate well, keep the patient informed, show the patient respect, and help the patient to like you. If something does go wrong, the patient with whom there is established rapport is the least likely to prosecute. One patient said about a court appearance, "They never listened to me in the hospital. Now they will have to."

Maintaining confidentiality is absolutely essential to building rapport. A patient is unlikely to sue over a breach of confidentiality alone, but if a maloccurrence should then arise, the patient will be much more likely to sue. For example, a physician who tells an acquaintance of a patient that the patient had cancer is unlikely to be sued. But, if the physician fails to diagnose that cancer until it is too late, the patient is much more likely to sue.

Good Standards of Practice

The essence of malpractice prevention lies in an honest, open, and communicative relationship with the patient. With such a relationship, much litigation could be prevented.

Documentation forces a review of the health professional's own actions. If doubt arises, the health professional must discuss it with the patient and must offer an opinion about calling in a consultant. The health professional or the patient may call in the consultant, and the consultation also should be discussed. If, for example, a patient tells the dietitian that her urine sugars have been running high but her doctor said not to change the insulin, then the dietitian must contact the doctor and document that contact.

Follow-up of the patient adds another dimension to the patient's care. Things may be seen in a different perspective during follow-up. Patients also feel more cared for if there is a follow-up telephone call or appointment. The patient also then has a chance to bring up any residual or hitherto unmentioned gripes, as well as to let the health professional know how treatment is progressing.

Abandonment is more a problem for diagnostic and assessment health professionals like physicians, dentists, psychologists, and visiting nurses. These health professionals are expected to be reasonably available, and if they terminate care of a patient without making reasonable alternative arrangements for care, the patient can charge them with abandonment.

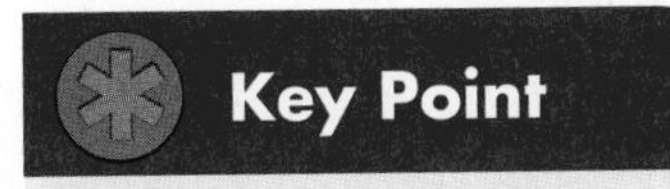

Abandonment unavailability or improper discontinuation of medical care.

If health care providers are contacted by an attorney about anything other than a worker's compensation or auto accident claim, it is probably safest to contact their own malpractice insurance company or attorney. Sometimes letters are sent simply as a way of fishing for incriminating information. Other than for a worker's compensation or auto accident claim, do not respond to telephone calls from attorneys without first consulting an attorney.

Summary

The right of practice is a privilege the would-be health professional must earn. Where licensure is involved, the scope of practice is legally protected. Only those who have prepared by virtue of educational training, who have not committed a felony, who have good character references, and who have proper clinical training may be licensed. Certification and registration also offer access to professional status and privileges.

Accreditation is a process of approving educational training programs for health professionals. The power inherent in this approval process has made accreditation a historically political tool.

Legal controls like licensure work best in tandem with the ethical controls of the various health professional associations. Weaknesses in each may be compensated for by the other. Still, there remains work to be done as each state struggles to deal appropriately with issues of interstate licensure.

Malpractice requires not only an unexpected event but also proof that there was deviation from the standard of care and that mental or physical harm resulted. The four Ds describe the criteria that must be satisfied to prove negligence in civil court (i.e., *d*ereliction of *d*uty *d*irectly causes the *d*amage). Abuses in the courtroom show how care must be taken in a relationship with a patient. It is this relationship that not only prevents malpractice but also makes us more professional. The most common cause of suits is a lack of relationship or breakdown of the relationship between patient and health professional. Communication and documentation are the cornerstones of preventing malpractice suits.

Chapter Review

Key Term Review

Abandonment: Unavailability or improper discontinuation of medical care.

Accreditation: Formal approval of an institution or educational program given by an outside agency.

Certification: A testament that an individual has attained qualifications for a specified part of his or her occupation.

Civil court: Court that handles actions by private litigants.

Criminal court: Court in which government prosecutor prosecutes defendant for crime.

Deep pocket: Person or institution with lots of money or high malpractice insurance.

Defendant: Person being sued.

Expert witness: Professional with education, training, skill, or experience in specific field beyond that of normal people.

Flexner Report: Abraham Flexner's report on the quality of medical education (1910), which led to accreditation.

Four Ds of malpractice: *D*ereliction of *d*uty *d*irectly causes *d*amage.

Jury system: A system in which a jury of peers rather than a judge decides the outcome of a case.

Licensure: Mechanism designed to assure patients that the care they receive from a professional meets a reasonable standard

Litigant: Person bringing a lawsuit.

Maloccurrence: Untoward event (not necessarily actionable).

Malpractice: Maloccurrence that is actionable.

Negligence: Unintentional tort that reasonable person would not have committed or omitted.

Persistent vegetative state: Unresponsiveness of a patient to mental or verbal stimuli without signs of higher brain function; the patient is kept alive artificially.

Plaintiff: Person who brings a lawsuit.

Rapport: Sympathetic connection to patient established by genuine interest and correct body language.

Registration: A term often used interchangeably with both licensure and certification.

SOAP: Method of record-keeping; acronym stands for *s*ubjective, *o*bjective, *a*ssessment, *p*lan.

Standard of care: Degree of care and competence expected of a particular professional.

Statute of limitation: A statute that says that legal action cannot be brought after a certain period (e.g., five years).

Tort: Civil wrong (excluding breach of contract) against person or property that causes injury.

Chapter Review Questions

1. Identify factors leading to the right to practice.
2. Describe what actions you might take and/or your duty to take action when you suspect that a colleague has a drinking problem.
3. It has been suggested that mandating continuing education programs might serve as a means of improving protections of relicensure. Describe the pros and cons of this suggestion.
4. What are the four Ds of malpractice?
5. Give examples of errors of omission and commission as malpractice.
6. What is the difference between malpractice and maloccurrence?
7. Why may allied health professionals assume greater liability for malpractice in the future?
8. List the benefits to society of the current malpractice climate.
9. List the costs to society of the current malpractice climate.
10. What is the most common reason that a maloccurrence is taken to court?

Case Study Critical Thinking Questions

1. Refer to Case Study 13.1. Should Ricardo have his license removed?
2. Refer to Case Study 13.1. Should Ricardo be forced to attend continuing education classes?
3. Is there any evidence that making people attend classes makes them a better practitioner?
4. It was found out by chance that Ricardo (Case Study 13.1) had a cousin who was practicing in Canada and that he had made copies of his degrees and licenses and was an impostor. Has Ricardo done any harm?
5. Refer to Case Study 13.2. What systems can you think of to prevent Jake from moving from state to state to continue using his position to manipulate women?
6. Refer to Case Study 13.2. If the women are willing to have sex with Jake, what is wrong with that?
7. Refer to Case Study 13.3. Why was Julia so angry?
8. Refer to Case Study 13.3. Why wouldn't Julia sue the physician and get a lot more money? Why did she not discuss it with the physician first?
9. Refer to Case Study 13.3. Why did Julia not try to persuade the physician to fire Sharon?

References

1. Department of Health and Human Services. www.hhs.gov
2. Summary of HIPAA privacy rules. www.hhs.gov/ocr/privacysummary.pdf
3. Allied Health Careers and their salaries. www.ama-assn.org/ama/pub/category/2322.html
4. Website for OSHA. www.osha.gov
5. Medical ethics. www.ama-assn.org/ama/pub/category/2512.html
6. Malpractice. www.texashste.com/documents/curriculum/professional_liability_and_medical_malpractice.pdf
7. Malpractice risk for physicians employing allied health professionals. www.ncbi.nlm.nih.gov/pubmed/1181497
8. Article about high Cesarean section rates. www.childbirthconnection.org/article.asp?ck = 10456

Additional Readings

1. *1998 Hospital Accreditation Standards.* Joint Commission on Accreditation of Healthcare Organizations, 1998. Pozgar, George D. *Legal Aspects of Health Care Administration,* 2nd ed. Aspen Law & Business; 1999.
2. Lecca, P. J., Valentine, P., Lyons, K. *Allied Health: Practice Issues and Trends in the New Millenium.* Binghamton, NY: Haworth Press Inc., 2003.
3. Lewis, M. *Medical Law, Ethics, & Bioethics for the Health Professions.* Philadelphia: F. A. Davis Company, 2007.
4. Sloan, F. A., Chepke, L. M. *Medical Malpractice.* Cambridge, MA: MIT Press; 2008.
5. Wischnitzer, S., Wischnitzer, E. *Top 100 Health Care Careers: Your Complete Guidebook to Training and Jobs in Allied Health, Nursing, Medicine, and More.* St. Paul, MN: Jist Publishing, 2005.
6. Bonner, T. N. *Iconoclast: Abraham Flexner and a Life in Learning*. Baltimore: Johns Hopkins University Press, 2002.

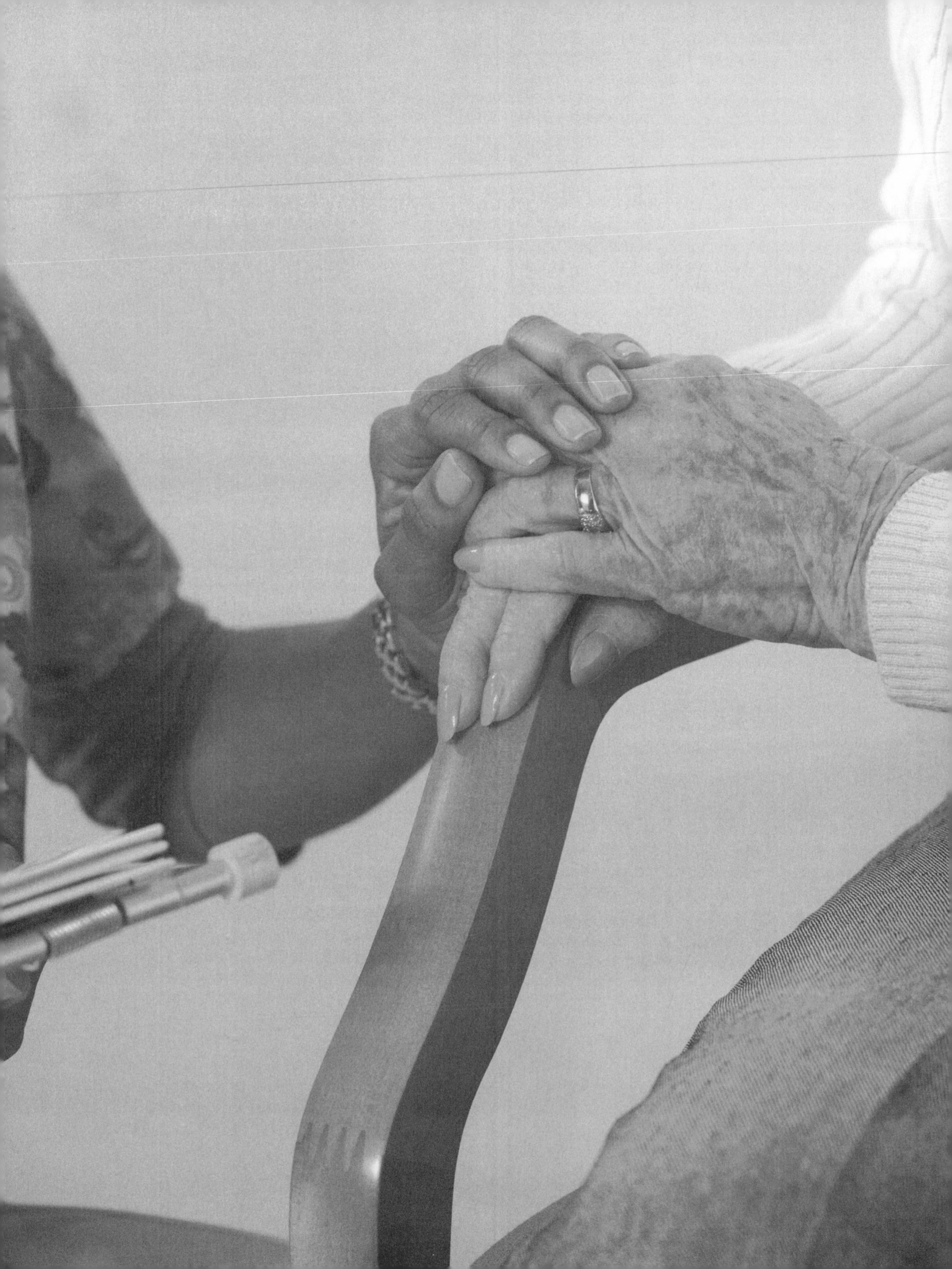

Multicultural Health Issues

Learning Outcomes

After reading this chapter, you should be able to:

14.1 Recognize the influence of historical events on racial, ethnic, and cultural issues in the United States and describe "culture."

14.2 Discuss cultural and familial influences on health and the importance of provider competence.

14.3 Discuss the term *ethnocentric* and analyze the effects of 9/11 on Americans' ethnocentricity.

14.4 List three forms of alternative medicines and describe controversial alternative beliefs.

14.5 Describe the impact of cultural identification on mental health.

14.6 Recognize the impact of demographics on U.S. health care.

14.7 Describe individual and institutional responsibilities in equal treatment, and incorporate knowledge of case studies on interracial body language.

14.8 Analyze strategies for health care improvements on the basis of ethnic disparities.

Key Terms

Alternative medicine
American Indian or Alaskan Native
Asian or Pacific Islander
Attribution theory
Black
Complementary medicine
Culture
Culture-bound
Culture-bound syndrome
Cultural competence
Cycle of poverty
Diversity
Ethnic incidence of disease
Ethnocentric
Family system approach
Formulation
Hispanic
Immediacy behaviors
Impression formation
Indian Removal Act
Indigenous
Individual discrimination/racism
Institutional discrimination/racism
Integrative medicine
Internment camps
Multicultural
Planned Approach to Community Health (PATCH)
People of color
Stereotyping
Trail of Tears
Tuskegee Airmen
U.S. demographics by 2050
Values
White

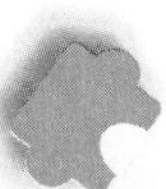

Historical Overview

"We are the World" is certainly a true descriptor of the ethnic and cultural composition of the continental United States. One-third of the population is expected to be people of color by 2020 and more than half by 2050; it is little wonder the U.S. population is known as a "melting pot." Few American people are "pure-blooded." Those who think they are 100 percent English, Italian, Puerto Rican, Ethiopian, Turkish, or Cantonese may not know enough about their ancestors to be certain of this. Conquering peoples traditionally mixed their genes with those of the lands they were in. It is safe to say that most Americans share bloodlines with more than one cultural or ethnic group.

The United States was involved with slavery from its inception as a nation, with some founding fathers among the slave owners. This is the most profound ethnic and cultural abuse in U.S. history. Following the Civil War, the struggle of African Americans has persisted at one level or another, a struggle that is examined throughout this chapter. One other early cultural shame to befall this country occurred 50 years after its birth. It was the ultimate American attack on an **indigenous** culture and began in 1828 when then President Andrew Jackson signed into law the **Indian Removal Act**. According to this bill the North Georgian Cherokee Nation, which had built its own roads, schools, and churches and had adopted a representative form of government, with its people living well as farmers, ranchers, and even plantation owners, was to be forced off its lands. The natural resources and the hard work of the Cherokees had made the land too highly sought after by white settlers. This controversial legislation was contested for 10 years, with protests from men such as Davey Crockett, Daniel Webster, and Henry Clay, but ratification of removal was finally passed by a single vote. Thus in 1838 the **Trail of Tears** began with the forced march of all Cherokees from their North Georgia homes to land in Oklahoma that had been deemed worthless. This march caused indescribable hardships and the death of at least 4,000 (out of 17,000) natives along the route.

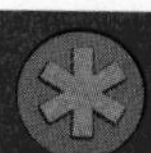

Key Points

Indigenous native.

Indian Removal Act Congressional act forcing North Georgian Cherokee Nation to relocate to Oklahoma.

Trail of Tears forced march of Cherokee Nation from Georgia to Oklahoma during which 4,000 out of 17,000 Natives died.

Dispossession of indigenous lands and slavery continued despite the country having been formed only 50 years earlier on the concept that "all men are created equal." In more recent times the United States instituted certain laws making it more difficult for people of color to obtain voting rights.

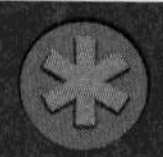

Key Point

Tuskegee Airmen first African American pilots in the U.S. Army Air Force.

CASE STUDY 14-1

During World War II African American soldiers did not serve in the same units as white soldiers. Additionally, there were no African American pilots until President Franklin D. Roosevelt ordered the opening up of this specialty area to all troops. Pilot-training officers gave more difficult tests to African American candidates than to whites. Eventually, however, a few good African American men were accepted to train and were qualified to fly and went on to distinguish themselves as heroes, coincidently protecting the lives of white bomber pilots. They were known as the **Tuskegee Airmen**, and they broke the color barrier for other pilots.

Even following the war, racism was still part of U.S. institutions. Whites-only restaurants, water fountains, and schools continued to divide this nation by color into the 1960s. Stories from 50 years ago still carry heavy messages of pain and despair in families where an African American grandfather was afraid to look at a white woman he might pass on the streets for fear of being lynched by an overreacting white mob. Stories of the Ku Klux Klan (KKK) still surface, demonstrating that hatred and bigotry are alive in pockets of this country despite improved laws and education. Even a country that has elected an African American man as president will find acts of terror inflicted on other African Americans, solely on the basis of skin color, because of ignorance and misplaced anger. African American people who have been raised around white Americans can generally all too easily recount stories of discrimination in societal situations such as in the job market, at swimming pools, and in everyday encounters. Health care professionals need to rise above such discriminatory actions and live by a code that guarantees respect for **diversity** and for different values. Diversity is the inclusion of people from different geographical locations, differing ethnic backgrounds and cultures, different physical abilities and genders, and differing beliefs and practices. According to the Society of Counseling Psychologists, July 2009, health professionals must train within **multicultural** communities that contain people of diverse racial, ethnic, and socioeconomic backgrounds; national origins; religious, spiritual, and political beliefs; physical abilities; ages; genders; gender identities; sexual orientations; and physical appearance. Multicultural is defined as inclusive of many cultures and connotes an appreciation of this cultural diversity.

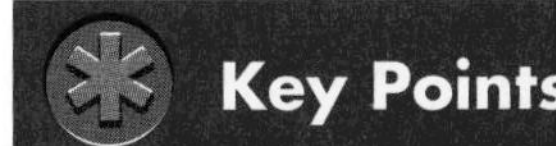

Diversity inclusion of people from differing backgrounds and cultures.

Multicultural valuing and inclusive of diverse cultures.

Racism is a serious psychologic and social problem. The daily occurrence of racism has profound ramifications on the health of millions in the United States. It has been said that it will not lessen until those in positions of power speak out to stop it, that silence is an inherent part of the problem.

Terms Evolve throughout History

Throughout history many different terms have been used to describe various pockets of the U.S. population. Several of these descriptors, and accompanying limited explanations, follow and may be helpful for health professionals in reading the literature and in navigating cultural competence.

According to J. Delgado, the delivery of quality health services to any population is "about being proficient in the art of listening and communicating with patients from a variety of backgrounds; understanding that health occurs in a holistic environment; incorporating an understanding of a person's unique family, work, spiritual and physical environment into health services" (National Alliance for Hispanic Health, 2001). Delgado goes on to say there must be assurances that institutional structures of health services act to encourage rather than discourage access to care.

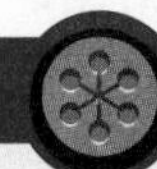

Fast Fact

- **American Indian or Alaskan Native**
  A person who has origins in any of the original peoples of North America and who maintains cultural identification through tribal affiliation or community recognition.
- **Asian or Pacific Islander**
  A person having origins in any of the original peoples of the Far East, Southeast Asia, the Indian subcontinent, or the Pacific Islands. This area includes, for example, China, India, Japan, Korea, the Philippine Islands, and Samoa.

(continued)

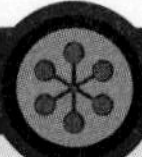

Fast Fact (continued)

- **Black**
  A person having origins in any of the black racial groups of Africa.
- **Hispanic**
  A person who is from Mexico, Puerto Rico, Cuba, Central or South America, or another Spanish culture. The current usage of the term *Hispanic* in the health literature is driven by Directive 15 of the Office of Management and Budget (OMB). This directive was issued in 1978 to increase the availability of data on persons of Hispanic origin and to encourage uniform collection and reporting of data on different racial and ethnic groups by federal agencies.
- **White**
  A person having origins in any of the original peoples of Europe, North Africa, or the Middle East.

These OMB categories assist with the collection of data but have also introduced problems inherent in all linear definitions.

- The term "Hispanic" is used simplistically, referring broadly to all populations with ancestral ties to Spain, Latin America, or the Spanish-speaking Caribbean. Such uncritical ethnic labeling can and may obscure the diversity of social histories and cultural identities that characterize these populations and, in turn, can influence health behaviors, the way care is accessed, and ultimately, health outcomes. Alternatively, subcategories based primarily on national origin, such as Mexican American, Puerto Rican, Central and South American, and Cuban, have been increasingly utilized to provide a more refined level of categorization. In this manner, one can distinguish, for example, between the access to care issues likely to be faced by Puerto Rican communities covered by U.S. entitlement programs and those encountered by Central and South Americans, some of whom may be fleeing a war-torn countryside and who, because of these circumstances, might be undocumented." (Eli, 1991)
- How does one describe those many Americans of mixed ancestry? While the government has said a person with even one drop of "black" blood is black, this definition does not fit well with current times. That is why, in this chapter, the descriptor **people of color** is used. It is meant to be inclusive, emphasizing common experiences of racism. *People of color* is preferred to both nonwhite and minority, which are also inclusive, because it frames the subject positively; *nonwhite* defines people in terms of what they are not (white), and *minority,* by its very definition, places the subject in a subordinate position. "Person of color" has a positive connotation and has often been preferred by people of color in the United States. (http://en.wikipedia.org/wiki/Person_of_color)
- Some native peoples may find the terms "Indian" or "Eskimo" derogatory as they are the first people of the land in recorded history. It is advisable to inquire how a group wishes to be identified before making assumptions.

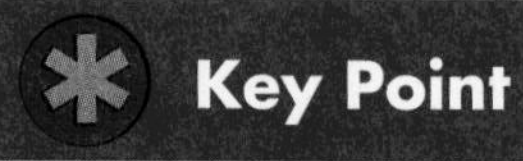

Key Point

People of color inclusive and positive term used in place of the terms *minority* and *nonwhite.*

What Is Culture?

Culture consists of beliefs, practices, values, religions, and languages. *A Primer for Cultural Proficiency: Towards Quality Health Services for Hispanics* (National Alliance for Hispanic Health, 2001) quotes Ian Robertson's description of culture as including sports, body adornment, cooking, cooperative labor, courtship practices, dances, feasts, folklore, food taboos, funerals, gift-giving, sexual taboos, laws, music, myths, toilet-training, tool making, religion, and medical beliefs and practices. An individual might, for example, speak Spanish but not understand the special meaning in the Mexican culture of Cinco de Mayo. Language proficiency certainly helps cross-cultural communication, but knowledge of the culture itself is also essential.

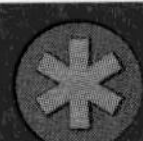

Key Point

Culture composite of beliefs, practices, religions, and languages that make up a group of people.

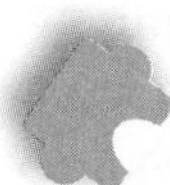

Cultural Considerations

Chapter 1 reviewed issues concerning sensitivity in communications, especially in nonverbal behaviors such as proxemics, haptics, oculesics, and adornment. This chapter takes a broader view of multicultural issues. Health professionals need to become educated to the needs and beliefs of populations differing from their own. They need to take individuals' cultural differences into consideration when assessing and treating them. Without knowledge of clients' cultures, it is far more difficult to treat them and even more difficult to expect that an impact has been made through the health care (perhaps cross-cultural) interaction. Will clients comply with health advice? Do they value and follow the necessary health care directions, or is there a combined cultural exchange that will permit them to feel their beliefs are also sound? Does the provider even know if clients are at a stage or point in their thinking at which they are open to change (see the section Motivational Interviewing in Chapter 9)?

A study published by *The American Journal of Psychiatry* found that individuals of Hispanic ancestry were more likely to discontinue use of antidepressants during the first 30 days of treatment (54 percent) than were individuals of non-Hispanic ancestry (41 percent)(Olfson, Marcus, Tedeschi & Wan, 2006). Since complying with prescribed medications is often essential to improvement and wellness, these statistics signal a more challenging road to alleviating suffering among those who are highly predisposed to give up on medications.

The ideal health professional might look like the client and share the same language and cultural beliefs and practices. Unfortunately, this is not always possible. The class might wish to take a survey of class members to find out how many have seen health professionals who come from a background that differs from their own. It may also be important to consider gender in understanding a "shared background." For example, do many women feel better understood by a female provider? Or would this only be the case for certain types of health needs?

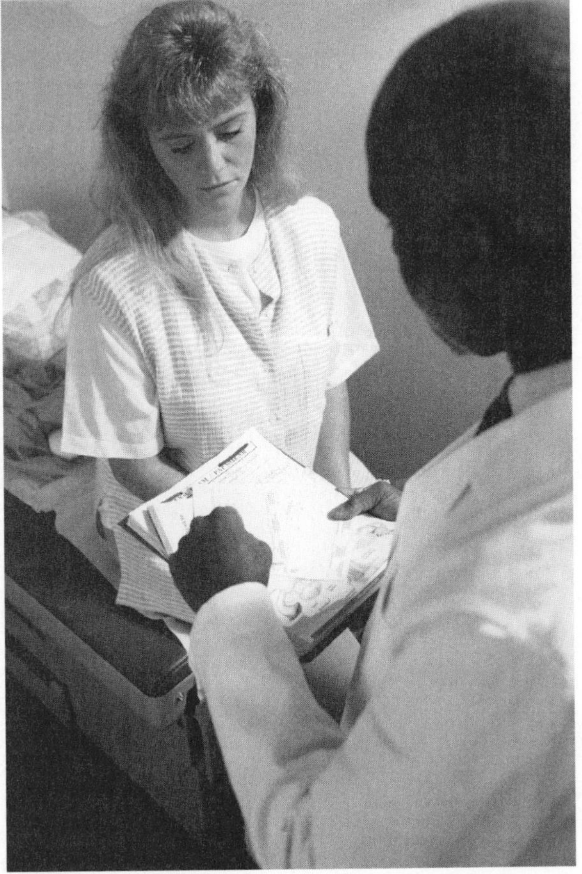

What issues may arise when the health professional and the patient are from different ethnic backgrounds? Different genders?

Might this preference be influenced by ethnicity and religion? Are there men and women who would NOT want to be treated by a woman doctor but expect that the nurse will always be female?

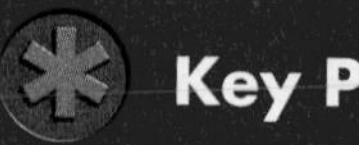

Key Points

Culturally competent ability to work within the cultural norms of another group.

Culture-bound pertaining to a belief that the values of our own culture is superior to others.

Culturally competent education for health professionals is based on learning an appreciation for the **values** of other cultures. All human beings are, to some extent, **culture-bound**, meaning that they believe the values of their own collective group are superior to those of other groups (see the section Ethnocentrism). When faced with the values of those from other cultures, you should suspend judgment and make an effort to understand those values. For example, in the United States it is generally accepted that "lean is healthy" whereas those in other cultures, especially those that have experienced great poverty and famine, may believe that "plump is healthy and wealthy." In the United States there is a tendency to embrace "change" as equaling growth and believe change is positive. Many people from other cultures have a far stronger belief in "tradition." Other mainstream values focus on belief in "personal control," which can be contrasted with strong belief in "fate." Although Americans may tend to feel superior when examining values of others, how does this "superiority" measure up against the American culture of "materialism" versus that of "spiritualism" so often expressed by those from a different value system?

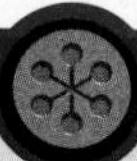

Fast Fact

Beliefs and Values Commonly Held in U.S.	Values Common in Other Cultures
1. Lean is healthy	1. Weight gain shows prosperity
2. Change is positive	2. Traditions are most important
3. Self-determination	3. "Fate" or God's or Allah's will
4. Materialism	4. Spiritualism

Some classes will wish to try the following workshop before moving on. It is included here so that instructors and students alike may see the goals and the exercise and decide together whether to implement it in class.

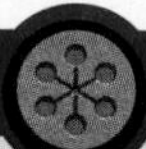

Racism Awareness Workshop

Goals of workshop: (1) to stimulate students to be aware of the many manifestations of racism that are built into U.S. institutions or core thoughts; (2) to experience an activity from the perspective of another culture, income, or ability level; (3) to be open about discrimination students have observed.

Instructors might begin this workshop with a basic discussion of the paragraph in this chapter that reads: *Racism is a serious psychological and social problem. The daily occurrence of racism has profound ramifications on the health of millions in the United States. It has been said that it will not lessen until those in the majority speak out to stop it, that silence is an inherent part of the problem.* Move further by reviewing the workshop goals with the class. If there are white class members, will they admit to any personal thoughts they have held that are racist? Do nonwhite groups have racial beliefs about others, about themselves?

(continued)

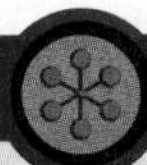

Racism Awareness Workshop *(continued)*

Students sit in a circle and are each given a roll and a half of pennies. Place a metallic bowl in the center of the circle. The instructor begins by naming a holiday or cultural tradition he or she celebrates and tosses in a penny. Each member of the class who celebrates that holiday also tosses in a penny. Next, move to the first person on the instructor's right or left. Ask that person to name a holiday or tradition which he or she celebrates and then continue around the circle with coins being tossed in by those who also celebrate the same traditions. Once all members of the class have had a turn (twice if a small group), check to see who has the most coins missing and who has the least. Process this in terms of cultural similarities and differences.

Now that the class has used this icebreaker, return to a more serious discussion of how we act in accordance with racial lines. Review the racial polarizing that occurred around reactions to the O. J. Simpson verdict; look at voter profiles for Barack Obama—to what extent did America follow racial lines, and to what extent were these lines blurred? Discuss Tiger Woods as well and what it means to be biracial in this society? Ask students if they ever tell racist jokes? Do they listen to racist jokes? Encourage the class to move away from these hurtful practices. End with the following 15-minute written exercise: "What I might do to decrease racism." For homework, if no realistic danger can be anticipated, ask students to invite a fellow classmate from a different cultural group to attend a service or cultural meeting with them. Each student should write a one-paragraph description of this experience, either a paragraph about being the outsider being invited in and possibly being "the only" one of their group present, or a paragraph about being the inviter who sees any possible reaction of his orher group. How do students feel in each situation? In communities where cultural and racial mix are very well-blended or conversely too homogeneous, assign students to spend 24 hours with a disability—use of a wheelchair, crutches, very dark glasses, or patch over one eye—and to attend all events with an aide; or to watch TV but not have volume on; or to demonstrate no ability to understand the language while shopping for one item in a department store. Continue to process this even into the next class session.

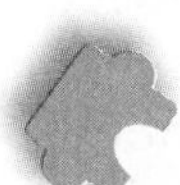

Cultural and Familial Influences

There are important universal truths to bear in mind, especially those related to patient care. All human beings feel pain, grief, and loss. All human beings have fears and an instinct toward self-preservation, love their young, and desire dignity and respect (recall Maslow's hierarchy). Sometimes people who have been abused and/or who may be mentally ill or addicted to drugs behave counter to these universal truths. They are not subhuman but in need of understanding and treatment. Sometimes these problems are associated with the **cycle of poverty**. Often they are also associated with an ethnic group who may live in these conditions of poverty. However, the problems of some should not be generalized to the total population. The cycle of poverty refers to those who are born into poverty having difficulty getting out of this socioeconomic condition. The impoverished may experience life models and role models that teach them more about "staying down" than getting out. Teenage pregnancy is one of the chief ways that the cycle is replicated. For example, a child born to a teenage mother who drops out of school to raise her child with the help of state assistance may repeat the same pattern.

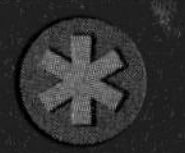

Key Point

Cycle of poverty the difficulty of breaking away from poverty when that is all one has ever known.

Some Pacific Islanders, Nomadic tribes people, and Baltic Pakistanis have a reputation for lateness or missing appointments, which health care professionals may attribute to the wrong commonality among them. But imagine coming from a culture in which you never wore a watch or saw a clock until you were an adult? The concept of an "appointment time" might have little value.

Lateness can symbolize hostility or resistance, but it may also mean "I had to wait for the babysitter to get off the school bus," or "I'm not familiar with the strict following of a schedule." When clients exhibit chronic lateness or appointment skipping, it is hard on everyone else. However, education, not anger, is the way to get the behavior to change. It will take more of your time, but teaching the client how to keep an appointment is part of teaching them how they will get well. It might also be necessary to find "open time" when such clients may come for treatment in a more open-clinic format.

Many Spanish-speaking families hold their children so dear that others might judge them to be "spoiling" that child, especially when the child is a young adult. Not holding the "child" accountable for certain actions, wanting to give him or her everything, and wishing to have all offspring at family functions at which alcohol and eating high-fat meals are the tradition is common to many Hispanic families. This makes treatment for conditions like obesity, diabetes, and substance abuse very difficult as the client must learn about the consequences of these actions so intrinsic to and accepted by the family.

What other cultural values can the class think of that are important to large segments of the population but may result in negative health care consequences within a paradigm of Western medicine?

Understanding Differences

Some of what accounts for the statistics provided in this chapter is socioeconomic status rather than strictly the influence of genetics or culture, unless "poverty" is defined as a culture. Both genetics and culture play a part, but to what degree remains as yet undetermined. Being overweight does affect African American men and women over *all* socioeconomic levels. Women of color with low incomes, particularly Mexican American women, appear to have the greatest likelihood of being obese; obesity is 13 percent more likely if they are living below the poverty line than above it.

It might be postulated that people without means would weigh less because food is expensive, but actually the opposite is true. Pasta, rice, beans, fatty meats, and sweets may fill stomachs when there isn't enough money for lean meats, fruits, and fresh vegetables; sugar and flour are cheaper than are salads and fish. Also, those living in an impoverished environment may be working more than one job or performing exhausting physical labor. This work might not offer the best form of exercise, but few people can get to a gym if they lack funds and are worn out just earning a living. Lack of sleep also adds to weight increase.

Incorporating the Family

Just as the Centers for Disease Control and Prevention (CDC) suggests working with community leaders when approaching solutions to community

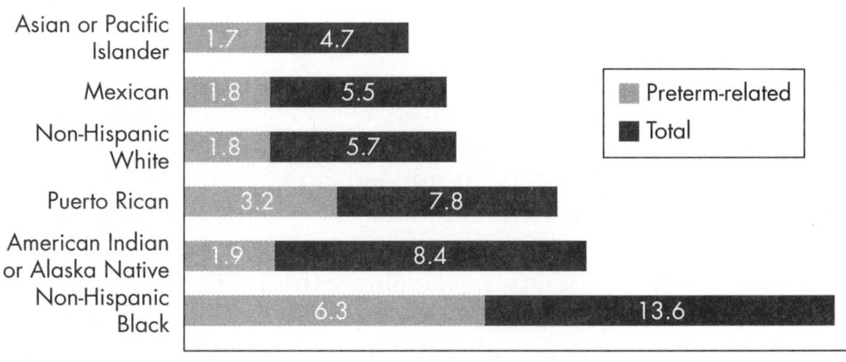

Infant Mortality Rates in 2004 by Race and Ethnicity

health issues, there needs to be a **family system approach** to cultural issues. Getting to know cultures means getting to know the families within those cultures; working with them to address health concerns, and letting them teach us about themselves and their needs. Breaking into the family system allows us to help a growing sphere of individuals and work with the family to support themselves instead of leaving individuals feeling isolated within the mainstream culture. In many communities, being accepted by a nuclear family means that you are then valued by the family's aunts, uncles, and cousins. Soon understanding spreads, and the needs and gaps may be bridged.

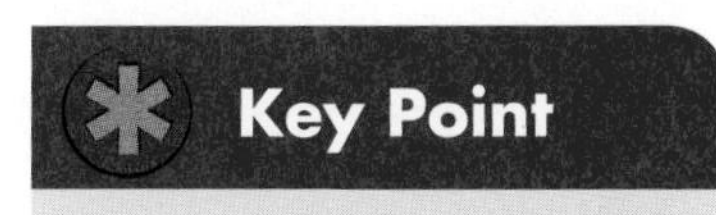

Family system approach Working within entire family systems to bridge cultural barriers and to have a broader impact on health care.

Churches or other places of worship where families congregate may be ideal places to appeal for help in attacking a health problem that is stronger in a particular community or cultural group. A congregation will feel safer dealing with outside help than will an individual, and a congregation knows the needs of its members. Churches in many communities run support groups for those with diabetes, for example. Church members may have the expertise to work with health issues. Or they may ask a trusted "outsider" to come in and speak or work with their families and friends, to listen, to value who they are, and to respond realistically and with compassion. This takes time, as trust and changing human behavior usually come around slowly.

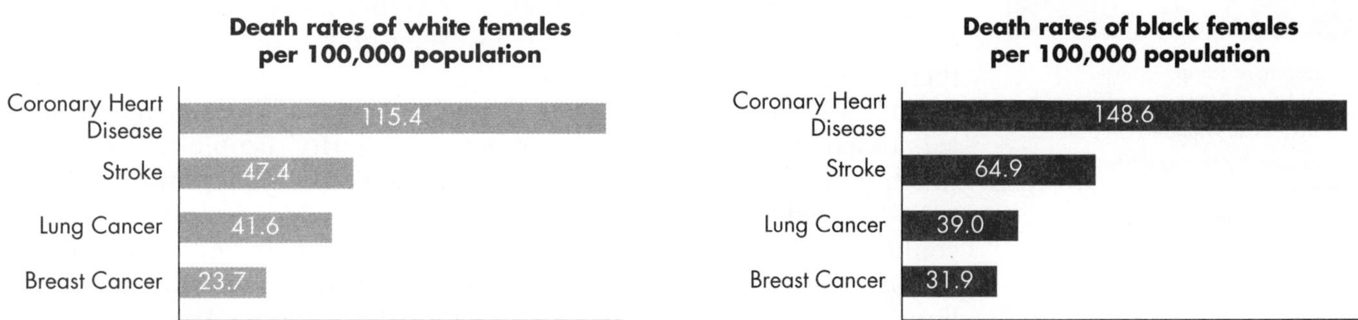

Death Rates for Coronary Heart Disease, Stroke, Lung, and Breast Cancer for White and Black Females

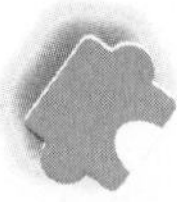

Ethnocentrism

As stated earlier, learning about other cultures best takes place when training or living occurs within those cultural communities. Yet it is possible to learn by reading, traveling, being open-minded, and communicating with those from diverse backgrounds. The National Alliance for Hispanic Health (2001) cautions, however, that in understanding culture there is also the tendency of every human society to develop **ethnocentrism**—judging other cultures by one's own. Beyond this, ethnocentrism means one sees his or her own standards as true and universal and the other culture may be just tolerated or seen in a negative light.

Key Point

Ethnocentric characterized by a strong belief in people who are ethnically the same as yourself to exclusion of others.

September 11, 2001

When planes crashed into the twin towers of the World Trade Center in New York City on September 11, 2001, the world changed in many significant ways. The loss of life and the horror of seeing innocent Americans and others die while engaged in peaceful routine activities scarred their families and people all over the world who watched the television footage again and again in repeated broadcasts. The grief and anger of America and her allies is still palpable today, and these innocent people will not be forgotten.

Some Americans felt vulnerable. People feared flying, and the airline industry suffered staggering economic losses. The Office of Homeland Security was born, and travel in America became more expensive, more time consuming, and hopefully safer.

But as America mourned the losses and celebrated the heroes, especially the New York City Fire Department, a natural reaction to loss emerged. Americans were angry for so cruel and cowardly an attack. And, with the enemy difficult to identify and capture, some Americans became outwardly ethnocentric, that is, focused on their own ethnic groups and suspicious of others, especially those from cultures associated with the terrorist acts.

It was unsafe for a time for Muslim women to appear alone wearing the burkha or chador or even simple head scarves that identified their faith. All followers of the Koran were seen as the enemy, even if they were born in the States. Hatred and stereotyping ran wild.

Similarly, in the 1940s, after Japan had bombed the U.S. port of Pearl Harbor in Hawaii, Japanese Americans were forced into **internment camps**. They were deprived of their dignity, livelihoods, and freedom simply because of their ancestry. They lost their quality of life, and many lost their possessions and businesses.

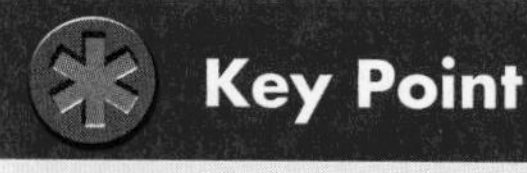

Internment camps camps consisting of poorly constructed barracks surrounded by barbed wire, sentry posts, and armed guards, to which over 100,000 Japanese Americans, mostly American citizens, were shipped during World War II.

After 9/11, feelings ran high and many individuals committed egregious acts based on fear. Yet, other courageous "majority" people spoke against this treatment; some non-Muslim women took to dressing in hijab attire (that dictated by traditional Muslims) so that misguided angry individuals could not tell a true Muslim from someone sympathetic to their plight. Enough rational minds prevailed, and the duration of this acting out was limited by comparison to the treatment of the Japanese Americans. Still, these wounds remain tender, and some segments of the country remain cautious of those who dress and pray differently than they do.

Alternative Medicine

A number of medical practices from other parts of the world have migrated to this country along with the populations from those areas. Certainly, western medicine itself is based on scientific practices from all over the globe. **Alternative medicine** is treatment methods that are popular, usually among a lay group, who believes these practices assist healing without necessarily having scientifically proven evidence for the group's beliefs (thus they are "alternatives" to mainstream medicine). The term *alternative medicine* evolved to become the term **complementary medicine**, which now combines complementary and alternative medicines (CAM). **Integrative medicine** combines conventional medicine with the safest forms of CAM and treats the mind, body, and spirit simultaneously. As these alternative methods have continued, they have become more accepted, not only by their communities of origin but also by the mainstream population, and they often find their way into conventional medical practices. Some western physicians, for example, now recommend yoga to their patients as a way of improving balance and relaxation.

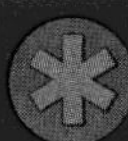

Key Points

Alternative medicine treatment not based on scientifically proven methods, often eschewing surgery or drugs, and used *instead of* conventional medicine.

Complementary medicine alternative medicine used together with conventional medicine—sometimes called CAM (Complementary and Alternative Medicine).

Integrative medicine the combination of conventional and alternative medicine for which there is some evidence of safety and efficacy.

One very popular form of CAM is acupuncture. Acupuncture is a technique of placing fine needles into parts of the human body that have been mapped, according to Chinese theory, as corresponding to special points. Theoretically these points lie along "meridians" that affect the vital energy flow of the body. It could be that needles placed in the feet actually affect a flow to relieve headaches, for example. Although no research has concluded the scientific bases for the effectiveness of acupuncture, well-respected and established medical entities such as the Mayo Clinic (2007, 2008) report reliable positive outcomes for the treatment of pain and nausea and reference the use of acupuncture in treating both cancer and asthma for such symptoms.

Another popular form of alternative medicine is Chinese herbology, which is part of traditional Chinese medicine (TCM). Chinese herbology is the art of combining medicinal herbs, which become a "cocktail" tailored to an individual patient. Thus, ginger might be the key ingredient used to help stomachaches, but the practitioner of herbology designs a remedy using many herbs along with the ginger. The medicine addresses the *yin* and the *yang* of the patient's condition. That is, some ingredients cancel out the toxicity or side-effects of the main ingredient, and others act as catalysts or enhance the potential of the main ingredient.

While western medicine focuses on the effect of a main ingredient, TCM treats the individual patient and concerns itself with the balance and interactions of all the ingredients in its medicinal cocktail.

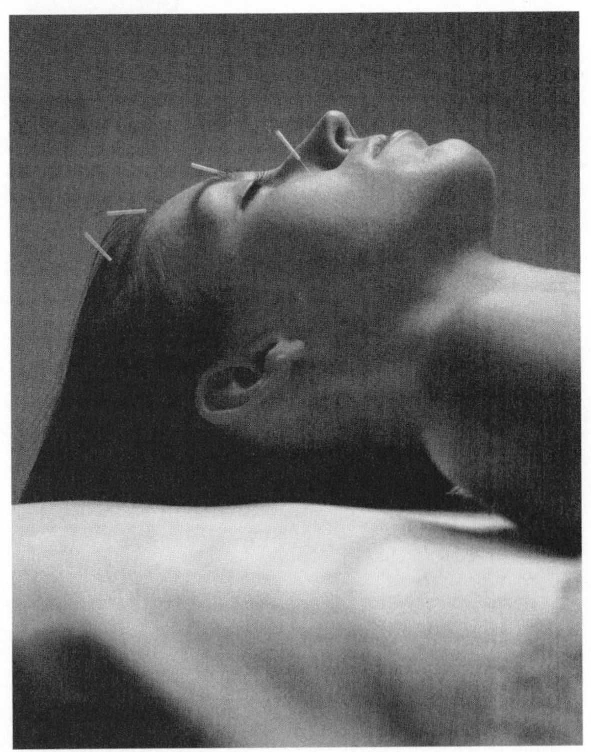

Woman receiving acupuncture

Ayurveda is a form of traditional Indian medicine. In Sanskrit the word *ayurveda* means *life* and *science,* It is an ancient practice that has resulted in identification of medicinal and surgical procedures. Ayurveda believes in five elements forming the universe—earth, water, fire, air, and space—and six elements forming the human body—

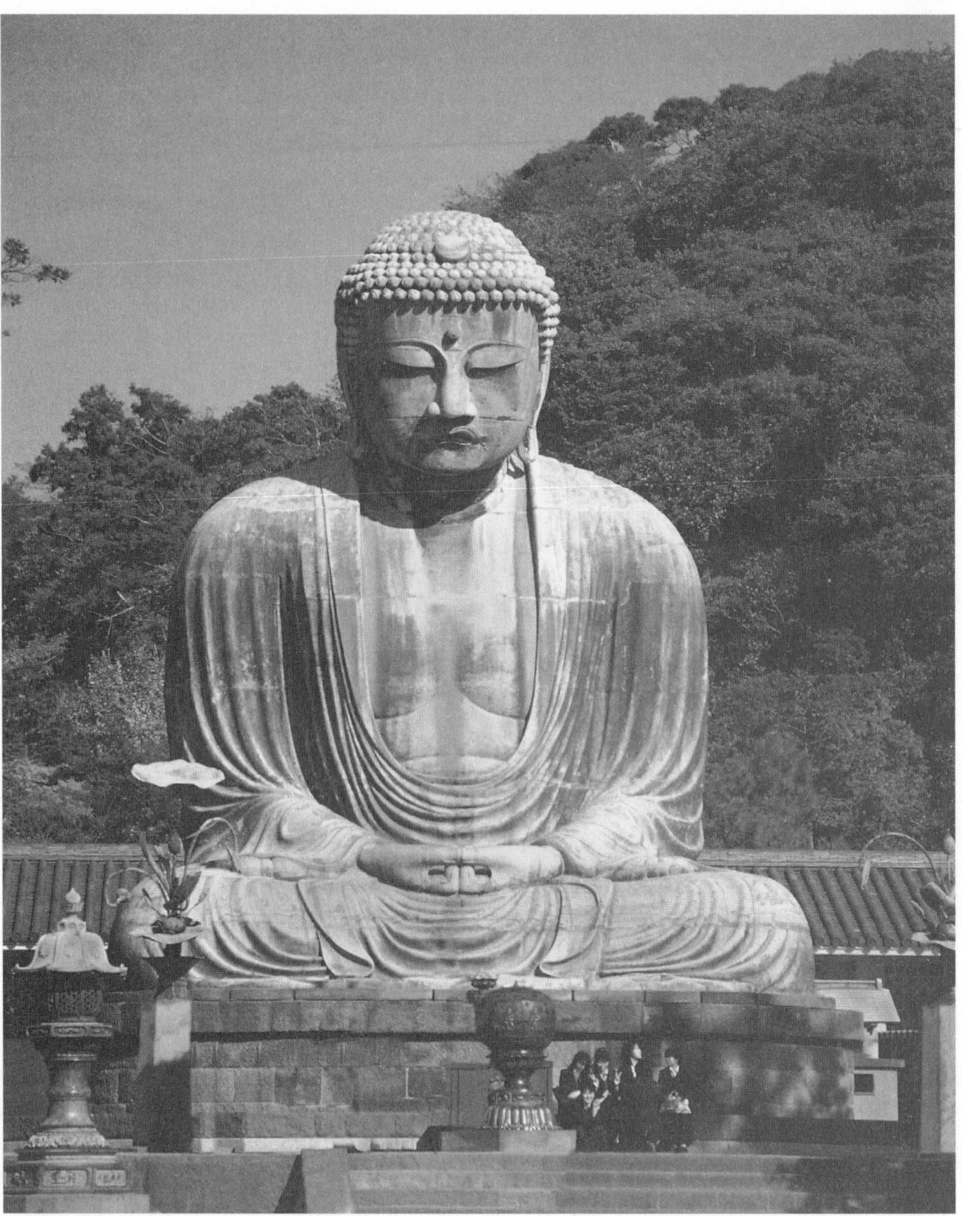

People in front of a statue of Buddha

blood, flesh, fat, bone, marrow, and semen. Exercise, digestion, yoga, and meditation are essential to the metabolic health of the body, which requires herbs, massage, and yoga for wellness.

Ayurvedic medicine is made from vegetables, including some spices that are common in curried foods, such as cardamom and cinnamon. This medicine has many goals, from stimulating digestion to decreasing heart pain or actually treating hypercholesterolemia. The influence of Buddhism is seen in the emphasis of Ayurveda on staying within limits of reasonable balance.

Hot and cold paradigms refer to the four body humors—yellow bile, black bile, phlegm, and blood—which believers postulate must be balanced or illness will result (Maurer and Smith, 2004). Practitioners use food that is hot, cold, wet, or dry to create this balance. An example of the use of hot and cold paradigms is the treatment of someone with a blood-related problem: As blood is considered hot and wet, the treatment should be cold and dry. These beliefs are held throughout various cultures, including many which are Hispanic. The caution here is to know that certain foods or medicines will be refused if they do not appear to restore the correct balance.

Fire cupping, or simply cupping, is a form of alternative medicine that is used by many Asian, Eastern European, and Middle East cultures. It is based on beliefs held by the ancient Greeks that temperature and health is related to a balance of the humors similar to Ayurvedic medicine. At one time the "hot cups" aided the bloodletting necessary to remove bad blood, which would then return the body to good health. In more contemporary uses and in TCM, cupping is simply a form of applying acupressure by creating a vacuum on the patient's skin in an area thought to need relief. It is typically used for the treatment of respiratory diseases and musculoskeletal pain. This is not a method that should be tried at home by amateurs because of the potential risk of burns. The basic principle is that a vacuum is created when fire in a glass cup is placed flush against a patient's skin and, as the oxygen is consumed, a partial vacuum is formed, pulling out the skin and simulating acupressure. Baby oil is often massaged into the skin before treatment as this affords a better seal.

Controversial Alternative Beliefs

In addition to these methods, there are "alternative medicines" that most members of western society not only oppose but world health organizations are attempting to combat as they cause undue risks and pain in the name of religious or philosophical beliefs. These practices encompass a wide range of processes, such as scarification, in which the skin is cut, branded, burned, or designed in accordance with a belief that certain life markers should be visible on the body. These scars may denote moving from childhood into adulthood or demonstrate emotional scars tied to grief. Scarification may also be performed on newborns in the belief that producing scars on newborns helps prevent vision problems and related illness. Whereas these beliefs may seem barbaric on initial examination, youth in western cultures now tattoo and pierce their bodies with less provocation.

Another practice that is so physically dangerous that many do not survive the infections it causes is female genital circumcision. This is a tradition in many Muslim cultures as a means of guaranteeing husbands that their brides are virgins. The clitoris is removed often through cutting with crude, dull instruments under nonhygienic circumstances, and then the labia are coarsely sewn shut. The clitorectomy is performed in the belief that this will prevent the young woman from desiring sexual activity whereas the labia are closed to prevent a male from penetrating the hymen. Traditionally this is performed on a very young girl prior to any likely sexual activity. If she survives the procedure, she will then have the stitches removed upon her wedding day. Not only is the performance of this procedure risky and painful, but the young woman experiences excruciating menstrual periods once her cycles begin because the flow is so confined by the stitches. There are funds established to help correct these procedures, but first a woman must immigrate to a country where such funds are available, and then she must overcome her guilt and shame to seek the help and challenge the beliefs under which she was raised.

Reconciling Differences

CASE STUDY 14-2

The Jehovah's Witness religion believes that the Bible prohibits them from receiving blood transfusions even in the case of an emergency. Hospitals often must have liaison committees that function to provide support to members of this faith. This places a burden on the medical professionals who cannot administer care as they deem necessary but must allow for their patients' religious beliefs to be honored even though death might ensue. Several alternative procedures have been accepted by Jehovah's Witnesses as a compromise, such as equipment being used for recirculation of the patient's own blood during surgery (accommodating differences). Among the current doctrine statements for this practice are the beliefs that blood is sacred to God, blood means life in God's eyes, blood is used for the atonement of sins, and faith must be expressed that Jesus Christ shed blood to redeem the faithful. As a number of diseases have been passed on through blood transfusions, including the human immunodeficiency virus (HIV) in the 1980s, there is even more reason to *not* judge other's values too quickly.

Health professionals cannot be too quick to judge or condemn practices simply because they do not conform to western medical beliefs. Western medicine is not itself totally evidence-based, and much of this body of knowledge was gleaned from once "alternative methods." Many alternative methods are helpful in easing pain even if the psychologic factor is the key ingredient for their success. Patients will not do well if their dedicated beliefs are not acknowledged and alternatives found to honor their doctrines, such as has been done for Jehovah's Witnesses. Certainly some practices are a violation of human rights, and health providers must take measures to counter these dangerous methods, but health providers must not dismiss all practices as barbaric simply because they are not understood or common in this country.

When you are treating patients from differing backgrounds, a significant goal is to use some of their cultural traditions along with modern medicine. For example, give approval for the use of certain herbal teas by older Chinese patients or incorporate "hot and cold" remedies into the regimen for patients who believe that diseases fall into categories that require treatment with one temperature or another.

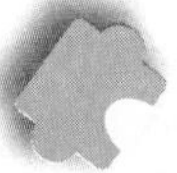

Culture and Mental Health

Sensitivity to mental health practices is also important as lack of sensitivity will fail to comfort or heal. In 2000 the American Psychiatric Association published a "Text Revision" edition of the *Diagnostic and Statistical Manual of Mental Disorders*, or DSM-IV. This textual revision contains in Appendix 1 an outline for cultural formulation of diagnoses and a glossary of terms used by large segments of people living in the United States but whose cultures lend themselves to different views of health and illness; these are the mental health equivalents of "alternative medicine." Familiarizing yourself with some of these terms and concepts will assist in understanding the client and more readily alleviating physical and mental stress.

Formulation refers to the health professional taking the individual's ethnic and cultural context into account when "formulating" a diagnosis. Determine the individual's reference group: What language do they think or feel in? If recent immigrants or ethnic minorities, how involved do they remain with their culture of origin or how involved are they with the ways of a nonmainstream group? Understanding the intensity of their cultural differences may enhance proper and accurate diagnosis.

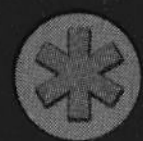

Key Point

Formulation mental health professional's taking into account the ethnocultural issues in formulating a DSM diagnosis.

Culture-bound syndromes refer to symptoms that appear in clusters and are named or labeled by a cultural group in a way that is not traditional in American health care. They are usually recurrent patterns of behavior connected to troubling experience. A few examples follow:

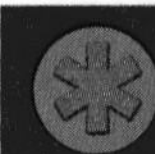

Key Point

Culture-bound syndromes syndromes occurring within a culture and not found in traditional American health care.

- Amok: A dissociative episode characterized by periods of brooding, violent outbursts, and aggressive or homicidal behavior precipitated by a slight insult and persecutory ideas, amnesia, and exhaustion. They appear as brief psychotic episodes. Originating in Malaysia, they are similarly found among those from Laos, the Philippines, Polynesia (where the syndrome is called cafard or cathard), Papua New Guinea, and Puerto Rico (where the syndrome is called mal de pelea), and among the Navajo (who call the syndrome iich'aa).
- Ataque de nervios: An idiom of distress reported among Latinos from the Caribbean but also seen among many Latin American and Latin Mediterranean groups. Common symptoms include crying, shouting, trembling, and attacks of heat in the chest and head, with a dissociative experience including seizures and fainting. These have similarities to panic attacks but span a broad number of anxiety, mood, dissociative, and somatoform Disorders.
- Boufee deliante: A syndrome found among West Africans and Haitians. It refers to a sudden outburst of agitated, aggressive, and confused behavior.
- Nervios: Refers to a state of vulnerability to stress and is thought to be brought about by difficult life circumstances. Symptoms include "brain aches," irritability, stomach and sleep disturbances, tearfulness, and dizziness. The term is used broadly and may resemble adjustment, anxiety, depression, dissociative, somatoform, or psychotic disorders. It is common among U.S. and Latin American Latinos.
- Rootwork: A set of cultural interpretations ascribing illness to hexing, sorcery, or witchcraft, with symptoms of acute anxiety and gastrointestinal complaints, weakness, and a fear of being poisoned. "Root doctors" from a similar healing tradition may "remove the hex." It is found in the southern United States among both African and European Americans and those from Caribbean societies.
- Shenjing shuairuo: A condition found in China. It is characterized by physical and mental fatigue, dizziness, headaches, and other pain. It often includes sleep problems and memory loss plus irritability, excitability, and sexual dysfunction. It appears similar to DSM IV criteria for mood or anxiety disorders and is included in the *Chinese Classification of Mental Disorders* (CCMD-2).
- Taijin kyofusho: Culturally distinctive phobia in Japan resembling social phobia in DSM-IV. Individuals have an intense fear of their

bodies, body parts and functions, appearance, and odor and movement. This syndrome is included in the official Japanese diagnostic system of mental disorders.

There is no reason to memorize these syndromes, but it is important to become familiar with their existence and the existence of other problems found within cultures so that the correct culturally sensitive and appropriate approach may be made. Health professionals need to treat all fairly and equally and work harder to be culturally competent in mental as well as physical health matters.

Changing Demographics

The history of employment needs in the United States, of famines and wars in other parts of the world, and of the location of indigenous peoples have led to pockets of ethnicity and a blending of cultures which vary throughout this country. Rapid growth among Spanish-speaking populations challenges our eastern cities and southwestern communities to provide care and education in Spanish as well as English. Because of the former mill complexes, a majority of their students (56 percent at this writing) in small cities such as Willimantic, Connecticut, come from Spanish-speaking homes. Certainly this is commonplace along the southwestern borders of the United States (see Box 14.4).

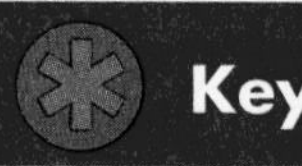

Key Point

U.S. demographics by 2050 white 40 percent, Hispanic 30 percent, Black 15 percent, Asian 12 percent.

According to the U.S. Census Bureau (reported in 2008), within a generation no single race will make up a "majority population" in the United States. By 2050 54 percent of the nation is predicted to be "minority," thus demanding a new view of these terms. The Hispanic population is expected to triple from 46.7 million in 2008 to 132.8 million by 2050. That means that the U.S. population will be 30 percent Hispanic by that date. Because of an anticipated higher death rate among whites predicted for the 2030s, followed by a slight population growth in 2040, whites will move from a current U.S. population of just under 200 million in 2008 to 203.3 million in 2050. The black population will grow from 41 million in 2008 to 65.7 million in 2050 to equal 15 percent of the U.S. population. Asian populations will more than double during this time, going from 15.5 million to 40.6 million, or approximately 12 percent of the total U.S. population.

U. S. Demographics by 2050

U.S. Race	2008 (millions)	2050	2050%
• White	• 199.8	• 203.3	40*
• Hispanic	• 46.7	• 132.8	30
• Black	• 41.1	• 65.7	15
• Asian	• 15.5	• 40.6	12

* "Others" must also be factored in/those who identify with multiple races/and discrepancies of rounded figures account for less than 100 percent total.

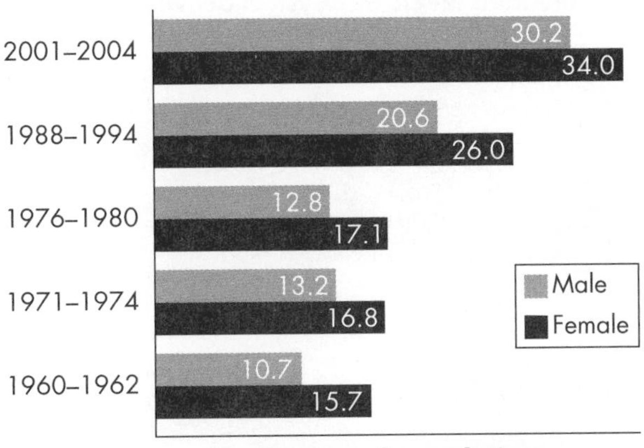

We can readily observe America is getting heavier but there are cultural differences.

> **Key Point**
>
> **Ethnic incidence of disease** incidence of disease in ethnic groups (diabetes over age 20: whites 6.6 percent, Asian 7.5 percent, Hispanic 10.4 percent, black 11.8 percent).

Impact of Ethnicity on Risk Factors

As cultural numbers shift so do risk factors; health care needs to be prepared to accommodate these changes. Let us take yet another look at diabetes. Consider that mainstream Americans value a "long life" whereas other cultures place more value on the "quality of life." The statistics of the American Diabetes Association, the American Heart Association, and the CDC show the incidence of both diabetes and obesity by ethnic background in the United States. This is an example of the **ethnic incidence of disease**. Please note that the increase in the body mass index of Americans has directly paralleled the increase in diabetes (as noted earlier). There is a definite cause-and-effect relationship between the two: that is, the heavier Americans become, the more Americans develop diabetes. And the younger

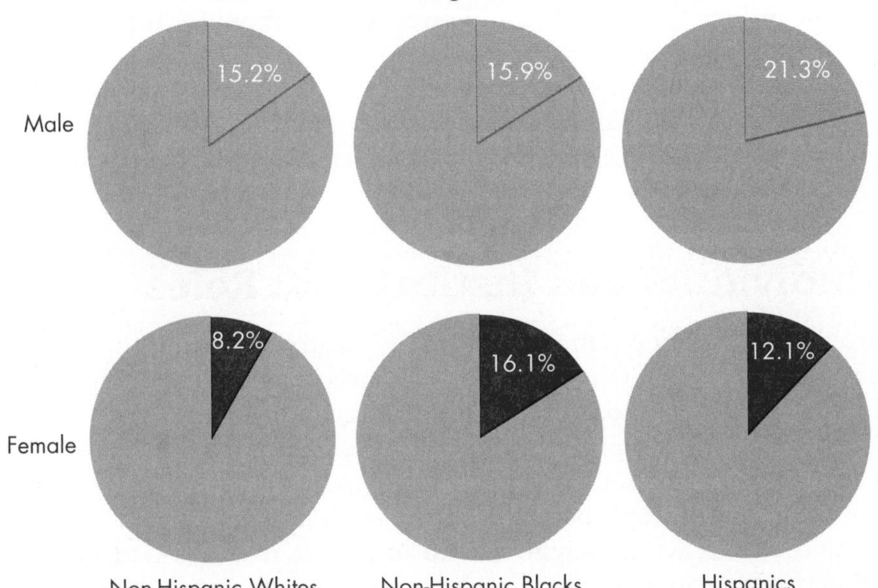

Surprisingly, Hispanic males have the highest percentage of overweight. Discuss and contrast with the next table.

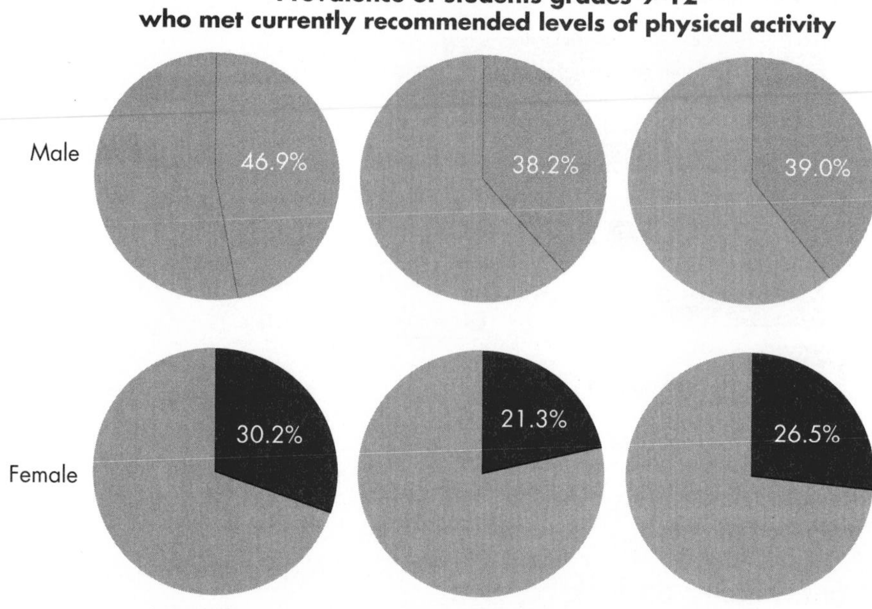

Patterns established in youth influence health throughout our lifetime.

obesity arises in the individual, the earlier is the onset of type 2 diabetes (related to metabolic disease rather than strictly to pancreatic beta cell failure as in type 1). The incidence of obesity is higher among African Americans and Hispanics than it is among white Americans; therefore the incidence of diabetes is also higher in these segments of the population.

After adjustment for population age differences, the 2004–2006 national survey data for people over age 20 diagnosed with diabetes by race/ethnicity is ranked as 6.6 percent non-Hispanic whites, 7.5 percent Asian Americans, 10.4 percent Hispanics, and 11.8 percent non-Hispanic blacks. Among the Hispanic groups the breakdown in rates is 8.2 percent for Cubans, 11.9 percent for Mexican Americans, and 12.6 percent for Puerto Ricans.

Review these tables carefully to determine the effects of exercise, gender and race on overweight. What are the surprises and where are intervention strategies most needed? Keep this table in mind when reading the section titled "Strategies for Improvements."

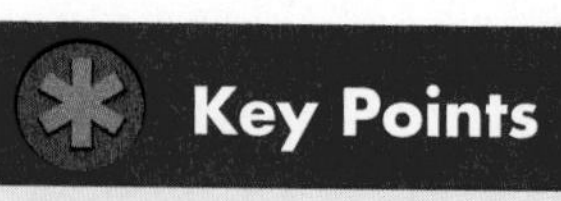

Individual discrimination discrimination by one individual.

Institutional discrimination discrimination by an institution (e.g., U.S. government).

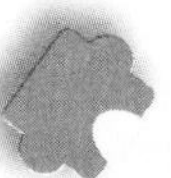

Individual and Institutional Roles

The current majority population finds many cultural forms of discrimination that are acceptable: One example is a Christmas holiday break from school. Whereas legally those with non-Christian beliefs may take time for their own holidays, their practices are not generally built into the school year. It is important to note, therefore, that there are two primary types of discrimination: **individual discrimination**, such as a realtor not wanting to show homes in a white neighborhood to people of color, and **institutional discrimination**, in which discrimation results from a governmental policy— either federal, such as the U.S. military with the earlier example of the Tuskegee Airmen, or local, as in the adoption of a school calendar treating Christian traditions as holidays. Health care professionals may need to be sensitive around institutionally imposed discrimination (later in this chapter there is a discussion of making change even here) and working to ensure that as individuals we commit no acts of discrimination. Further, relating to patients by showing knowledge of their language and celebrations is part of cultural competence.

Individual Considerations

A key to examining how to treat individuals equally and fairly involves accepting that one's own biases are often hidden from oneself. Individuals are taught subtly, at an early age, to react to people differently by how they look.

Perceiving Others: Impression Formation and Attribution Theory

Impression formation looks at how individuals make their first judgments of others. What sort of information is used? A great deal of information is taken in: age, gender, disability or fitness, race, hairstyle, glasses, manner of dress, height, physical attractiveness, cleanliness. On the basis of these factors and previous experiences, others are judged as intelligent, well off financially, friendly, or dishonest. The mind couples characteristics together so that a friendly person is rarely perceived as dishonest (think about the smiling man getting more tickets from strangers in Chapter 1). Or an attractive person is seen as kind whereas a large muscular man may be seen as threatening or mean.

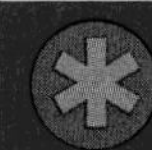

Key Point

Impression formation the way we make our first judgments of others.

Attribution theory is a theory that, based on a perceived impression of another person, we come to a quick conclusion of what this other person is likely to do. Unfortunately, impressions are sometimes formed with very little or no direct evidence about the other. In 1985 Heilman and Stropek published their study on the judgment of the ability of alleged vice presidents based on their photographs. Raters believed that the more attractive a man was, the higher was his ability, but the women who were judged to be most able were the least attractive. This can be carried further; once an initial impression is formed, conclusions are likely to be drawn about other traits of that individual. This also accounts for how **stereotyping** works: We associate a string of traits with one piece of information—perhaps someone who likes to read is seen as automatically more intelligent than someone who states he plays football. Think of Superman wearing a suit and glasses to disguise his superior physical abilities.

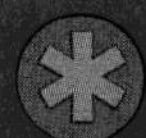

Key Points

Attribution theory theory that we draw quick conclusions about person's likely actions on the basis of perceived impressions.

Stereotyping associating a string of traits with an individual or group, generally on the basis of a single factor about that individual or group.

In a classic 1974 study, Word, Zanna, and Cooper examined the problems of impression formation. They found several things:

- It is problematic to rely heavily on a schema that states, "If this, then that" without real evidence.
- Impression formation relies too heavily on first impressions.
- Actor and observer differences may occur because of a situation that is observed under special circumstances rather than because of behaviors that really reflect on dispositions (we see someone on a very "bad day" for him or her or a very "good day," but neither is an accurate picture of his or her typical day or reactions to others).
- Most critically, expectancies influence behaviors, or *we see what we expect to see.*

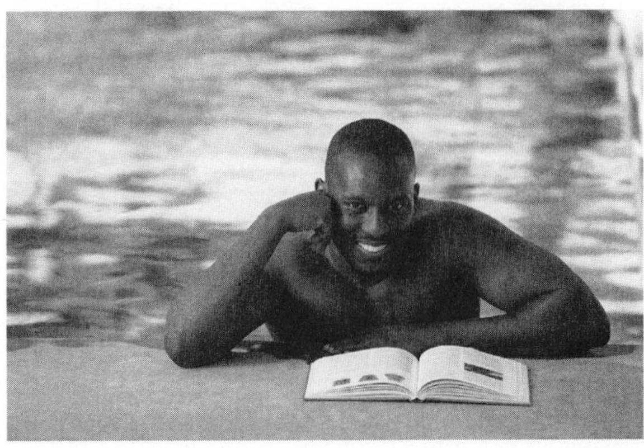

Is this man judged to be studious or athletic—or perhaps both?

Body Language between the Races Experiment

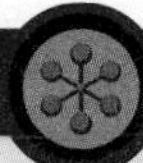

Experiment:
White males were told they would be interviewing candidates to select a teammate for a subsequent, competitive task. When they were interviewing African Americans, they sat further away, held shorter interviews, and demonstrated fewer immediacy behaviors (moving closer while talking, maintaining eye contact, and leaning forward while interacting) than when they interviewed white males.

A second experiment was conducted within this study. White male interviewees were actually part of this second experiment (confederates), and they were prompted to make fewer **immediacy behaviors** in their interviews. When this occurred, they were reported to be less competent, less composed, and less liked—the same report that was given of the African American interviewees! Interviewers sent off a less friendly message to African Americans and then judged them as unfriendly and less competent.

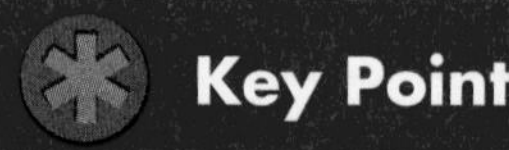

Immediacy behavior body language that conveys attention and interest, such as moving close and maintaining eye contact while talking.

How has the passing of time between 1974 (when this experiment was first published) and now influenced its outcomes? Would the reactions differ today? Think back to Chapter 1; these stereotyping thoughts play out even when communicators are trying to control or mask their hasty, often subconscious, conclusions. Body language or nonverbal behavior will send its own signal. In interracial communications what is felt will come through; this underscores the importance of working on ourselves toward a goal of true sensitivity and understanding.

Working to eliminate prejudice and discrimination from one's own behaviors also requires examination of the health care disparities that abound as a result of institutional discrimination. For example, figures for HIV infection and incidence released by the CDC for 2006 demonstrate a more pervasive spread of this devastating disease than had been expected. Not too surprisingly, the increases in HIV are demarcated along ethnic lines.

Of those infected with HIV, 45 percent are African American; 35 percent are white, 17 percent are Hispanic, and 3 percent are other. Because of the greater population of whites in the general population, the CDC reported in 2008 that the incidence in African Americans is 7 times higher and 3 times higher in Hispanics than in whites (cases per 100,000).

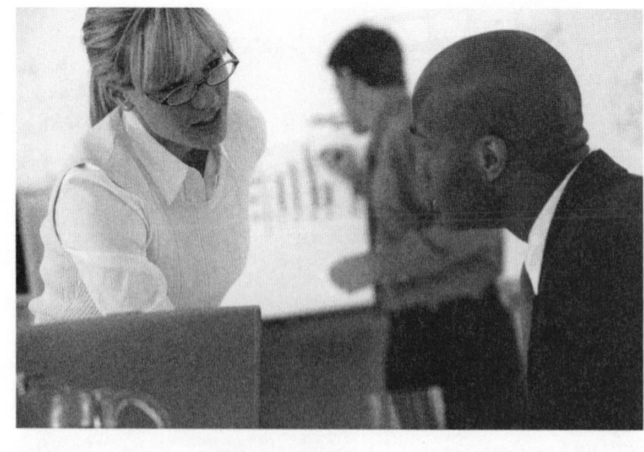

Individuals can make a difference and influence the institutions in which they work.

Institutional Racism

It is hard for individuals to change systems and institutions, but it is possible. Think of the work of Dr. Martin Luther King, Jr. in the United States, Mother Theresa in Calcutta, and Father Damien with the "lepers" in Hawaii. Look at more ordinary heroes such as Richard Pimentel, whose life is portrayed in the 2007 film *Music Within*, or Greg Mortenson, who has devoted his life to building schools in remote areas of Pakistan as described in the *New York Times* bestselling book *Three Cups of Tea*. Each one of you may have an opportunity to influence systems simply by virtue of the work done within them. These opportunities generally present themselves to those who are in management positions when mission statements are written or strategic plans are formulated; organizations that serve the public need to strive to reach those in greatest need even if they are the most reluctant consumers. Laws and policies favoring the dominant culture, and conversely *not* addressing the disparate needs of the remaining ethnic/cultural groups, are the essence of the term **institutional racism**. The Indian Removal Act is one early example of institutional racism created by federal law. Would you have voted with President Jackson or held the value of human rights high as did Crockett, Webster, and Clay?

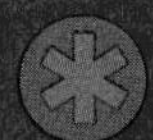

Key Point

Institutional racism discrimination against a racial group by an institution.

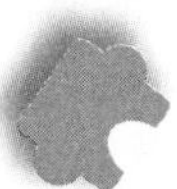

Strategies for Improvements

The CDC offers a model for public health changes across multiple cultures. It is referred to as **Planned Approach to Community Health (PATCH)**. Essentially, it bases its approach on good strategic planning within the communities needing the most assistance. Strategies include partnerships with community leaders, development of community ownership of the program(s), and finding a way to personalize the delivery of the program. The groups begin by working together to determine what the community's health priorities are as those living within the communities have first-hand knowledge. Community leaders and other members of the health care team then work to develop an intervention or implementation plan complete with timetables so that progress may be gauged and evaluated.

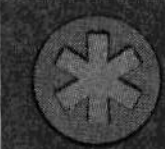

Key Point

PATCH an acronym for Planned Approach to Community Health, strategies to change public health across cultures.

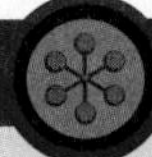

According to the American Cancer Society Surveillance Research from 2007:

- White women have a higher incidence of breast cancer (131 per 100,000 people) than do African American women (112), Asian American and Pacific Islander women (91), American Indian and Alaska Native women, (74) and Hispanic/Latina women (93).
- More African American women die of breast cancer (34 per 100,000) than white women, who have the next highest mortality (25 per 100,000).
- The sad explanation for this is that African American women are diagnosed at a more advanced stage.

How may outreach be improved for early detection of breast cancer in the African American population? Think about steps to take that would change later diagnoses. A possible strategic plan would include the following: goals, objectives, community input and review, and a written action plan with not only a timetable but also individuals to be held responsible for each step.

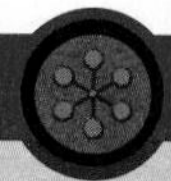

Another factor that influences the mortality of African Americans is reported in a 2007 study by Ioana Popescu, MD, MPH, of Iowa City VA Medical Center and the University of Iowa. When treated in hospitals that provide angioplasty and bypass surgery, African Americans with heart attacks receive these services far less than do white Americans (34 percent versus 50 percent). Further, if treatment occurs at facilities that do not offer these services, African American patients are less likely to be transferred than are white Americans (25 percent versus 31 percent).

An understanding of this may help all health professionals improve education of heart attack patients and especially those who are from underserved groups. *Failure to adequately address these issues keeps the disparity in place or institutionalizes it.*

Summary

This chapter provided a brief historical perspective on ethnic, cultural, and racial issues within the United States. Further, it defined the term culture to include beliefs, practices, religion, language, music, sports, laws, taboos, and much more beyond ethnic identity. The considerations raised may also be applied to gender differences and to those with disabilities. The cultural and familial influences on health and developing an appreciation of the importance of cultural competence among providers was also discussed.

An overview of ethnocentricity was also provided. This helps the reader to accept that the values and practices of others may hold more merit than on first examination. Additionally, an overview of popular complementary and alternative medicine practices and mental health concerns was presented. A few examples of practices that are deemed unacceptable by reason of the unnecessary harm they cause were also discussed. It is believed that all of health care profits by learning from other cultures even though the practices of these cultures may be non–evidence-based. It is also imperative to understand the belief systems of our clients in order to reach them for appropriate treatment that they will accept. This is part of becoming culturally competent.

This chapter synthesized the impact of demographic trends and how the needs of current and future populations will require specific consideration for both physical and mental health issues. Graphs and tables were used to provide statistics that will help health care providers to focus on the health risks most particular to certain sectors of our population. A classic experiment was also discussed to demonstrate the impact of body language on interracial interactions, with questions as to how this experiment might be replicated today.

Most importantly, this chapter challenged the reader to look at his or her own ability to make a difference—individually and through institutions. The chapter borrowed from social psychology to examine how individuals make generalizations through impression formation and attribution theory. The chapter then discussed strategies for making a more meaningful impact on the health care needs of Americans irrespective of race, ethnicity, color, religion, language, gender, disability, sexual preference, or gender identity. Making such an impact will require that providers become involved with the communities they wish to serve.

Chapter Review

Key Term Review

Alternative medicine: Treatment not based on scientifically proven methods, often eschewing surgery or drugs, and used *instead of* conventional medicine.

American Indian or Alaskan Native*: A person who has origins in any of the original peoples of North America and who maintains cultural identification through tribal affiliation or community recognition.

Asian or Pacific Islanders*: A person having origins in any of the original peoples of the Far East, Southeast Asia, the Indian subcontinent, or the Pacific Islands. This area includes, for example, China, India, Japan, Korea, the Philippine Islands, and Samoa.

Attribution theory: Theory that we draw overall conclusions solely on the basis of first impressions.

Black*: A person having origins in any of the black racial groups of Africa.

Complementary medicine: Alternative and conventional medicine used together.

Culture: Composite of beliefs, practices, religions, and languages that make up a group.

Culture-bound: Pertaining to a belief that the values of your own group are superior to other groups.

Culture-bound syndromes: Syndromes occurring within a culture and not found in traditional American health care.

Cultural competence: Ability to transcend one's own cultural values and to work within the cultural norms of another group.

Cycle of poverty: The difficulty of breaking away from poverty when that is all one has ever known.

Diversity: Inclusion of people from different geographical locations, differing ethnic backgrounds and cultures, different physical abilities and genders, and differing beliefs and practices.

Ethnic incidence of disease: Incidence of disease in ethnic groups (e.g., diabetes over age 20: whites 6.6 percent, Asian 7.5 percent, Hispanic 10.4 percent, blacks 11.8 percent). (American Diabetes Association Web site)

Ethnocentric: Characterized by a strong belief in people who are ethnically like yourself to the exclusion of other ethnic groups.

Family systems approach: Working with entire families as a means to bridging cultural barriers and to broadening the impact of health care interventions.

Formulation: Taking individuals' ethnic and cultural background into account, especially when "formulating" a mental health diagnosis.

Hispanic*: A person who is from Mexico, Puerto Rico, Cuba, Central or South America, or another Spanish culture.

Immediacy behaviors: Body language that conveys attention and interest, such as moving closer to an individual and maintaining eye contact during a dialogue.

Impression formation: The way we make first judgments of others.

Indian Removal Act: Under President Andrew Jackson, the Congressional Act that forced the North Georgian Cherokee Nation to relocate in Oklahoma.

Indigenous: Native.

Individual discrimination/racism: A personal belief or bias against a group/race that differs from one's own race.

Institutional discrimination/racism: Treatment by a group holding majority power over differing ethnic/racial groups that promotes the values of the group in power.

Integrative medicine: The combination of conventional and alternative medicine for which there is evidence of safety and efficacy; it focuses on mind, body and spirit.

Internment camps: Camps consisting of poorly constructed barracks surrounded by barbed wire, sentry posts, and armed guards, to which over 100,000 Japanese Americans, mostly American citizens, were shipped during World War II.

Multicultural: Inclusive of and valuing many cultures and cultural diversity.

Planned Approach to Community Health (PATCH): CDC's model for strategically planning for work within communities.

People of color: Inclusive term emphasizing common experiences of racism. It frames the subject positively unlike the terms *nonwhite,* which defines people in terms of what they are not (white), and *minority,* which places the subject in a subordinate position. The term has a positive connotation and has often been preferred by people of color in the United States.

Stereotyping: Associating a string of traits with an individual or group, generally on the basis of a single factor about that individual or group (i.e., all men are…)

Trail of Tears: The forced march of 17,000 members of the North Georgian Cherokee Nation from their land in

Georgia to unwanted land in Oklahoma, resulting in the death of 4,000 along the way.

Tuskegee Airmen: First African American pilots in the U.S. Army.

U.S. demographics by 2050: White 4 percent, Hispanic 30 percent, black 15 percent, Asian 12 percent

Values: Beliefs that hold meaning to an individual or group and by which the individual or group tries to guide decisions.

White*: A person having origins in any of the original peoples of Europe, North Africa, or the Middle East.

* Federal definitions formulated in 1978 for the collection of comparative differential data.

Chapter Review Questions

1. What will be the population mix of the United States in 2050? How will you want your ethnic group described?
2. Describe the "ideal" health practitioner to provide care to a middle-aged female person of color.
3. How does racism hurt us all?
4. What was the immediate impact of 9/11 on ethnic interrelationships within the United States?
5. If you believe that lean is healthy, how would you go about convincing a 50-year-old obese male with diabetes that he needs to drop pounds if he comes from a background where eating defines family life and a large build is highly valued?
6. If racial lines are used to set up interviewers versus interviewees, as in the classic experiment cited in this chapter, describe how you believe the outcome would differ today.
7. What are the problems with "attribution" judgments?
8. How might you as an individual make significant change in this country?
9. Discuss culture-bound syndromes and their influence on mental health.

Case Study Critical Thinking Questions

1. Refer to Case Study 14-1. Who were the Tuskegee Airmen, and what impact do they have on society today?
2. Review Case Study 14-2 regarding Jehovah's Witnesses and blood transfusions. Imagine now that you are a devout Jehovah's Witness and you must explain to health professionals why your child, who has just been injured in an auto accident, may NOT have a transfusion. Then switch the argument, placing yourself as the health professional arguing for the transfusion. Finally, imagine that this takes place in mid-1980; what are the possible ramifications of each position? What would be different with the argument today and why?

References

1. Bertrand, M., Mullainathan, S. "Are Emily and Greg More Employable than Lakisha and Jamal? A Field Experiment on Labor Market Discrimination." *American Economic Review,* 94: 991–1013; 2004.
2. Council of Counseling Psychology Training Programs. "Counseling Psychology Model Training Values Statement Addressing Diversity. *The Counseling Psychologist* 37:5; 2009.
3. Danner, M. *The Massacre at El Mozote*. New York: Vintage Books/Random House, 1993.
4. Davis, K. *Don't Know Much About History.* Harper Collins, 2003.

5. Dirie, W., Miller, C. *Desert Flower*. New York: William Morrow and Co., 1998.
6. Dunlap, E., Tourigny, S. C., Johnson, B. D. "Dead Tired and Bone Weary: Grandmothers as Caregivers in Drug Affected Inner City Households." *Race and Society* 3 (2):143–163; 2000.
7. Eli, G. "Access to Health Care for Hispanics." *JAMA* Jan. 9, 1991.
8. Feagin, J., Vera, H., Batur, P. *White Racism*. New York: Routledge, 2001.
9. Mauer, F., Smith, Claudia. Chapter 9. *Community/ Public Health Nursing Practice*. Philadelphia: Elsevier Saunders, 2004.
10. Mayo Foundation for Medical Education and Research. *Acupuncture: Ancient Practice Finds Place in Western Medicine*. Rochester, MN: Mayo Clinic, 2007.
11. Mayo Clinic. "Mayo Clinic Study Shows Acupuncture and Myofascial Trigger Therapy Treat Same Pain Areas." *Sci News*, May 13, 2008.
12. National Alliance for Hispanic Health (Foreword by J. Delgado). *A Primer for Cultural Proficiency: Towards Quality Health Services for Hispanics*. Washington, DC: Estrella Press, 2001.
13. Norton, M., et al. "Colorblindness and Interracial Interaction: Playing the 'Political Correctness Game.'" *Psychol Sci* 17: 949–953; 2006.
14. Olfson, M., et al. "Continuity of Antidepressant Treatment for Adults with Depression in the United States." *The Am J Psychiat* 163:1, 95–108; 2006.
15. Popescu, I., Vaughan-Sarrazin, M., and Rosenthal, G. "Differences in Mortality and Use of Revascularization in Black and White Patients with Acute MI Admitted to Hospitals with and without Revascularization Services. *JAMA* 297:2489–2495; 2007.
16. Sommers, S., and Norton, M. "Race and Jury Selection." *Am Psychol* 63(6):527–539; 2008.
17. Taylor, R. L., ed. *Minority Families in the United States*. Upper Saddle River, NJ: Prentice Hall, 2002.
18. Word, C. O., Zanna, M. P., Cooper, J. "The Nonverbal Mediation of Self-Fulfilling Prophecies in Interracial Interaction." *J Exp Soc Psychol* 10:109–120; 1974.
19. Zack, N., Shrage, L., and Sartwell, C. ed. *Race, Class, Gender and Sexuality*. Blackwell Publishers Ltd., 1998.
20. www.cdc.gov
21. www.rice.edu/projects/HispanicHealth/Courses/mod1/hispanic-sk.html
22. http://en.wikipedia.org/wiki/Person_of_color

Additional Readings

1. Brooks, G. *Nine Parts of Desire*. New York: Anchor Books/Doubleday, 1995.
2. Civil Rights Act of 1964, 42 U.S.Code, sec. 2000d (1988).
3. Crouch, S., and Benjamin, P. *Reconsidering the Souls of Black Folk*. Philadelphia: Running Press, 2002.
4. Fumia, M. *Honor Thy Children*. Berkeley, CA: Conari Press, 1997.
5. Mortenson, G., and Relin, D. O. *Three Cups of Tea*. New York: Penguin Books, 2006.

Glossary

A

Abandonment unavailability or improper discontinuation of medical care.

Absolute total, all or nothing.

Abuse willful infliction of physical or mental pain through acts of commission or omission.

Acceptance fifth Kübler-Ross stage of loss: resignation with fate, return to realistic existence.

Accreditation formal approval of an institution or educational program given by an outside agency.

Acronym series of capital letters standing for a phrase.

Adaptive regression ability to take on the child role when ill as a patient.

Addiction physical and/or psychologic dependence on a substance (often leading to drug-seeking behavior).

Additive effect the cumulative effect of sedatives (e.g., alcohol, benzodiazepines, barbiturates, sleeping pills, inhalants, anesthetics).

ADL acronym for activities of daily living.

Adornment and appearance dress, appearing clean, jewelry, tattoos, piercings.

Advance directives living will and designation in writing of a health care agent made while person is competent in case unable to express his or her wishes in the future.

Aerobic exercise exercise that uses large muscle groups and increases oxygen flow.

AIM counseling technique using awareness, information, and motivation as tools.

Alcoholics Anonymous (AA) informal meeting society for recovering alcoholics wanting to achieve and maintain sobriety. AA uses a 12-step program to help people stay off alcohol and believes that complete abstention is the only way.

Alcoholism chronic consumption of alcohol that continues despite significant interference with a person's physical, economic, or social health.

Alternative medicine treatment not based on scientifically proven methods, often eschewing surgery or drugs, and used instead of conventional medicine.

Americans with Disabilities Act (ADA) law administered by EEOC (Equal Employment Opportunity Commission) prohibiting employers from discriminating against the disabled.

American Indian or Alaskan Native a person who has origins in any of the original peoples of North America and who maintains cultural identification through tribal affiliation or community recognition.

Amniocentesis medical procedure in which amniotic fluid is removed from abdomen of pregnant women. Tests run on this fluid indicate certain health characteristics of the fetus.

Anger second Kübler-Ross stage of loss: unreasonable anger directed at self or others.

Anima inner self theorized by Jung.

Antagonists opponents, against good.

Appraisal-focused coping alteration of value or view of stress; for example, use of humor to cope.

Asian or Pacific Islander a person having origins in any of the original peoples of the Far East, Southeast Asia, the Indian subcontinent, or the Pacific Islands. This area includes, for example, China, India, Japan, Korea, the Philippine Islands, and Samoa.

Assault verbal abuse or threats of physical abuse.

Atmosphere for communication being at the correct distance from the patient, usually at arm's length and without barriers.

Attribution theory theory that overall conclusions we draw are based solely on first impressions.

Autonomy the individual right of a patient to exercise own judgment.

B

Baby boomers people born between 1946 and 1964 as a result of post-WWII marriage boom.

Bargaining third Kübler-Ross stage of loss: delaying tactic to put off need for acceptance.

Battery actual physical violence, involving physical contact with other person.

Behavioral observation studying the patient's nonverbal behavior, specifically, eye contact, facial expressions, appearance, posture, and proximity.

Behaviorism school of psychology focusing on patient behavior.

Beneficence the use of a professional's expertise for patient well-being.

Black a person having origins in any of the black racial groups of Africa.

BMI an acronym for body mass index, a number that expresses degree of body fat.

Body image mental picture of self including value judgments or psychologic distortions.

Body schema child's ability to use herself or himself as a reference for understanding the world sense of self.

Bonding close mutual attachment between two people (e.g., maternal or paternal bond, male or female bond).

Boundaries (1) a mental or physical line delineating territories between two people that cannot be crossed, especially with gender or cultural differences; (2) limits, professional distance.

C

CAGE a mnemonic for the following questions: Have you ever felt: (1) you should *c*ut down your drinking, (2) *a*nnoyed by others' comments about your drinking, (3) *g*uilty about your drinking, (4) you needed an *e*ye opener (drink on rising in the morning)? Even one positive answer is significant.

Cartesian dualism a philosophy that postulates that body and mind are two separate entities.

Case conference ad hoc meeting of health care professionals focusing on a specific patient at a specific time.

Case manager a person appointed to handle a specific patient.

Certification a document that attests that an individual has attained qualifications for a specified part of his or her occupation.

Chronemics use of time, pausing, waiting, speeding up.

Chronic suicide chronic self-destructive behavior.

Civil court a court that handles actions by private litigants.

Closed-ended question a question that can be answered simply and that does not encourage further discussion.

Cognitive of thought, factual knowledge, thinking skills.

Cognitive behavioral therapy (CBT) a kind of psychotherapy that deals with thought processes, beliefs, and responses to influence problematic emotions or behaviors.

Cognitive dissonance the theory that the human mind seeks harmony in making choices and thus will rationalize the advantages to the choice made.

Cognitive impairment loss or absence of intellectual capacity.

Collaborator a person working with another person to a common end for material information or to transfer patient care.

Collective unconscious according to Jung, the preprogrammed unconscious with which all humans are born.

Comfort Measures Only treating for comfort only—no attempts to prolong life (i.e., quality, not quantity, of life).

Communication sequence paraphrasing (with use of nonverbal language), then empathizing, then asking open-ended questions.

Compensation overcompensation, addressing a problem by excelling at it.

Competence the ability to perform according to the standards of the profession.

Competent mentally capable of understanding relevant risks, benefits, and alternatives.

Complementary medicine alternative and conventional medicine used together.

Complex group of ideas with common feeling or tone (e.g., inferiority complex).

Compliance following directions, especially as given by health care provider for patient health.

Conditioned reflex a learned response to a stimulus.

Confabulation cover-up in which the patient fabricates or makes up events.

Confidentiality keeping information private.

Conservator person appointed by probate court to take care of financial and/or personal decision-making for an incompetent person.

Consultant temporary adviser on current problems.

Contingency management specific rewards given or withheld contingent or dependent upon specific behavioral changes.

Countertransference health professional's nonprofessional feelings toward a patient.

CPOE acronym for computerized physician order entry, the part of the clinical information system that replaces written orders for physician, nurses and allied health professionals.

Criminal court court in which a government prosecutor prosecutes defendant for crime.

Crisis intervention brief therapy to resolve a major crisis in a patient's life.

Culture composite of beliefs, practices, religions, and languages that make up a group.

Culture-bound belief that the values of your own group are superior to other groups.

Culture-bound syndrome syndromes labeled by a culture and not found in traditional American health care.

Cultural competence ability to transcend one's own cultural values and to work within the cultural norms of another group.

Cycle of poverty the difficulty of breaking away from poverty when that is all one has ever known.

D

DARE acronym for Drug Abuse Resistance Education.

Decorum term used for the medical etiquette of the Hippocratic Oath.

Deep pocket person or institution with lots of money.

Defendant person being sued.

Defense mechanism (1) psychological method of reducing psychic pain from mental conflict. (2) psychological means of avoiding conscious conflict.

Degree a step in a series.

Dementia chronic diffuse mental deterioration in a conscious patient, manifested primarily by memory loss and secondarily by behavioral and emotional changes.

Denial (1) defense mechanism in which painful truths are denied. (2) first Kübler-Ross stage of loss: bereaved client uses denial as defense mechanism. (3) psychological mechanism in which conflict in mind is resolved by denial of that conflict.

Depression fourth Kübler-Ross stage of loss: actual grief from loss.

Developmental assessment evaluation by professional to determine child's personal-social, fine motor, gross motor, and language abilities.

Developmental delay delay in any one of key milestones—it may be necessary to label child as delayed to get services.

Developmental milestones usual age ranges for the child to sit, walk, talk, copy shapes, etc.

Dialysis circulation of blood through a machine to get rid of waste chemicals and return blood to body—typically takes several hours three times a week for maintenance, or may be needed only during serious illness, replacing kidney function.

Differentiate make distinct, make separate.

Disability physical or mental impairment that interferes with normal life.

Discreditable description of person with hidden social stigma.

Discredited description of person with obvious social stigma.

Discrimination unfair treatment of person on the basis of group, class, or category to which that person belongs rather than on individual merit.

Disengagement theory theory that the elderly sever friendships as part of a more general disengagement from society.

Disorientation a loss of memory for time, person, and place.

Displacement putting (usually) negative feelings on someone or something other than cause.

Distant relative syndrome a syndrome in which distant relative visits create a whirlwind of criticism about a previously stable patient's care because she or he does not understand the gestalt.

Diversity inclusion of people from different geographical locations, differing ethnic backgrounds and cultures, different physical abilities and genders, and differing beliefs and practices.

Downregulation decrease in number of receptors (e.g., for dopamine) on surface of cell, making it less sensitive to further stimulation (e.g., by dopamine).

DSM IV TR (Diagnostic and Statistical Manual, fourth edition with text revision) classifies psychologic diseases using five axes: Axis I, clinical syndrome; Axis II, personality disorder; Axis III, physical disease; Axis IV, severity of stress; and Axis V, level of functioning.

Dyad a couple, a group of two.

E

Eclectic using many different theories to make decision.

Ego the realization of a person's conscious mind as a unique individual.

EHR acronym for electronic health record, information technology replaces old paper physician or hospital chart.

Electra complex Freudian theory that penis envy causes a girl to be sexually attracted to her father.

Emotional augmentation a lowered threshold for action when a person is concerned about something.

Emotion-focused coping coping with stress by trying to "let one's feelings out" or using relaxation techniques rather than a direct attempt to change the stress object.

Empathize to convey understanding of another person's feelings.

Environmental conditions the world around us.

e-prescribe electronic means to write prescriptions direct to pharmacy.

Eros life instincts.

Ethics a set of standards and codes held as essential by professionals for the welfare of their patients and their professional standing.

Ethnic incidence of disease the incidence of disease in a particular ethnic group (e.g., diabetes over age 20: whites 6.6%, Asian 7.5%, Hispanic 10.4%, black 11.8% [American Diabetes Association Web site]).

Ethnocentric characterized by a strong belief in people who are ethnically like yourself to the exclusion of other ethnic groups.

Etiology cause.

Etiquette 19th century medical code used to guide professional conduct without relying on the term *morality,* based on the presumption of "an upright man instructed in the art of healing."

Expert witness professional with education, training, skill, or experience in specific field beyond that of normal people.

Exploitation taking advantage of another person, usually financially.

Extrovert a sociable and outgoing person.

F

Family systems approach working with entire families as a means to bridging cultural barriers and to broadening the impact of health care interventions.

Feeling words words that express emotional feelings rather than just cognitive thoughts.

Fetal alcohol syndrome a syndrome that occurs in babies of mothers who drink excessively during pregnancy.

Flexner Report Abraham Flexner's report on the quality of medical education (1910), which led to accreditation.

Food pyramid a pyramid-shaped diagram that shows the consumer how much of each food group is advised.

Formal network a team that is apparent and obvious, for exchange through defined relationships in an organized structure.

Formulation taking individuals' ethnic and cultural background into account, especially when "formulating" a mental health diagnosis.

Four Ds of malpractice *d*ereliction of *d*uty *d*irectly causes *d*amage.

G

Gastric feeding tube plastic tube usually placed through the abdominal wall into the stomach for artificial feeding.

Genetic counseling the assessment of genetic risk by a professional, who presents the statistics in a cogent way to the individual.

Genetic programming inherited characteristics carried by our genes.

Gestalt form of therapy that treats the patient as a whole and focuses on current feelings.

Giving feedback a procedure that includes starting with the positive, being specific, focusing on behavior, knowing one's motives, and being immediate and private.

H

Haptics touch.

Health not simply the absence of disease but a state of complete physical, mental, and social well-being.

Health care agent person named in advance to have power of attorney for health care decisions if patient becomes incompetent.

Hierarchy of basic human needs human needs in order of priority as theorized by Maslow.

Hippocratic Oath oath sworn to by new physicians declaring that they place the welfare of their patients first and will do no harm.

HIPAA (Health Insurance Portability and Accountability Act) legal standard to protect the privacy and security of patient information, applied especially when insurance reimbursements and information are exchanged.

Hispanic a person of Mexican, Puerto Rican, Cuban, Central or South American, or other Spanish culture.

HIT acronym for health information technology, the use of computers in medicine.

Hospice (1) supportive medical and home care focusing on dying with dignity; an organization that helps the dying and their families. (2) support program for terminal patients emphasizing comfort and home care.

I

Id mass of undifferentiated instincts in newborn child.

Ideal communication model an ideal for communication that includes the following attributes: professionally attired; arm's length from the patient; private setting; relaxed, attentive posture; friendly expression and tone; hold patient's gaze; focus on patient's body language and reflect conflict.

Identification unconscious transfer of outside character traits into one's own mind.

Identity differentiation and separation from parents.

Illness behavior ways different people respond when suffering the same symptoms.

Immediacy behaviors body language that conveys attention and interest, such as moving closer to an individual and maintaining eye contact during a dialogue.

Impression formation the information people use to make first judgments of others.

Incidence of illness the frequency with which an illness occurs (e.g., heart disease, cancer, and strokes are the top three causes of death).

Incontinent Unable to control flow of urine or feces, resulting in urination or defecation at any time.

Indian Removal Act under President Andrew Jackson the congressional act that forced the North Georgian Cherokee Nation to relocate to Oklahoma.

Indigenous native.

Individual discrimination/racism a personal belief or bias against a group/race that differs from feelings about one's own race.

Inferiority complex strong feeling of inferiority with undue pessimism.

Influencing response responses of health professionals that influence or may lead the patient toward action.

Informal network team that is hidden, with no set rules or procedures to follow, no permanent structure.

Informed consent "knowing" permission—patient reasonably informed about the pros and cons of a test or treatment.

Institutional discrimination/racism treatment, by a group holding majority power over differing ethnic/racial groups, that promotes the values of the group in power.

Institutional review boards independent ethics committees that oversee medical research on humans.

Integrative medicine medicine that combines conventional medicine and alternative medicine for which there is evidence of safety and efficacy and focuses on mind, body, and spirit.

Interdisciplinary communication communication between members of different health specialties.

Internment camps camps in which Japanese-Americans were imprisoned during World War II—over 100,000 Japanese-Americans, mostly American citizens, were rounded up and shipped eventually to these camps, which consisted of poorly-constructed barracks surrounded by barbed wire, sentry posts, and armed guards.

Interoperability the ability of one computer system or network to interact with another.

Intervention stepping into health problem issues in order to facilitate change.

Intradisciplinary communication communication between members of the same health specialty.

Intravenous (IV) within a vein—intravenous medicines and fluids are administered through a plastic tube put in the veins and taped to the skin.

Introvert shy and introspective.

Institutionalization the placement of a person in an institution, where that person eats, sleeps, and spends working time (or what should be working time).

Intubate put tube hooked up to machine called a ventilator down the windpipe to keep breathing going.

Inversion when a person does the opposite of what he or she wants.

J

Jury system a legal system in which a jury of peers rather than a judge decides the outcome of a case.

Justice a sense of fairness.

K

Kinesics body motions such as shrugs, foot tapping, drumming fingers, clicking pens, winking, facial expressions, and gestures.

L

Lack of biological adaptability decreased ability as one ages to change physically, socially, or psychologically.

Leading response advice giving, questioning, and influencing—when communication turns to counseling, the health professional makes several types of leading responses.

Legacy a system whose design contains hardware and software elements that may be unsupportable in later years when more advanced systems replace it.

Liberated minor child under 18 who is emancipated (i.e., free of parental control or power) and may assume most of legal responsibilities of an adult.

Libido sexual instinct

Licensure mechanism designed to assure patients that the care they receive from a professional meets a reasonable standard.

Life instincts sexuality and self-preservation instincts as theorized by Freud.

Lifestyle factors how we choose to live.

Litigant person bringing a lawsuit.

Living will written document expressing patient's wishes on resuscitation, intubation, and artificial hydration or nutrition.

Locomotion walking, jumping, swaying, and moving in a wheelchair.

Lonely immigrant syndrome a syndrome in which an immigrant substitutes medical care for lack of socialization.

M

Maloccurrence untoward event (not necessarily actionable).

Malpractice maloccurrence that is actionable.

Masculine protest natural tendency of people to move from passive, or feminine, role to aggressive, or masculine, role.

Mental incompetence person's inability to make decisions in his or her own best interest.

Metabolic syndrome generally the combined occurrence in one individual of any three of the following: obesity, diabetes, high cholesterol, and high blood pressure.

Model a person whom a child looks up to and imitates.

Moderation Management (MM) organization that believes that problem drinkers can continue to drink in a controlled fashion but, if they fail, suggests AA.

Motivation drive toward a particular action.

Motivational interviewing specific technique to motivate client that uses client's own motivation to change and pushes the client to articulate ambivalence, using nondirective and empathic eliciting style.

Multicultural inclusive of and valuing many cultures and cultural diversity.

N

Negative euthanasia tacit noninterference with the process of death.

Negativism resisting direction from others, which leads to separation and understanding self-determinism.

Neglect willful infliction of physical or mental pain through acts of omission.

Negligence unintentional tort that reasonable person would not have committed or omitted.

Neonate an infant in the first four weeks after birth.

Networking marshalling people, systems, agencies or resources that a specific person needs at a specific time.

Neurotransmitter chemical substance released from a nerve ending to stimulate other nerves.

Neutral position of behavior the body's *natural* position (e.g., hands relaxed at sides is a neutral position; other positions would be purposeful and have some meaning).

Nonmalfeasance above all else, doing no harm.

Nonverbal behavior body language that reveals patient's underlying feelings.

Nonverbal language composite of eye contact, facial expressions, appearance, posture, and proximity.

Nonverbal message communication without the use of language, the most powerful way of communicating with patients. A relaxed yet steady gaze is ideal eye contact. Facial expression and professional appearance are the key to sending the correct message. Adopt a relaxed posture with hands relaxed.

O

Obesity BMI over 30.

Oculesics eye contact.

Oedipus complex Freudian theory that a boy is sexually attracted to his mother and sexually jealous of his father.

Olfactics smell.

ONDCP acronym for Office of National Drug Control Policy.

Open-ended question a question that cannot be answered simply but encourages further discussion.

Overweight BMI over 25.

P

PACS acronym for Picture Archiving and Communication System, which stores and retrieves imaging studies on computer.

Paraphrase repeating message in different words.

Parasuicide mentally allowing death when death need not occur; includes chronic suicide, giving up, and dying of a broken heart.

Parental expectations discrepancy between expectation and reality, gradually adapted to.

Parental responsibility issues trust, driving, drinking, drugs, sex, birth control, venereal disease.

PATCH CDC's acronym for Planned Approach to Community Health, a strategic plan for work within communities. .

Patient's Bill of Rights list of patient's rights.

People of color inclusive term, with a positive connotation, emphasizing common experiences of racism. It frames the subject positively whereas *nonwhite* defines people in terms of what they are not (white), and *minority* places the subject in a subordinate position. "Person of color" has often been preferred by people of color in the United States.

Persistent vegetative state the state of a patient unresponsive to mental or verbal stimuli without signs of higher brain function who is kept alive artificially.

Persona front person puts on for the world.

Physical dependence physiologic need for a substance resulting in a withdrawal syndrome when substance is ended.

Plaintiff person who brings a lawsuit.

Polysubstance abuse use of two or more different substances of abuse—very common.

Positive euthanasia actively taking a life.

Positive regard deeply caring, nonjudgmental, supportive approach to patient, which makes him or her feel special.

Positive reinforcement constant focus on identifying appropriate behavior and praising the child for this behavior while avoiding castigating child for negative behavior.

Posture body position, stance.

Power of attorney the granting of power by a competent person to another to make specified decisions on the first person's behalf.

Prejudice prejudgment about a person.

Primary gain psychologic advantage that illness itself creates.

Primary prevention action taken to prevent or delay the onset of a disease.

Primary relationship closest person with whom you presently choose or are forced to relate.

Primary sex characteristics reproductive organs.

P.R.N. abbreviation for pro re nata, Latin for if necessary.

Problem drinkers people with high alcohol consumption who may stop of their own volition without medical treatment, peer group support, or a spiritual awakening. May progress to alcoholism.

Problem-focused coping learning more about the stressor and then taking direct action to cope with the stress (i.e., changing one's lifestyle to cope with a disease or quitting a problematic job).

Professional responsibility acceptance by health professionals of the consequences of their own actions.

Proxemics nearness to, distance from, or position in relation to another.

Psychologic dependence addiction to a substance leading to a psychologic withdrawal.

Psychologic treatment motivational interviewing; CBT; group and family, individual, and multiple approach models.

Psychosocial stress stress most commonly caused by death of loved one, divorce or separation, jail and illness.

R

Rape sexual penetration or its reasonable intent, without the subject's consent.

Rapport sympathetic connection to patient established by genuine interest and correct body language.

Rationalization defense mechanism in which individual makes unacceptable events acceptable through psychologic argument.

Receiving feedback thanking the giver, paraphrasing the giver, seeking clarification, and discussing how you can change.

Referral source person who may supply information or care for the patient.

Registration often used interchangeably with both licensure and certification.

Regression assuming childlike behavior.

Reinforcement praising child for success, which builds child's self-esteem.

Repression pushing painful thoughts into the unconscious mind.

Resistance mentally holding off painful reality.

Restraint limitation of physical or verbal activity by chemicals (sedating drugs) or physical items (tying patient down).

Resuscitate squeezing the heart and inflating and ventilating the lungs with chemicals given intravenously after patient has stopped breathing; also called cardiopulmonary resuscitation, or CPR.

Risk–benefit ratio weighing relative gain over possible loss.

Rogerian approach nondirective or client-centered counseling.

Role all behaviors expected from a person who occupies a particular position and status.

S

Sanctions penalties for noncompliance.

Secondary gain a consequence of illness that has a bonus aspect for the patient.

Secondary prevention action taken to delay or prevent complications once a disease process has begun.

Secondary sex characteristics changes in shape, body hair, and voice that accompany primary sex development and that occur at puberty

Sedentary inactive.

Self-efficacy belief in self.

Senescence aging, growing old, study of aging.

Separation anxiety the anxiety of a young child when separated from a person or thing to which it has strong emotional attachment, usually a parent but sometimes objects (e.g., security object).

Sickness role adaptive regression of a significantly ill patient in order to accept treatment.

Silence long pauses, withholding information, secrecy.

SOAP acronym for subjective, objective, assessment, plan, a method of record-keeping.

Sound symbols grunting, ahs, pointed throat clearing.

Stages of loss Kübler-Ross' five stages of bereavement: denial, anger, bargaining, depression, and acceptance.

Standard of care degree of care and competence expected of a particular professional.

Statute of limitation a deadline for legal action (e.g., five years).

Stereotyping association of a string of traits with an individual or group, generally on the basis of a single factor about that individual or group (i.e., all men are ...).

Stigma feeling of social disgrace connected with a social impairment.

Stigmatized adolescents adolescents who are often rejected by peers.

Stress external forces that lead to distress.

Sublimation a socially acceptable outlet for a socially loaded problem.

Substance abuse significant distress, manifested by three of the following: a failure to fulfill school, work, or parenting obligations; hazardous use (e.g. driving); recurrent substance-related legal problems (e.g., DUI); and continued substance use despite persistent or recurrent social or interpersonal problems.

Substance dependence significant distress manifested three of the following: tolerance, withdrawal; increasing consumption; desire to quit; excessive time spent on abuse; fewer social, occupational, or recreational activities; and continued use despite knowing physiologic and psychologic effects.

Substance use disorder a disorder that includes substance abuse and, more seriously, substance dependence.

Superego conscious mind responsible for adult mind.

Suppression the conscious rather than unconscious pushing away of painful thoughts.

Symbolism the representation of one idea by another (e.g., money for love).

Sympathy shared feelings of pain over a loss, best used in a social context.

T

Task focus outcome toward which team is working.

Team leader person appointed to head a team.

Teens of divorce adolescents whose parents have divorced and who have difficulty because of lack of security, mistrust of family ethic, uncovered repressed anger, playing parents off against each other, and loneliness.

Thanatology the study of death.

Thanatos death instincts.

Tobacco dependence continued consumption of tobacco that the patient cannot control, despite significant physical, economic, or social side effects.

Token economy usually in-patient reward tokens for desirable behaviors that patient can use for desirable commodity—a form of behavior modification.

Torts (1) laws that define what constitutes a legal injury and establish the circumstances under which one person may be held liable for another's injury; torts cover intentional acts and accidents. (2) civil wrong (excluding breach of contract) against person or property that causes injury.

Trail of Tears the forced march of 17,000 members of the North Georgian Cherokee Nation from their land in Georgia to unwanted land in Oklahoma, resulting in the death of 4,000 along the way.

Transactional analysis psychotherapy in which people assume different roles and play games in their interactions.

Transference identification of the health professional with someone else by the patient.

Transtheoretical model of change (TTM) a model that divides people into six categories: precontemplation, contemplation, recognition/preparation, action, maintenance, and relapse.

Treating addiction detoxification, psychologic treatment, medications.

Treatments of alcoholism motivational interviewing, cognitive behavioral therapy, Alcoholics Anonymous, individual and group therapy, medication.

Turf territorial rights within an area of expertise.

Tuskegee Airmen first African American pilots in the U.S. Army.

Type A personality a personality type characterized by a sense of time urgency, striving for perfection, and difficulty in accepting things if they are not the way the person wants them.

Type B personality a personality type that is easygoing, accepts people and events as they are without frustration, and feels no compulsion to compete.

U

U.S. Demographics by 2050 whites 40 percent, Hispanic 30 percent, black 15 percent, Asian 12 percent.

V

Values beliefs that hold meaning to an individual or group and by which they try to guide their decisions.

Visceral fat fat in and around organs, especially intraperitoneal (liver, kidneys, omentum, mesentery, and bowels) but also the heart.

Vocalics tone, timbre, volume.

W

White a person having origins in any of the original peoples of Europe, North Africa, or the Middle East.

Photo Credits

CHAPTER 1

Opener © Image Source Photography, Veer, Inc./RF
page 6 © Big Cheese Photo/Jupiter Images/RF
page 7 © Mel Curtis/Getty Images/RF
page 8 Image Source/Jupiter Images/RF
page 9 © David Buffington/Getty Images/RF
page 11 © Stockdisc/PunchStock/RF

CHAPTER 2

Opener © Image Source Photography, Veer, Inc./RF
page 25 © Michael Matisse/Getty Images/RF
page 34 © Pure Stock/RF
page 36 © BananaStock/PictureQuest/RF
page 38 © Creatas/PunchStock/RF

CHAPTER 3

Opener © Image Source Photography, Veer, Inc./RF
page 46 © Nova Development/RF
page 49 © Digital/RF

CHAPTER 4

Opener © Image Source Photography, Veer, Inc./RF
page 62 © Corbis/Alamy/RF
page 68 © Photodisk/SuperStock/RF
page 71 © Royalty-Free/Corbis
page 74 © Stockbyte/PunchStock/RF

CHAPTER 5

Opener © Image Source Photography, Veer, Inc./RF
page 84 © Photodisk/SuperStock/RF
page 87 © Creatas/PunchStock/RF
page 95 © The McGraw-Hill Companies, Inc./Rick Brady, photographer

CHAPTER 6

Opener © Image Source Photography, Veer, Inc./RF
page 103 © 2009 Jupiter Images Corporation/RF
page 107 © Dynamic Graphics/Creatas/PictureQuest/RF
page 115 © Rubberball Productions/RF

CHAPTER 7

Opener © Image Source Photography, Veer, Inc./RF
page 140/top © Royalty-Free/Corbis/RF
page 140/bottom © LifeART/Fotosearch/RF

CHAPTER 8

Opener © Image Source Photography, Veer, Inc./RF
page 152 © Comstock/PunchStock/RF
page 156 © Jess Alford/Getty Images/RF
page 158 © Getty Images/RF
page 168 © image100/Corbis/RF

CHAPTER 9

Opener © Image Source Photography, Veer, Inc./RF
page 183 © Getty Images/Mark Thornton/RF
page 189 © Photodisc Collection/Getty Images/RF
page 190 © Geoff Manasse/Getty Images/RF
page 195/top left © Purestock/SuperStock/RF
page 195/bottom left © Rubberball/Getty Images/RF
page 195/middle bottom © Rubberball Productions/Getty Images/RF
page 195/bottom right © BananaStock/age fotostock/RF
page 195/top right © Digital Vision/PunchStock/RF
page 195/top middle © Comstock/Alamy/RF

CHAPTER 10

Opener © Image Source Photography, Veer, Inc./RF

page 216 © Comstock Images/PictureQuest/RF

page 219 © BananaStock/PictureQuest/RF

page 223 © Comstock Images/PictureQuest/RF

CHAPTER 11

Opener © Image Source Photography, Veer, Inc./RF

page 230 © Image Source Photography, Veer, Inc./RF

page 237 © Royalty-Free/Corbis

CHAPTER 12

Opener © Image Source Photography, Veer, Inc./RF

page 259/top © Scott T. Baxter/Getty Images/RF

page 259/bottom © Medioimages/Photodisc/Getty Images/RF

page 262 © Barbara Penoyar/Getty Images/RF

page 266 © BananaStock/PunchStock

page 269 © Keith Brofsky/Getty Images/RF

page 272 Armed Forces Institute of Technology/RF

CHAPTER 13

Opener © Image Source Photography, Veer, Inc./RF

page 280 © Stockbyte/PunchStock/RF

page 289 © Tim Pannell/Corbis/RF

page 296 © Stockbyte/PunchStock/RF

CHAPTER 14

Opener © Image Source Photography, Veer, Inc./RF

page 307 © Getty Images/RF

page 313 © Anthony Saint James/Getty Images/RF

page 314 © Royalty-Free/Corbis

page 321 © Veer/RF

page 322 © Comstock/PictureQuest/RF

Index

D

E

F

G

H

M

N

O

P

Q

R

S

T

U

V

W

Y

Z